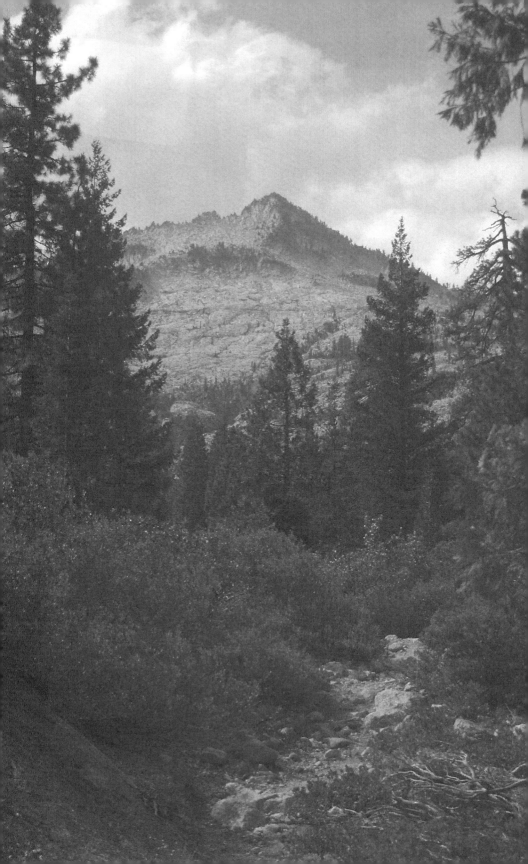

Trinity Alps & Vicinity

A HIKING AND BACKPACKING GUIDE

Including Whiskeytown,
Russian Wilderness,
and Castle Crags Areas

Mike White

 WILDERNESS PRESS ... *on the trail since 1967*

BERKELEY, CA

Trinity Alps and Vicinity: A Hiking and Backpacking Guide
Including Whiskeytown, Russian Wilderness, and Castle Crags Areas

1st EDITION 1983
2nd EDITION 1986
3rd EDITION 1994
4th EDITION 2004
5th EDITION 2010

Copyright © 1994, 2004, 2010 by Mike White

Front cover photo copyright © 2010 by Martin Beebee / Alamy
Interior photos by author and Luther Linkhart
Maps: Mike White
Cover design: Scott McGrew
Book design and layout: Larry B. Van Dyke
Book editor: Laura Shauger

ISBN 978-0-89997-501-6

Manufactured in the United States of America

Published by: **Wilderness Press**
 1345 8th Street
 Berkeley, CA 94710
 (800) 443-7227; FAX (510) 558-1696
 info@wildernesspress.com
 www.wildernesspress.com
Visit our website for a complete listing of our books and for ordering information.

Cover photo: Trinity Alps Wilderness with Mt. Shasta in the background
Frontispiece: Mt. Hilton from Boulder Scramble Trail (Trip 32)

SAFETY NOTICE: Although Wilderness Press and the author have made every attempt to ensure that the information in this book is accurate at press time, they are not responsible for any loss, damage, injury, or inconvenience that may occur to anyone while using this book. You are responsible for your own safety and health. The fact that an activity or a trail is described in this book does not mean that it will be safe for you. Be aware that trail conditions can change from day to day. Always check local conditions, know your own limitations, and consult a map.

To the memory of Luther Linkhart,
who was the Trinity Alps first and foremost author,
and who provided me with a great foundation
upon which to begin my writing career

✳

Acknowledgments

As for all my book projects, support and encouragement from my wife, Robin, is absolutely essential—all my efforts would be fruitless without her help. I would also like to thank those friends who joined me on the trail for the updates during the 2008 season: Keith Catlin, Tic Long, and Bob Redding. Roslyn Bullas has always provided invaluable oversight for all of my projects for Wilderness Press, and Laura Shauger proved once again to be an excellent editor.

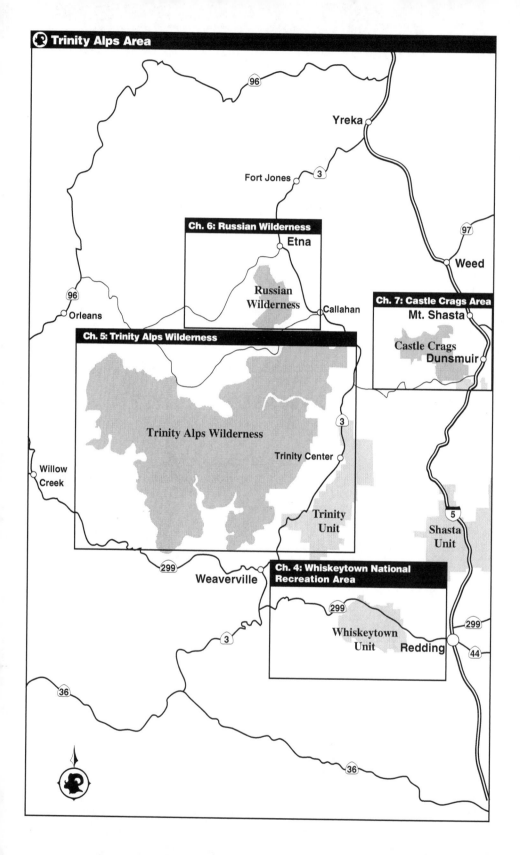

Trinity Alps Area

96

Yreka

Fort Jones   3

Ch. 6: Russian Wilderness

Etna

97

Weed

Russian
Wilderness

96

Orleans   Callahan

Ch. 7: Castle Crags Area

Mt. Shasta

Castle Crags
Dunsmuir

Ch. 5: Trinity Alps Wilderness

Trinity Alps Wilderness   3

Trinity Center

5

Shasta
Unit

Willow
Creek

Trinity
Unit

Ch. 4: Whiskeytown National
Recreation Area

299   Weaverville

299

Whiskeytown
Unit   Redding

299

44

3

36

36

Contents

Preface to the Fifth Edition

On June 21, 2008, a flurry of lightning strikes swept across California in a nearly unprecedented fashion. In and around the Trinity Alps, several small fires started by those strikes merged and grew into devastating forest fires combined under the names of the Alps, Lime, and Iron complexes. These fires burned for several weeks ultimately laying claim to a total of nearly 170,000 acres burned. Along with the forest destruction and an eventual cost of nearly 150 million dollars to fight, the Trinity Alps fires decimated the usually bustling summer recreation and tourism season. Throughout most of July, the town of Weaverville resembled an apocalyptic war zone rather than the usual tourist hamlet of the region. Even greater losses occurred in the toll of human lives, as a helicopter crash on August 7 killed seven Oregon firefighters, the pilot, and a U.S. Forest Service employee (four others were seriously injured but survived). Another firefighter died of injuries sustained while working on the Iron Complex in late July.

These fires resulted in vastly diminished opportunities to gather updated field information on many of the trails in the Trinity Alps. While I successfully hiked all of the new trails included in this guide within the Whiskeytown, Russian Wilderness, and Castle Crags areas in 2008, I was unable to complete fieldwork for many of the trails in the Alps directly because of the fires and indirectly because of the resulting poor air quality from smoky skies. In addition, inadequate funding has kept the Forest Service from performing necessary maintenance on some of the lesser-used trails in the Alps, particularly in the western half. Many of the trails within the New River watershed have not been maintained for years and are now considered unmaintained trails. Consequently, hikers should be prepared for less-than-perfect conditions in some areas and should check with the Forest Service about the current status of trails before embarking on any of these trips, especially in the western part of the Trinity Alps. Because of the absolute necessity of dedicating government personnel to the fighting of the 2008 fires, information on the conditions of the trails I was unable to hike was almost impossible to obtain. However, most of the trails in the eastern half of the Trinity Alps Wilderness should present little, if any, problems for hikers, backpackers, or equestrians.

The greater Trinity Alps region remains one of my all-time favorite hiking areas, as the diversity of terrain, vegetation, and wildlife is difficult to match just about anywhere else in the West. The significant distance from any major metropolitan center ensures that devotees won't overrun the area in the near future, providing a wealth of opportunities for achieving solitude and serenity. These attributes and many more make the area well deserving of your time and interest.

Summary of Trips

TRIP NUMBER AND NAME	MILEAGE	DAYS	ELEVATION CHANGE
Whiskeytown National Recreation Area			
1. Kanaka Peak Loop	6.5	1	3600'
2. Brandy Creek Falls	3	1	700'
3. Boulder Creek Falls	2.4	1	400'
4. Whiskeytown Falls	3.4	1	1040'
Trinity Alps Wilderness			
5. Stuart Fork to Emerald, Sapphire, and Mirror Lakes	29	4–7	4240'
6. Stuart Fork to Alpine Lake	17.4	2–4	3800'
7. Deer Creek and Four Lakes Loop to Long Canyon	25	5–8	11,545'
8. Granite Peak	10	1	4450'
9. Long Canyon, Lake Anna, and Billy Be Damn and Echo Lakes	12	2–4	9155'
10. Granite Lake and Bear Basin Loop	17.2	3–5	7955'
11. Deer Flat, Thumb Rock, and Landers Creek Loop	19.7	3–5	11,850'
12. Boulder Lake to Poison Canyon and Lilypad Lake	9.2	2–4	2780'
13. Boulder, Lion, Foster, and Sugar Pine Lakes	21	3–5	11,200'
14. North Fork to East Fork Coffee Creek Loop	27.5	3–7	12,035'
15. Union Creek and Dorleska Mine to Big Flat	10.3	2–5	5125'
16. South Fork Coffee Creek Loop to Trail Gulch and Long Gulch Lakes	17	3–5	9135'
17. Adams Lake	4.6	1	1160'
18. Caribou Basin and Sawtooth Ridge	16.6 or 13.6	2–5	3910' or 5100'
19. Sunrise Basin, Horseshoe Lake, and Ward Lake Loop	19.5	3–5	10,560'
20. Stoddard Lake, Doe Lake, and Eagle Creek	19.1	3–5	13,250'
21. Big, Little, and Wee Bear Lakes	9.4	2–3	3200'
22. Tangle Blue Lake	6.6	2	940'
23. Pacific Crest Trail: Scott Mountain Summit to Carter Meadows Summit	18.4	3–5	6785'

TRIP TYPE	DIFFICULTY	SEASON	FISHING
Loop	Moderate to difficult	April to early June and late September to November	
Out-and-back	Moderate	April to early June and late September to November	
Out-and-back	Easy	April to early June and late September to November	
Out-and-back	Moderate to difficult	April to early June and late September to November	
Out-and-back	Moderate	Mid-June to mid-October	•
Out-and-back	Moderate	Mid-July to late September	•
Point-to-point	Moderate	Early July to early October	•
Out-and-back	Difficult	Early July to mid-October	
Loop	Difficult	Early July to mid-October	•
Loop	Moderate	Mid-July to mid-September	•
Loop	Difficult	Mid-July to late September	•
Out-and-back	Moderate	Mid-July to mid-October	•
Point-to-point	Difficult	Late July to mid-September	•
Loop	Moderate	Mid-July to mid-October	•
Point-to-point	Easy	Late June to mid-October	•
Loop	Easy to moderate	Mid-July to mid-September	•
Out-and-back	Moderate	Late June to early October	•
Out-and-back	Moderate	Mid-July to late September	•
Loop	Difficult	Mid-July to late September	•
Point-to-point	Moderate	Early July to mid-October	•
Out-and-back	Moderate	Late June to early October	•
Out-and-back	Moderate	Mid-June to mid-October	•
Point-to-point	Moderate to difficult	Early July to early October	•

TRIP NUMBER AND NAME	MILEAGE	DAYS	ELEVATION CHANGE
24. Mavis, Fox Creek, and Virginia Lakes	9.4	2–3	1460'
25. Hidden Lake	1.8	1–2	450'
26. Trail Gulch and Long Gulch Lakes	8.4	1–2	5330'
27. China Gulch to Grizzly Lake	14	2–5	5540'
28. High Point to Rock and Red Cap Lakes	7.6	1–3	5560'
29. Salmon Summit Trail to Red Cap Lake	8.2	1–3	3920'
30. East Weaver and Rush Creek Lakes	8	1–3	3720'
31. Canyon Creek and El Lakes	16.6	2–5	3810'
32. Canyon Creek to Boulder Creek Lakes	14.8	1–4	2987'
33. North Fork Trinity River to Grizzly Lake	35	4–7	4650'
34. North Fork Trinity River to Papoose Lake	25	3–6	3695'
35. New River Divide Loop	20.5	3–4	9880'
36. Green Mountain Trail to North Fork Trinity River	17.6	3–5	10,875'
37. New River and Slide Creek to Historic Mining District and Eagle Creek	24	3–6	7740'
38. New River and Virgin Creek to Salmon Summit and Devils Backbone	40	5–9	22,120'

Russian Wilderness

TRIP NUMBER AND NAME	MILEAGE	DAYS	ELEVATION CHANGE
39. Waterdog and Russian Lakes	9	1–2	1600'
40. Bingham Lake	2.5	1	780'
41. Big Duck, Little Duck, and Horseshoe Lakes	13	1–3	3465'
42. Paynes Lake	4.2	1–2	2100'
43. Taylor, Hogan, and Big Blue Lakes	8.6	1–2	3000'

Castle Crags Area

TRIP NUMBER AND NAME	MILEAGE	DAYS	ELEVATION CHANGE
44. Root Creek	2.2	1	250'
45. Crags Trail to Castle Dome	6	1	2635'
46. Flume Trail, PCT, and Bobs Hat Trail Loop	7	1	2800'
47. River Trail	3	1	50'
48. Castle Lake Trail to Mount Bradley Lookout	11	1–2	2400'

TRIP TYPE	DIFFICULTY	SEASON	FISHING
Out-and-back	Moderate	Early July to mid-October	•
Out-and-back	Moderate	Late June to mid-October	•
Loop	Moderate	Early June to early October	•
Out-and-back	Moderate to difficult	Mid-July to late September	•
Out-and-back	Moderate	Late June to early October	•
Out-and-back	Easy	Late June to mid-October	•
Out-and-back	Moderate to difficult	Early July to mid-October	•
Out-and-back	Moderate	Early July to mid-October	•
Out-and-back	Moderate to difficult	Early July to mid-October	•
Out-and-back	Moderate	Mid-July to early October	•
Out-and-back	Moderate	Mid-July to early October	•
Loop	Moderate	Early July to mid-October	•
Point-to-point	Moderate	Mid-July to mid-October	
Loop	Difficult	Mid-May to early November	•
Loop	Difficult	Mid-July to early October	•
Out-and-back	Moderate	Mid-June through October	•
Out-and-back	Moderate	Mid-June through October	•
Out-and-back	Moderate	Late June through October	•
Out-and-back	Difficult	July through October	•
Out-and-back	Moderate	July through October	•
Out-and-back	Easy	April through November	
Out-and-back	Difficult	Mid-April through mid-November	
Loop	Moderate	April through November	
Out-and-back	Easy	Late March through November	•
Out-and-back	Moderate to difficult	Mid-June to mid-October	•

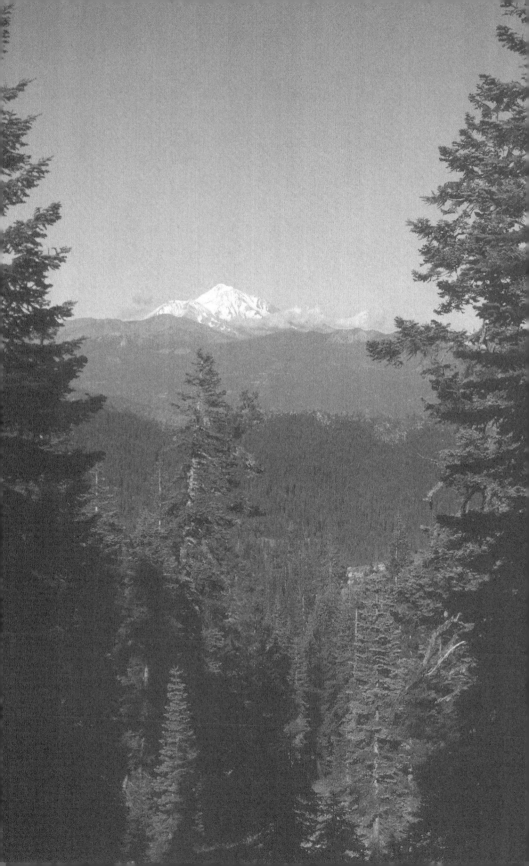

CHAPTER 1

Introduction to the Area

I magine for a moment that you're driving north on Interstate 5 south of Redding, California, on a glorious spring day, after a north wind has cleared the air above the upper Sacramento River Valley—a day when you can see for a distance of more than 100 miles. As the freeway crests a ridge, the frosted cone of Mt. Shasta directly north suddenly enthralls you and your passengers, the majestic peak towering into the sky above the surrounding lowlands. Over to the northwest, a row of snow-capped peaks above the lower ridges behind Redding intrigues you. Most of your riders may be surprised to see snowy mountains toward the Northern California coast, but a few in the know may recognize the Trinity Alps, and soon regale the group with interesting accounts of past experiences in one of the state's most diverse mountain ranges. With the possible exception of fishing stories, they are probably telling the truth.

The Trinity Alps, along with the nearby Whiskeytown Unit of Whiskeytown-Shasta-Trinity National Recreation Area, Russian Wilderness, Castle Crags Wilderness, and Castle Crags State Park, all within a remote and diverse range known as the Klamath Mountains, make up the scope of this book. This range of approximately 8,300 square miles encompasses a large area of northwestern California and southwestern Oregon, extending from the Sacramento Valley all the way north to the Willamette Valley. The area is deeply dissected by rivers, with the Trinity Alps Wilderness, Russian Wilderness, and Whiskeytown NRA drained by the Trinity, Scott, and Salmon rivers, and Castle Crags drained by the upper Sacramento River.

The Trinity Alps form the centerpiece of this guide, an area of approximately 525,000 acres of splendid wilderness and near-wilderness. The federally designated Trinity Alps Wilderness, set aside by the U.S. Congress in the California

Left: **Mt. Shasta from Eagle Divide**

1

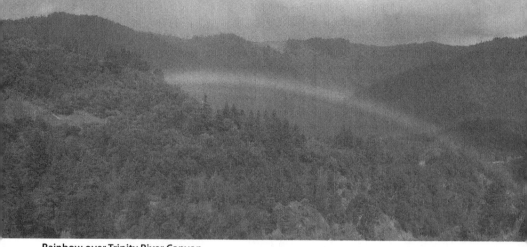
Rainbow over Trinity River Canyon

Wilderness Bill in 1984, contains a half million of those acres, an area of more than 780 square miles. The wilderness includes all of the 234,000 acres previously protected as the Salmon-Trinity Alps Primitive Area, plus, obviously, a great deal more land.

In comparison to the Sierra Nevada or Cascade Range, the Trinity Alps is a much smaller mountain range in both height and expanse. However, bigger is not necessarily better, as the Alps are filled with rushing streams, high waterfalls, gorgeous mountain lakes dimpled with trout rises, glaciated granite peaks, remnant glaciers, and cool, green forests—plus some unique features all their own.

What the Alps don't have, at least to the extent of other popular mountain ranges in the state, is hordes of people. Positioned in remote northwestern California, hundreds of miles away from any large population centers, only a few areas in the Alps tend to attract crowds. Part of the purpose of this guide is to inform the reader about some of the lesser-used places that, in many cases, can handle more visitors than some of the more popular areas.

Whiskeytown Unit is one of three parcels of land surrounding artificial reservoirs built as part of the Central Valley Project in the 1960s comprising the Whiskeytown-Shasta-Trinity National Recreation Area. Whiskeytown Lake is a 3,250-acre reservoir that doesn't suffer the effects of drawdown like Shasta and Clair Engle lakes, which makes Whiskeytown a popular summertime destination for boaters and water skiers. Encompassing nearly 42,500 acres, the land around the reservoir boasts 24 trails well-suited for dayhiking and mountain biking. With elevations ranging from 1200 feet at the lake's surface to 6029 at the summit of Shasta Bally, summertime temperatures can be quite hot during the typically sunny afternoons. Therefore, spring and fall tend to be the most pleasant seasons for trail users. Four of Whiskeytown's trails are included in this guide, three to picturesque waterfalls and one to the view-packed summit of Kanaka Peak.

The Russian Wilderness, also set aside by Congress in 1984, is much smaller than the Trinity Alps, at a mere 12,000 acres. However, within that more diminutive acreage is a biological diversity that makes the area very unique.

The concentration of 17 distinct conifer species in the Duck Lake Botanical Area distinguishes the Russian Wilderness as one of most biologically diverse areas in the world. In addition, some smaller plants here grow nowhere else in the world. The area straddles a divide between the Scott and Salmon rivers, and elevations range from a little more than 5000 feet to 8196 feet at the summit of Russian Peak. This compact wilderness also boasts 22 lakes and numerous trails, including a section of the famed Pacific Crest Trail.

The 4,000-acre Castle Crags State Park and adjoining 10,500-acre Castle Crags Wilderness combined are the final backcountry area covered in this guide. Situated along a stretch of the upper Sacramento River and just off Interstate 5, the park is open all year to campers, picnickers, sightseers, and recreational enthusiasts. Ranging in elevation from around 2000 to 3000 feet, the lands within the park are towered over by the Castle Crags, a series of dramatic, granite spires, some of which exceed 6000 feet in elevation. With 22 miles of trail, Castle Crags State Park offers plenty of opportunities for hikers. Castle Crags Wilderness, also set aside in 1984, contains the namesake crags and surrounding higher-elevation backcountry. Nearly 28 miles of trails, including a 19-mile section of the Pacific Crest Trail, offer opportunities to visit a wide variety of terrain, including high-elevation lakes, flower-covered meadows, and the crags themselves. While defined tread leads to the base of the crags, a more intimate visit requires basic off-trail skills.

The Klamath Mountains yield their inner secrets and pleasures only to hikers, backpackers, and equestrians willing to head out on 500-plus miles of trail. Automobile-bound visitors to resorts near the lakes and rivers see only a fraction more of the mountains than they would see from their car windows on Interstate 5. The general purpose of this book is to inform and inspire those willing to forgo the comforts of their vehicles to get out onto the trails.

Natural History and Environment

Geology

If you crumple a piece of paper into a ball, and then spread the paper out partway so it's still crumpled and creased in all directions, you would have an approximate model of the topography of the Klamath Mountains. Although the Trinity Alps do form a generally east-west divide and the Russians a north-south divide that separates the Scott and Salmon rivers, the area's contorted ridges, canyon, and peaks seem to run helter-skelter in all directions.

These mountains are only vaguely related, geologically, to the Coast Range to the west, and not related at all to the volcanic Cascades beginning with Lassen Peak and Mt. Shasta to the east. They are, in fact, the southern part of the Klamath Mountains, which include the Marbles and Siskiyous farther north. The Klamath Mountains harbor some of the oldest rocks in California. These

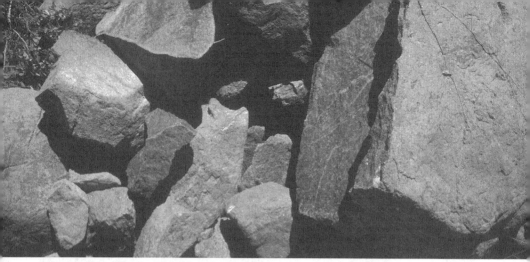

Metamorphic rocks are red only on the outside.

rocks originated as offshore sediments, largely volcanic in origin, which were repeatedly uplifted, folded, and combined with the granite bedrock below the seafloor, creating an amalgam of varied rock types formed at different times, by different means, and in different locations. In the process, tremendous pressures metamorphosed the deposits into uptilted and distorted strata of slate, quartzite, schist, gneiss, chert, and soapstone. Isolated pockets of unmetamorphosed sandstones, limestones, mudstones, and conglomerates can be attributed to later sedimentation and fallout from eruptions in a nearby volcanic chain. Geologists refer to this widely varied, complex, and mixed-up geology as the Klamath Knot.

There is no evidence of volcanic lava flows or eruptions with the Klamath Mountains. Granitic magmas did well up at various times, which accounts for the composition of most of the higher peaks in the area. Other igneous rocks, known as mafic and ultramafic, also squeezed up into faults and cracks in the earth's crust; the high iron content of much of this rock accounts for the weathered red- and rust-colored rock of many of the other high peaks in the region.

Further upheavals, lateral movements, and constant erosion over geologic time gave many of the lower ridges and canyons much of the same shape as they display today, but the higher peaks and ridges received their final contours during periods of glaciation. Although these glaciers ran down the canyons just a few miles, the massive sheets of ice removed cubic miles of rock from the higher areas, depositing the ground-up rock in the lower areas. Once the glaciers receded, they left behind many small cirque-bound lakes at the heads of U-shaped valleys, with fantastically carved divides between them. Moraines dammed some of the larger valleys, which formed large lakes and marshes that eventually became some of the present-day meadows; Morris Meadows in the Trinity Alps is an outstanding example. Continuing and ongoing erosion distributed glacial till farther down the canyons, putting the finishing touches on the landscape that is visible today. Elevations in this part of the Klamath Mountains range from 900 feet along the lower Trinity River to 9002 feet on top of Thompson Peak.

Climate

Although the Klamath Mountains are much wetter than the Sacramento Valley and many other regions of Northern California, they are not nearly as wet as locations along the Northern California coast. Precipitation varies greatly in this relatively small area, from as much as 80 inches a year on some of the higher, west-facing slopes to less than 20 inches in some of the lower east-side canyons. Much of the precipitation occurs as either rain or snow during the winter months. However, thunderstorms are not uncommon during the summer.

Temperatures vary more greatly than along the coast, or the Sacramento Valley, as well. Winter temperatures can be quite cold. Even Weaverville, at 2000 feet, receives some snow almost every winter. The snowpack at the higher elevations can build up to 10 to 20 feet, making it an important storage facility of water for the Central Valley Project. High-country trails are usually free of snow by late June, but snow may linger all summer on north-facing slopes following winters of heavy snowfall.

Summer daytime temperatures can be quite hot, exceeding 90°F even at 5000 or 6000 feet. Down in the lower canyons, 100-degree days are not uncommon. Day-to-night differentials can range up to as much as 45 degrees.

Average Monthly Weather Data for Weaverville

	JAN.	FEB.	MAR.	APR.	MAY	JUNE
Minimum Temperature (°F)	27.7	29.2	31.5	33.4	39.7	45.6
Maximum Temperature (°F)	49.0	54.6	59.8	67.4	76.9	85.8
Precipitation (inches)	7.1	6.1	5.5	2.3	1.3	0.6

	JULY	AUG.	SEPT.	OCT.	NOV.	DEC.
Minimum Temperature (°F)	49.9	48.4	42.4	35.5	32.6	27.6
Maximum Temperature (°F)	94.2	94.3	87.8	75.4	55.8	47.0
Precipitation (inches)	0.2	0.3	1.1	2.3	5.5	6.3

Plants

An amazing variety of plants grow within the Klamath Mountains. The varied geology, assisted by a relative lack of glaciation and volcanism, has produced one of the most unique floral provinces in the world, which botanists refer to as the Klamath-Siskiyou Ecoregion. At the intersection of five major biotic regions, Coast Range, Cascade Range, Great Central Valley, Sierra Nevada, and Great Basin, the area boasts more than 130 endemic plant species and the highest concentration of different conifers in the world. The range harbors about 3,500 different plant species, including some unusual meat-eaters.

The most obvious members of the plant community are the trees. The forests in the Klamath Mountains are marvelously diverse and include some of the largest individuals of some species seen in the U.S. Two unusual conifer species, weeping spruce and foxtail pine, are fairly common in the higher elevations, and rare elsewhere. Shasta red firs grow north of Redding, extending into southwestern Oregon.

The best way to categorize the forests and other flora of the Klamath Mountains is by plant communities. As in other mountain ranges, plant communities are determined primarily by elevation. However, many other contributing factors, including soil type, rainfall, wind, and exposure, make dividing lines rather indistinct. There is more intermixing of species between plant communities in the Klamath Mountains than in most other mountain ranges. Descriptions of six very general plant communities follow.

Mixed Low-Elevation Forest: This classification represents the low-elevation community up to approximately 3000 feet, including isolated riparian (streamside) communities that may be found as high as 6000 feet. The deciduous, broadleaf trees found here include alders, dogwoods, bigleaf maples, black oaks, hazelnuts, and Oregon oaks. Douglas fir is overwhelmingly the most common conifer in this community, but lesser amounts of ponderosa pines and Jeffrey pines also appear, as well as sparse stands of Digger pines on lower, dry slopes. Evergreens other than conifers include madrones, chinquapin, tanoaks, California live oaks, and canyon oaks.

Some bushes appear as trees in the lower riparian areas, including coast, red, and blue elderberries, along with ceanothus, dogwoods, hazelnuts, and manzanitas. Thick stands of chaparral extend over dry hillsides, with ceanothus and manzanita as the most common shrubs, and gooseberries, wild roses, and poison oak also present.

Poison oak grows in many forms, from low, spindly plants to tree-climbing vines, and is the bane of this plant community. Touching the plant produces a violent skin reaction in most humans and, when the plant is burned and the smoke inhaled, may cause serious poisoning requiring hospitalization. This noxious plant has shiny leaves in groups of three and is easy to identify and thereby avoid. The U.S. Forest Service has some helpful information (available at ranger stations) that can help you learn to identify this plant.

Mixed-Conifer Forest: The largest trees—sugar pines, ponderosa pines, Jeffrey pines, Douglas firs, white firs, and incense cedars—grow in this zone between 3000 and 6000 feet. Vine maples and mountain ash are occasional associates to the stately conifers. Black oaks and alders are also found in the lower realms of this zone. These magnificent forests are found on most of the trails you'll end up hiking in the Klamath Mountains.

Shrubs such as azaleas, raspberries, wood roses, and coast huckleberries carpet small openings in the forest. Pinemat manzanita and thimbleberries are common members of the understory. Large expanses of brush are uncommon at these elevations but where they do occur, huckleberry oaks and other scrub oaks, which do not appear at lower elevations, are the principal plants.

Red-Fir Forest: Red firs and their subspecies, Shasta red firs, occur almost equally in the Klamath Mountains between 5000 and 7000 feet. They often overlap considerably with conifers from the next lowest community, especially white firs. Slightly larger, beautiful cones distinguish Shasta red firs from the standard red firs, with longer bracts than scales, giving the cones a silver-flecked appearance.

At these elevations, western white pines begin to replace their close relatives, the sugar pines, while Jeffrey pines take over completely from their relatives, the ponderosa pines. Mountain junipers are not particularly common in the Klamath Mountains, but a few do show up here and there in this community. Pockets of mountain hemlocks and weeping spruces can be found at the upper limits of this zone on north-facing slopes and cirques. This zone is the highest with large stands of trees. Above these elevations trees grow alone or in small clusters.

Streams at these elevations may be lined with cottonwoods. Alders are reduced to the size of bushes and are usually associated with willows in wet areas. Different varieties of willows thrive at all elevations, but they are generally the size of shrubs here. Mountain ash and vine maple are also fairly common broadleaf shrubs in this region.

Some southern exposures at this level are covered with large areas of solid brush, referred to as mountain chaparral. Ceanothus, manzanita, chokecherry, serviceberry, tobacco brush, and huckleberry oak are the primary shrubs.

Subalpine Forest: Foxtail pines have found a home in the Trinity Alps at elevations ranging from 6500 to 8000 feet, along with smaller amounts of whitebark pines and mountain mahoganies clinging to the exposed and inhospitable ridgecrests. Somewhat surprisingly, Jeffrey pines, western white pines, and an occasional incense cedar persist in this zone, but usually in startlingly modified forms—stunted and contorted, pruned by the high winds, and bent over by the weight of winter storms. The only trees seemingly able to stand erect on top of these wind-swept ridges are whitebark pines and foxtail pines. Foxtail pines may sometimes be mistaken for firs at first glance, but they have bundles of five needles that grow tightly spaced all the way around supple branches that resemble small, green fox tails.

Mountain hemlocks grow in protected pockets on north-facing slopes, usually in protected areas away from the strongest winds. Weeping spruces

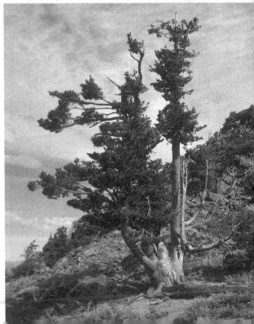

Whitebark pine on Scott Crest (Trip 23)

scattered around the higher lakes and cirques in the wettest and coldest places also tend to avoid the winds.

Mountain chaparral extends into the lower end of this community, with flattened mats of willow and pinemat manzanita making up the only persistent brush in the upper realms of this zone.

Mountain Meadow: There are meadows in the mixed low-elevation forest, but true mountain meadows begin in the mixed-conifer community and extend into the subalpine forest. The obvious plants in mountain meadows are grasses, sedges, and wildflowers, but shrubs are also present, along with two species of trees that thrive around the edges of meadows—lodgepole pines and quaking aspens. Neither tree is particularly common in this area, but they are a pleasant surprise when encountered.

Alpine: The handful of true alpine ecosystems that exist in this part of the Klamath Mountains are positioned around the highest peaks in the range, at elevations near 9000 feet. Trees are completely absent, and only a few shrubs and heaths hug the surface of small pockets of soil between the rocks. The most abundant plants are lichens, but a remarkable array of wildflowers burst into bloom during the very short frost-free period in late summer.

Wildflowers

More than 100 acres of wildflowers bloom in a solid mass in late July and early August on a northeast-facing slope at the head of Long Canyon in the Trinity Alps. Probably dozens of species are represented, but the most prominent are

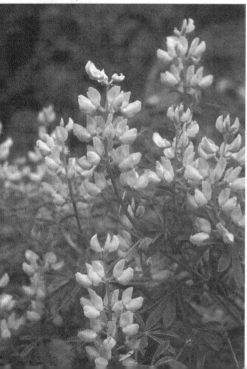

Yellow lupine

vivid red paintbrushes; blue, yellow, and purple lupines; white angelica; and creamy western pasqueflowers that turn into fuzzy white mops when they go to seed.

In a completely different location, under evenly spaced red firs on the south side of the Salmon River divide, the waxy white blossoms of queen's cups and twinflowers shine against the dark background of the forest floor.

The preceding two paragraphs only hint at the diversity of the hundreds of species of plants that thrive in this section of the Klamath Mountains. To name and describe them all would require an entire volume. Many people derive a great deal of pleasure from being able to identify, as well as admire, the many flowers they see. For such a purpose, *A Field Guide to Pacific States Wildflowers* by Theodore E. Niehaus, Roger Tory Peterson, and Charles L. Ripper (in the Peterson Field Guides series) is highly recommended.

You may be surprised by the sheer number of species you can identify here that are described in the guide as normally found somewhere else. This is because, as mentioned earlier, the Klamath Mountains are a meeting place for plant species from five biotic zones. At least one species, the California pitcher plant, found more often in the Trinity Alps than anywhere else, is rare and listed as being of special concern in California. Please do not pick any specimens, and be very careful not to damage the native flora.

Many locations and descriptions of wildflowers are noted in the trips at the points where they occur, but some general descriptions may be in order. The largest displays of flowers are found in mountain meadows. The species vary considerably with the type of meadow, elevation, and location. You'll find California pitcher plants in the wettest and steepest meadows at fairly high elevations, but they also may be found growing around the edges of ponds in the midst of small openings in the mixed-conifer and red-fir communities. Angelica and yampa bloom in most meadows, except for very dry meadows on flat ridgetops. Those high, dry, and often gravelly meadows support pussy paws, cat's ears, sulfur flowers, and cinquefoils. All of these represent only a small sampling of the marvelous variety of flowers you're apt to see in the meadows.

Streamside locations support a completely different group of wildflowers. Most showy among these are the head-high spikes of larkspurs and monkshoods. Marsh marigolds, but-

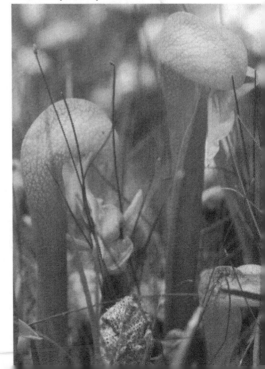

California pitcher plants

tercups, and Jeffrey's shooting stars bloom beside little rills at the higher elevations just after snowmelt. Later, and even higher, a dozen or more varieties of monkeyflowers display a wide range of colors beside seeps and springs, while edible swamp onions grow right in icy streams.

A surprising number of flowers bloom in the deep shade of the mixed-conifer community. Early in the season you may see woodland stars, milkmaids, and trillium. Later, the parasitic flowers, such as coral roots and pinedrops display their ghostly beauty on leafless forest floors. Mahonia and salal, usually considered more north Pacific Coast plants, grow under thick stands of Douglas firs. Washington lilies prefer a little more sun in openings in the low-elevation mixed forest, as do gilias, irises, and mints.

Other Plants

Ferns, mosses, and lichens are abundant in the Klamath Mountains, approaching rainforest proportions in some of the lower canyons and covering rocks and trees alike with a green mantle. In other low-elevation areas, gray strands of Spanish moss drape away from tree limbs, and staghorn lichens stand out from the trunks. At boundaries between meadows and forests in the mixed-conifer community, ferns grow to head height, crowding the trails. Acres of brake ferns cover some of the meadows at the red-fir level. A variety of lichens add their colors to the rocks higher up, and delicate five-finger ferns decorate dripping grottos.

Animals

Warm-Blooded Animals

A quite common, and wild, large, warm-blooded animal in the Klamath Mountains is the black bear. The area has seen a sizeable increase in the bear population in recent years, although you probably won't see one on your backpack, as these animals remain quite wary of humans. However, you should be prepared for the possibility of encountering a bear in the backcountry by following a few simple guidelines. At camp, effectively hang all of your food, trash, and scented items (toothpaste, sunscreen, etc.) from a stout tree limb out of a bear's reach, or, better yet, put all of that stuff in an approved bear canister. Wash your dishes, keep your camp clean, and don't prepare any food you can't eat. You may still hear a bear nosing around your camp in the middle of the night, searching for food but, with the proper precautions, at least you won't go hungry for the rest of your trip. More than likely, you will see bear scat on the trails as well as other signs, such as scratch marks on tree trunks, or torn-up logs, but people rarely see bears in this region.

Columbian black-tailed deer appreciate the pathways humans have constructed as much as the bears do, so you'll probably see their signs along the trail as well. You're apt to see does and fawns along the way and, if you are lucky, a buck or two. Every buck has been hunted after the first year of their life, so they're justifiably wary of humans. Noises around your camp at night are much more likely to be made by a deer than a bear. Deer are attracted to camp food, especially anything salty, and they also have been known to chew on anything that is sweat-soaked, such as clothing, pack straps, and boots. While setting up camp in Grizzly Meadows after the hot and sweaty climb from the China Gulch trailhead, I removed my soaking wet T-shirt and set it out on some bushes to dry. A short time later a deer wandered into camp and started chewing away on my shirt. When the deer finally finished, the T-shirt had a pattern of holes resembling a slice of Swiss cheese. Don't feed the deer—they become horrible pests once they've become accustomed to getting food from humans. Don't approach or try to pet one either—despite our Bambi-inspired feelings they are potentially dangerous, and they carry ticks and lice. Still, a doe and her twin fawns drinking out of a fog-shrouded stream at dawn is a most memorable sight. Mountain lions, the deer's only predator (besides humans), are very scarce in the Klamath Mountains.

The next largest mammal in the area is the resourceful coyote. Coyotes are rarely seen but more often heard on moonlit nights. Coyote calls, passed back and forth from ridge to ridge, are a thrilling wilderness symbol. Martens, fishers, and long-tailed weasels are also seldom-seen animals, although present in the Klamath Mountains in significant numbers.

Smaller warm-blooded animals of the rodent order swarm in some parts of the Klamath Mountains. Mice, chipmunks, and ground squirrels prosper in areas of high human visitation, partly because some people unwisely choose to feed them directly and partly because humans feed them indirectly with leftovers from horse feed, horse droppings, and garbage. There is a relationship between large rodent populations and healthy populations of rattlesnakes—the snakes move in to take advantage of the abundant food supply. In the less-traveled western Trinity Alps, there is a dearth of rodents when compared to more popular areas in the eastern Alps. Bears, bobcats, weasels, and coyotes may also have an impact on the absence of rodents in the western Alps.

One delightful rodent you're apt to see is the cheeky Douglas squirrel (also known as pine squirrel or chickaree). This rodent's strident scolding and frenetic activity in the mixed-conifer and red-fir forests are often a source of amusement to passersby. The Douglas squirrel is rarely a camp robber, but he may drop a green pine or fir cone uncomfortably close to you as you pass beneath his tree. The piles of cone scales and cones under trees usually belong to Douglas squirrels.

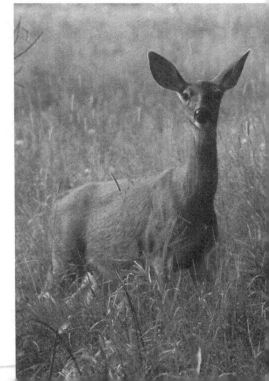

Black-tailed doe in Morris Meadow

The much larger gray squirrel, which lives in the mixed low-elevation forest, is very shy and seldom seen. Skunks, raccoons, ringtail cats, opossums, and foxes also frequent this community, rarely moving into the upper communities.

Oddly, the western states' largest rodent, the porcupine, is rare in this area, although quite common elsewhere in California. Bats are often seen around lakes and meadows after dusk, hunting for insects. Their marvelous flight rarely ceases to amaze visitors to their realm.

Birds

Nothing begins the day quite as well as birdsong outside your tent—unless you're exhausted from the previous day's hike and would like nothing more than to sleep in that morning. Unless the weather is horribly bad, you'll rarely be without that gentle awakener in the Klamath Mountains. Vireos, warblers, robins, and finches greet you in the mixed-conifer forest. Of course, you'll undoubtedly hear a few raucous jays as well. In the higher realms of the red-fir forest, you may hear a mountain bluebird, a golden-crowned kinglet, or a hermit thrush. The distant drumming of a pileated woodpecker, evidence that some creature can be so industrious early in the morning, isn't all bad. Hummingbirds are occasionally seen in some of the upper communities, no doubt drawn by the stunning wildflowers of midsummer. On the lower trails you're sure to find the dust wallows of California quail, and you may hear a mother quail calling to her chicks to freeze in their tracks. Even though you've just heard their peeping, you're unlikely to find a single chick after they become silent and motionless, as their camouflage renders them virtually invisible. Blue grouse also have excellent camouflage—you seldom see them in the grass and brush until they instantaneously explode from under your feet, doubling your heart rate.

Raptors are well represented at all elevations in the Klamath Mountains. Many species of hawks course the ridges in search of prey, and golden eagles nest in a few locations. Even bald eagles have been seen in recent years. A few ospreys nest along the rivers, and owls can often be heard at night as high as the red-fir forest.

Literally hundreds of avian species are represented in the Klamath Mountains. If you want to add to your list, pack along a copy of *Peterson Field Guide to Western Birds* by Roger Tory Peterson, along with a pair of binoculars. You're sure to find something new with each trip.

Cold-Blooded Animals

Reptiles and amphibians are common in all of the communities except alpine. Various snakes, such as rubber boas, garter snakes, gopher snakes, king snakes, and various water snakes are fairly common in all zones up to the subalpine.

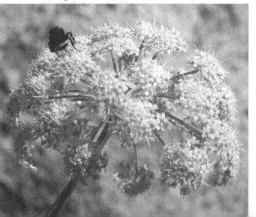

An angelica blossom and a bee

An area with as much water as the Klamath Mountains is bound to be home to a high number of water-loving amphibians. Red-legged and yellow-legged frogs thrive in the wet meadows and ponds in the mixed-conifer forest community. Higher up you may find tiny tree frogs. An amazing number of salamanders live in damp forest areas up to the subalpine level.

The amphibians that receive the most attention are the newts and salamanders that live in many of the middle- and lower-elevation lakes. Some of them are 8–10 inches long and bright red, quite startling as they come up to the surface to breathe when you're expecting trout.

Insects
Insects inhabit the Klamath Mountains in numbers similar to all other earthly paradises. Only a few of these numerous species of insects are problematic for humans and, of course, many of them can be quite interesting, if not beautiful creatures. Mosquitoes can be a considerable annoyance in many areas right after snowmelt. Repellents can be quite helpful during the day, and a screened tent can be a godsend at night.

Horseflies and deerflies are irritating later in the summer, but at least they go away at nightfall. During and immediately after wet springs, ticks can be a particular nuisance at the lower elevations, especially since they can carry Lyme disease or infections. Repellents sprayed on collars, cuffs, and pant legs should help, but the best way to deal with ticks is by inspecting your entire body daily. If discovered soon after it has attached, a tick can be removed by grabbing the body with a pair of tweezers and applying gentle traction until the pest is pulled out of your flesh. Once removed, thoroughly wash the affected area and watch for signs of infection or rash around the wound. If any unusual symptoms develop after a few days, seek medical attention.

Human History

Three natural resources have profoundly affected the human history of the Klamath Mountains, almost to the exclusion of any other factors. They are, in chronological order, gold, timber, and water.

The Wintu Indians
Gold meant very little to the Wintu Indians, who lived very well along the Trinity River and its tributaries for hundreds, possibly thousands, of years without any awareness that gold was even present. The Wintu had no use for gold, and they certainly had plenty of timber and water for their needs. As a matter of fact, they had just about everything else they needed. Deer and elk were plentiful, providing both food and clothing. Each autumn brought the return of salmon and steelhead up the river for harvest and, in most years, a bountiful crop of acorns. In the summer, berries and seeds were plentiful, along with small animals that they could snare. They built roofs for their homes of bark and rushes, and sedges and willows provided the materials for beautifully woven baskets.

Winters were bearable along the river, and the Wintu had very little reason to travel very high into the mountains, except to pass through on trading expeditions to the coast or Central Valley. What need had a Wintu for gold? Would gold keep a grizzly from attacking (they were still here in those days)? In the end, of course, gold destroyed the Wintu completely, as the people who came to the area in the 19th century wanted the gold and the Wintu were in the way.

From Trappers and Gold Diggers to Homesteaders and Loggers

Although Jedediah Smith, and possibly other trappers before him, may have visited the area, Major Pierson P. Reading received the credit for naming the Trinity River in 1845. Actually the river was named by mistake, as Reading thought the river emptied into the Pacific Ocean at Trinidad Bay, naming the river *Trinity* (the English translation of the Spanish word *Trinidad*). Four years later, two miners who were searching for a way to the ocean discovered that the river flowed into the Klamath River, not the ocean.

Going for the Gold

There is some conjecture that Major Reading discovered gold at the same time he discovered the Trinity River. However, that would have been three years prior to John Marshall's discovery of gold at Sutter's Mill. If Reading discovered gold on his first trip to the Trinity River, he was really good at keeping a secret. The big gold rush to the Trinity River didn't begin until late 1849 or early 1850.

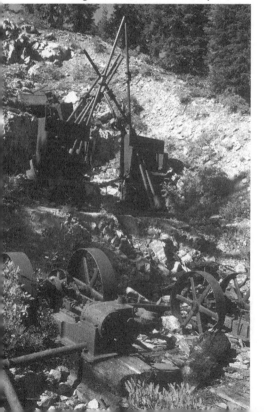

Steam engines at Dorleska Mine (Trip 15)

By the end of 1850, the gold rush on the Trinity River and its tributaries was in full swing. Weaverville had almost as many people living there as it does now. In contrast, Trinity Centre (original spelling) had many more people than it does today. Even in 1850, many of those people were Chinese immigrants. By 1853, close to 2,000 Chinese immigrants lived and worked in the Weaverville area alone. Their labor was a boon to the local economy: They worked cheaply and, if they mined their own claims, renegade whites promptly robbed them. Most important, they paid four dollars a head per month to the government for the privilege of digging, which went a long way toward supporting the public sector during the

1850s. Contrastingly, the whites paid nothing, despite the fact that they too were immigrants.

Tensions resulted in a one-day Chinese tong war in 1854, an uprising instigated and promoted by whites. The American and European gold seekers didn't allow the Chinese to use guns (white bystanders might get hit by stray bullets), so the "Hongkongs" and "Cantons" fought with knives, spears, and hatchets in a field near Weaverville. "Military advisers" for both sides cheered them on and bet on the outcome, with the "Cantons" eventually triumphant. However, many Chinese on both sides were losers, with 10 dead and two or three times more wounded. Surprisingly, there were no casualties among the "advisers."

More people swarmed over the area in the 1850s than have been there at any time since. In less than a decade most of the available placer gold had been mined, and the Chinese moved on to help build a section of the Transcontinental Railroad over the Sierra Nevada. Only the Weaverville Joss House, museum, artifacts, and miles of carefully stacked boulders the miners left along the streams remain to remind present-day visitors and residents of the former Chinese community.

The Wintu fared far worse than the Chinese. Estimated with a population of between 5,000 and 10,000 prior to the arrival of Europeans, the Wintu were nearly exterminated in the mid-1850s, leaving fewer than 1,000 members by 1910. Of the original nine bands of Wintu only three remain, and there are very few reminders of their former presence within the Trinity Alps.

After the placer gold had been diminished, gold mining became big business. Capital and corporations are required to finance giant dredges, excavate deep shafts and drifts, and build miles of ditches and flumes. Such large-scale mining continued in the area through the 1930s, the most obvious example of which is the La Grange Mine. Water was transported 29 miles from lakes at the head of Stuart Fork in the early 1900s to wash away a big part of Oregon Mountain west of Weaverville. The remains were deposited down Oregon Gulch toward Junction City, the scars still visible along a portion of Highway 299.

A few individual prospectors and small-scale placer miners have continued in the old way in an attempt to eke out an existence to the present day. One Mr. Jorstad, who lived in a cabin on the North Fork Trinity River, was an outstanding example until his passing in 1989. A new breed of gold miner has invaded the area more recently, using gasoline-powered Venturi dredges, wet suits, and snorkels to find gold in deep pools, areas that were out of reach to the old placer miners. Existing laws (primarily the 1872 Mining Law) and other regulations allow these miners to continue working existing claims within wilderness areas.

Ranchers

Along with the miners of the 1850s came a number of ranchers who homesteaded along the rivers, mostly in the area north of Lewiston known as Trinity Meadows, which now rests at the bottom of artificial Trinity Lake. Some of their descendants remain cowboys, still driving beef cattle to summer pasture in the Klamath Mountains.

Mr. and Mrs. Anton Webber, who traveled extensively in Europe, bought one of these ranches in 1922, and established the Trinity Alps Resort along the Stuart Fork. The Webbers are credited with naming the mountains the Trinity Alps, as they felt the mountains resembled the Austrian Alps that they had admired so much on their European travels.

Loggers and Lumbermen

The miners and early settlers, although profligate in their use, hardly made a dent in the vast supply of timber present in the mountains. However, with the coming of the railroad in the late 1800s, timber cutting began in earnest, and logging and running sawmills soon eclipsed mining as the main industry in the region.

Later improvements in transportation and mechanization increased the rate of cutting dramatically, pushing the cuts to the boundary of the former Salmon-Trinity Alps Primitive Area in many places. In spite of intense pressure on the Forest Service and Congress by timber interests, much of the wilderness was spared the loggers' axe. Checkerboard ownership (due to land grants from the federal government as an inducement to build the Central Pacific Railroad) of some of the land within the wilderness area was supposed to have been resolved by land trades and buyouts.

Dam Builders and Fishermen

Many acrimonious, and sometimes fatal, arguments took place among the early miners about water rights, but those disagreements paled in comparison to what happened when the Central Valley Project was pushed through at the insistence of Central Valley and Southern California water users. The CVP steamrolled right over Trinity County residents and the few conservationists existing in those days, diverting water from the Trinity River to points south.

Trinity, Lewiston, and Whiskeytown dams were completed in the early 1960s, drowning Trinity Meadows, among other things, and seriously damaging one of the finest salmon and steelhead fisheries left in California. In place of beautiful Trinity Meadows, and the opportunity to fish for salmon and steelhead, we now have the pleasure of water skiing on red-dirt-rimmed Trinity Lake. However, all is not lost, as the Trinity River Restoration Council (www. trrp.net) has spearheaded efforts to enhance the fisheries habitat and, after years of serious declines, salmon and steelhead runs at least have shown some hope in recent years.

Recreational Enthusiasts

Except for occasional horse-mounted hunting and fishing expeditions, recreational use in the Klamath Mountains increased with the improvements of surrounding roadways in the 1920s, and a number of dude ranches and resorts sprung up around Trinity Meadows, Trinity Center, and Coffee Creek. Horses

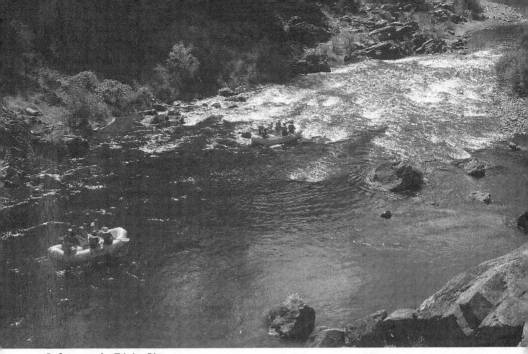

Rafters on the Trinity River

still carried most of the visitors to the backcountry until the late 1950s, when much improved equipment and freeze-dried food encouraged a backpacking boom. Today, backpackers far outnumber equestrians. Rafting on some of the major rivers in the area, such as the Klamath, Trinity, and upper Sacramento, has become a very popular outdoor activity as well.

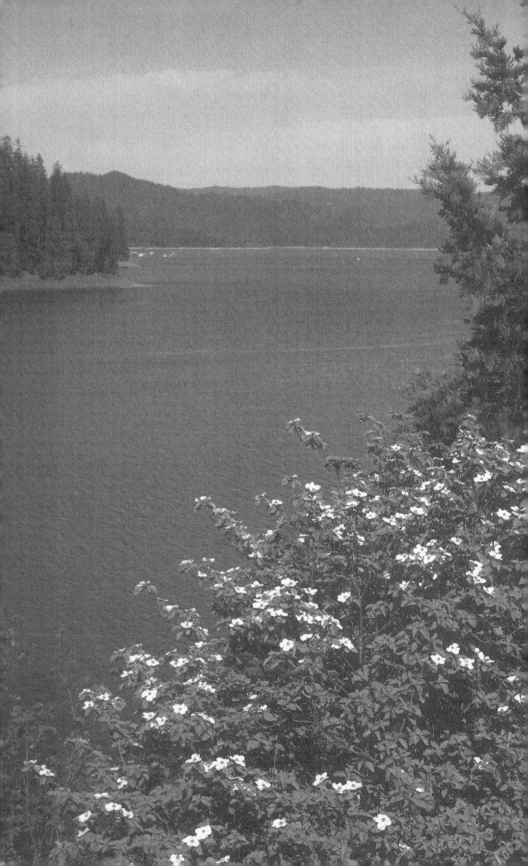

CHAPTER 2

Access, Facilities, and Supplies

As alternatives are fairly limited in this area, the private automobile remains the easiest mode of transportation for getting to the trailheads. Both Redding and Eureka have limited commercial airline service and rental cars available at both airports. Amtrak's Coast Starlight train stops in Redding, Dunsmuir, and Yreka, where picking up rental cars is also possible. Greyhound offers bus service between Arcata and Redding.

Highways, Cities, and Towns

Redding, Eureka, and Yreka are the closest cities of any substantial size to the areas covered in this guide. The small town of Weaverville is the point of departure for many of the trips in the Trinity Alps. The even smaller community of Etna serves the same purpose for most trips into Russian Wilderness. The Interstate 5 towns of Dunsmuir and Mt. Shasta are the closest communities to trailheads in Castle Crags State Park and Castle Crags Wilderness.

Cities and Towns Along State Highway 299:
Redding to Willow Creek

Redding is a little more than 200 miles north of the San Francisco Bay Area, 160 miles from Sacramento, and 545 miles from Los Angeles. The city straddles the Sacramento River near I-5 and the junctions of State Highways 229 and 44. Plenty of options exist in this town of 90,000 people for motels, restaurants, gas stations, grocery stores, and commercial campgrounds. The best place for

Left: Dogwoods and Trinity Lake

backpacking and hiking gear is Hermit's Hut at 3184 Bechelli Lane (888-507-4455, www.hermitshut.com). Shasta-Trinity National Forest Headquarters is located in Redding at 3544 Avtech Parkway (530-226-2500, www.fs.fed.us/r5/shastatrinity). The Whiskeytown Unit of Whiskeytown-Shasta-Trinity National Recreation Area is 8 miles west of Redding on Highway 299.

Weaverville is 45 miles west of Redding via Highway 299. From Weaverville, Highway 299 continues westbound toward Willow Creek and access to trailheads on the south side of the Trinity Alps, while State Highway 3 heads north from the center of town to access trailheads on the east side of the Trinity Alps.

Historic buildings dating from gold rush days line the main street of the quaint town, with exterior spiral staircases from arcaded sidewalks to second stories adding a charming touch. The Trinity County courthouse in the center of town is a fine brick building that's more than a century old. The old buildings in this part of town are filled with shops, art galleries, restaurants, and even a wine tasting room. The Weaverville Joss House State Historical Park boasts the oldest continuously used Chinese temple in the state. Close by, the J. J. Jackson Memorial Museum chronicles the early days of settlement and the subsequent mining boom.

This small town of 4,000 souls is the seat of government for Trinity County and boasts one of the few operating sawmills left in California. Weaverville's economic health depends on recreation and tourism, and so visitors have many options for motels, restaurants, gas stations, and stores.

Weaverville, California

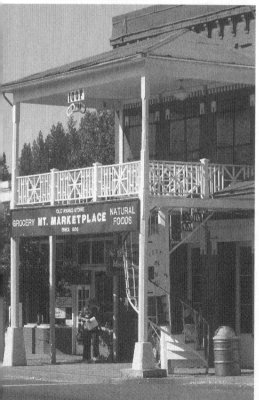

A pre- or post-trip meal at one of the many dining establishments lining Main Street, where Highway 299 runs through town, is a common practice. Although franchises have recently spread their tentacles into the area (Subway, Burger King, Round Table, and Starbucks), plenty of independent restaurants still remain, especially in the historic section. At the top of the food chain, La Grange Cafe (520 Main St., 530-623-5325) offers by far the best food in the old section of town, with moderately priced, slightly upscale lunches and dinners. The Garden Cafe (252 Main St., 530-623-2058) is my favorite for breakfast, especially when the weather is warm enough for outside dining on their patio. Sharing the downstairs of the same building with the Garden Cafe is La Casita (530-623-5795), a tiny Mexican restaurant with a fine menu and ample portions for those with a big appetite. Miller's Drive-In (901 Main St., 503-623-4585) is the place to grab an old-fashioned burger, fries, and shake—an unfortunately disappearing tradition in much of the franchise-driven U.S. Fresh and wholesome delicatessen fare is available from Trinideli just off the main drag (201 Trinity Lakes Blvd., 530-623-5856). Susie's Bakery (1260 Main St., 503-623-5223) is the town's traditional bakery, where you can pick up standard carbo-loading fare.

On the east part of town is the area's only bona fide shopping mall (housing the Starbucks, Subway, and Burger King, with Round Table directly across the street). The highlight for hikers is Top's Sentry Market, an excellent grocery store, especially well stocked with a diverse assortment of food products for a town of this size. About the only thing lacking from a backpacker's perspective is a selection of freeze-dried foods. A few doors from the grocery store, Dragonfly Outfitters is the closest thing to a camping store in Weaverville, which likely has a few necessary items for a hiking or backpacking trip, such as insect repellent or U.S. Geological Survey maps—just don't expect to find bigger gear like a pair of hiking boots, a tent, or a backpack.

The Forest Service has a district office west of the historic district on the south side of the highway at 210 Main Street. Self-issue wilderness permits, as well as information sheets about trails, campgrounds, and natural history, can be obtained from the display immediately outside the front door. During business hours you can usually get updated information from the rangers, as well as have the opportunity to purchase relevant maps and books.

Weaverville does not have any commercial campgrounds in town. However, the Forest Service's all-year East Weaver Campground is only a couple of miles north of the airport on East Weaver Creek Road (fee, water, vault toilets, picnic tables, and fire pits). There is an excellent Bureau of Land Management campground 7 miles west of town via Highway 299, 1 mile past Junction City (fee, water, flush toilets, picnic tables, and fire pits). In the opposite direction on Highway 299, 2.3 miles east of Douglas City, driving 4 miles on Steel Bridge Road (County Road 208) will get you to the BLM's Steel Bridge Campground (fee, no water, vault toilets, picnic tables, and fire pits).

Junction City, 8 miles west of Weaverville on Highway 299, with fewer than 750 residents, can hardly be considered a true city. This tiny town at the confluence of Canyon Creek, is the oldest settlement along the Trinity River and has the only full-fledged grocery store between Weaverville and western Trinity Alps trailheads. Numerous river resorts, RV parks, taverns, tackle shops, and rafting outfitters are strung out along the Trinity River downstream from Junction City, which is a noted salmon and steelhead fishery, as well as river rafting center.

Unless they're coming from the coast, most Trinity Alps hikers won't reach **Willow Creek,** a small town of less than 2,000 people at the junction of Highway 299 and U.S. Highway 96. The town does have gas stations, motels, and restaurants, and the Six Rivers National Forest has a district office on Highway 96, a quarter mile north of the Highway 299 junction.

Towns Along Highway 3: Weaverville to Yreka

Trinity Center is the only town on the shoreline of Trinity Lake, 30 miles north of Weaverville. Ending up at Wyntoon Resort instead is fairly easy if you miss the turnoff to Trinity Center, which is immediately south of the Swift Creek bridge. The present site of the town is not at all the original Trinity Centre of gold rush days, which lies beneath the waters of Trinity Lake. The only structure moved from the original site to the current location prior to the filling of the lake is the Odd Fellows Hall. Trinity Center has the only airstrip close to the eastern Alps, along with Jaktri Market, a grocery store with gas pumps and a small cafe next door. Lodging is limited to houseboat and cabins rentals. The seasonally open Scott Museum has an interesting collection of pioneer memorabilia.

Coffee Creek is a tiny community near the junction of Coffee Creek Road and Highway 3, about 40 miles north of Weaverville. The eclectic Forest Cafe is immediately east of the junction, while Coffee Creek Country Store, gas station, and laundromat are west of the junction, a short distance down County Road 136, and not far from a Forest Service guard station.

The very quiet community of **Callahan** is 3 miles north of Scott Summit and 65 miles from Weaverville. From Gazelle on I-5, Callahan is only 30 miles away on paved Forest Road 17. If you're traveling from Oregon, the best route to Callahan and vicinity is via Highway 3 from Yreka. About the only thing Callahan has to offer the tourist is an old-time general store.

Farther north on Highway 3 is the town of **Etna**, which after Callahan, feels like a bustling metropolis, despite the fact that fewer than 800 people live here. The lodging options in this town are limited to one small motel and a bed-and-breakfast. Fortunately the traveler has more options for grabbing a bite to eat (there's even a brewery here). Some supplies can be obtained at the local grocery or drugstore. A complex containing a gas station, convenience store, and campground is near the junction of Highway 3 and Sawyers Bar Road.

Farther north still, Highway 3 terminates at I-5 in **Yreka**, a substantial town of fewer than 7,500 people, with all the basic services, including most fast-food restaurants, motels, gas stations, and big-box store chains.

Cities and Towns Along Interstate 5: Redding to Yreka

Redding is described above in the Highway 3 section (see page 19). Heading north from Redding on Interstate 5 motorists pass Shasta Lake in the Shasta Unit of Whiskeytown-Shasta-Trinity National Recreation Area. Exits lead to resorts, marinas, general stores, motels, campgrounds, and a few cafes scattered around the lakeshore.

The first town of any substance you come to past the Castella exit to Castle Crags State Park is **Dunsmuir**, 185 miles north of Sacramento. The quaint old town of fewer than 2,000 souls is far enough off the freeway to avoid the look and feel of a town that exists solely for the impatient traveler in need of a tank of gas or a quick bite to eat. For a town of this size, Dunsmuir boasts a number of non-franchise restaurants well worth a visit. Cafe Maddelena, (5801

Sacramento Ave., 530-235-2725) a block east of the main drag, is an upscale eatery serving Mediterranean cuisine. Cornerstone Bakery and Cafe (5759 Dunsmuir Ave., 530-235-4677) is the place for a fresh and wholesome breakfast, or for pastries for the road. Sengthong's Restaurant (5841 Dunsmuir Ave., 530-235-1046) more than fills the bill as a good Thai restaurant. Lodging is available at a handful of motels in town and a couple of nearby resorts. Vacation rentals are also an option.

City of Mt. Shasta sits another 8 miles up I-5 from Dunsmuir. This town of about 3,500 residents formerly thrived on logging as the chief economic force but now depends mainly on tourism and recreation. Consequently, travelers will find plenty of gas stations, restaurants, and motels near the freeway exits and along the main road. Situated at the base of the Cascade Range volcano of Mt. Shasta, the town has a cosmic feel that attracts a large number of spiritually minded souls. Catering to the high number of recreational enthusiasts that the area draws, the town has a couple of outdoor stores where hikers and backpackers can find almost anything they need, including mountaineering gear, at The Fifth Season (300 N. Mt. Shasta Blvd., 530-926-3606), or Shasta Base Camp (316 Chestnut St., 503-926-2359).

Car Camping and Other Recreational Facilities

Campgrounds are plentiful and well placed in this area of Northern California. The Whiskeytown Unit of Whiskeytown-Shasta-Trinity-National Recreation Area has a couple fully developed campgrounds and four primitive campgrounds. You can obtain more information and pay fees at the visitor center immediately off Highway 299. Picnic sites and swimming areas are scattered around the shoreline of Whiskeytown Lake, but boating is the primary activity here, especially during summer (personal watercraft are prohibited). With a California license, anglers can fish for rainbow and brown trout; largemouth, smallmouth, and spotted bass; and kokanee salmon. For a dollar, recreational enthusiasts can pan for gold. Contact Whiskeytown National Recreation Area, P.O. Box 188, Whiskeytown, CA 96095. Call them at 530-242-3400 or visit www. nps.gov/whis.

The best car-camping campgrounds close to the Trinity Alps are found in the Trinity Unit of Whiskeytown-Shasta-Trinity National Recreation Area around Trinity and Lewiston Lakes. Information sheets listing the campgrounds and their amenities are available at any ranger station, Forest Service Information Station, or tourist information facility from Redding to Big Bar. At least 15 campgrounds are listed within the recreation area, but not all of them are open at all times. Most of these campgrounds charge a nightly fee.

Of course, you can do more than simply camp in the recreation area. Trinity Lake has picnicking and swimming sites scattered around its shore.

A particularly fine swimming area with dressing rooms and picnic tables is immediately north of the Stuart Fork, above the lake where Highway 3 crosses Stoney Creek. However, the water level is occasionally too low here to swim during dry years. Boaters can fish and water ski on Trinity and Lewiston lakes, and boat rentals are available at marinas.

National Forest campgrounds outside of the recreation area around the perimeter of the Trinity Alps are not as developed or well maintained as the recreation area campgrounds. With the exception of campgrounds on the upper section of Highway 3, such as Eagle Creek, Horse Flat, and Scott Summit, Shasta-Trinity National Forest campgrounds typically receive a fair amount of use. For more information, contact Shasta-Trinity National Forest, 3644 Avtech Parkway, Redding, CA 96002. Call them at 530-226-2500 or visit www.fs.fed.us/r5/shastatrinity.

Between the north side of the Alps and the south side of Russian Wilderness, within Klamath National Forest, several good campgrounds can be accessed from Forest Highway 93 between Callahan and Cecilville. As most of the land east of Russian Wilderness is private property, there are no Forest Service campgrounds accessed from Highway 3 between Callahan and Etna. The Sawyers Bar Road provides access to Idlewild Campground, the lone campground on the west side of Russian Wilderness. For more information, contact Klamath National Forest, 1312 Fairlane Road, Yreka, CA 96097. Call them at 530-842-6131 or visit them online at www.fs.fed.us/r5/klamath.

Castle Crags State Park offers a number of developed campsites and a half-dozen environmental sites. Only a handful of sites are suitable for RVs, which makes the park a great place for tent campers. Situated in a steep canyon of the Sacramento River near I-5 and a Southern Pacific Railroad line, the nearly constant drone of traffic and the occasional rumble from passing trains negates any sense of being away from it all. A general store with a small cafe and bar immediately outside the park adds to the civilized nature of the area. Along with the excellent hiking, visitors can fish in the nearby river. For more information, contact Castle Crags State Park, P.O. Box 80, Castella, CA 96017. Call them at 530-235-2684 or visit www.parks.ca.gov.

Outside of Castle Crags State Park, there are no-fee, primitive campsites around Castle Lake and Castle Creek on the north side of Castle Crags Wilderness. For more information, contact Shasta-Trinity National Forest, which is listed above.

Resorts, Bed-and-Breakfasts, and Pack Stations

Ownership, locations, and policies of resorts and outfitters are subject to frequent change—contact the appropriate Forest Service headquarters for a list of currently permitted concessionaires. I highly recommend that you begin any search for such services with the Shasta Cascade Wonderland Association.

This recreation and tourism agency maintains an information center at 1699 Highway 273, Anderson, CA 96007, just off I-5, about 10 miles south of Redding in the Shasta Factory Outlets Mall. Contact them by phone at 530-365-7500 or 800-4SHASTA, by fax at 530-365-1258, or online at www.shastacascade.com.

Resorts near Trinity Alps

The all-year Lakeview Terrace Resort in Lewiston overlooks Lewiston Lake and offers cabin rentals for a night, a week, or more. There is a small RV park at the resort as well. Boating and fishing are the main activities at this resort, but the 10 mile-per-hour speed limit on the lake makes kayaking or canoeing a viable option. For more information, call 530-778-3803, email the resort at lvtr@snow-crest.net, or visit them online at www.lakeviewterraceresort.com.

At a shady location along the Stuart Fork, a half mile up Trinity Alps Road from Highway 3, Trinity Alps Resort offers weeklong cabin rentals from Memorial Day weekend through Labor Day weekend. The resort is also available for private groups during the shoulder seasons of May and September. Reservations for the 43 cabins and 3 lodge rooms are hard to come by and usually need to be made a year in advance. The resort has a general store and the Bear's Breath Bar and Grill, which operates on limited days and hours. For more information, call 530-286-2205, or visit www.trinityalpsresort.com.

Trinity Center on the west shore of Trinity Lake has a couple of boat-oriented resorts. Pinewood Cove Resort offers cabins with full baths and kitchens for weeklong rentals between Memorial Day weekend and Labor Day weekend. Cabins can be rented for a two-night minimum during the off-season at reduced rates between mid-September and mid-May. For more information, call 530-286-2201, or visit www.pinewoodcove.com. Trinity Lake Resorts (formerly Cedar Stock Resort) has housekeeping cabins with full kitchens and baths for nightly or weekly rental periods (and houseboats for three- to seven-day rental periods). Timbers Restaurant is open from mid-May to the end of August on a limited basis (530-286-2225). For more information, call 800-255-5561, or visit www.trinitylakeresort.com.

Before Trinity Dam backed up the waters of Trinity River forming Trinity Lake, several old houses from the soon-to-be inundated community of Stringtown were relocated to dry ground in Enright Gulch west of the lake. Since the 1950s, Enright Gulch Cabins and Motel has provided travelers with housekeeping cabins on a weekly basis and motel units on a nightly basis from mid-May through Labor Day weekend. For more information, call 530-266-3600, or visit www.trinitycounty.com/enright.htm.

Bonanza King Resort is a half mile west of Highway 3 on Coffee Creek Road. The resort has seven cabins, with kitchens and full baths, available for rent on a weekly basis during the summer season, which runs from Memorial Day weekend to Labor Day weekend. The cabins are available on a two-night minimum basis during the rest of the year. For more information call 530-266-3305, or visit www.bonanzakingresort.com.

A dude ranch about 5 miles up Coffee Creek Road from Highway 3, Coffee Creek Ranch has a history dating back to the late 1800s and is run by the Hartman Family. Daily trail rides are a staple of the ranch and overnight trips can be arranged. The ranch is open from Easter to Thanksgiving. For more information, call 800-624-4480 or visit www.coffeecreekranch.com.

Trinity Mountain Meadow Resort is also on Coffee Creek Road, 18 miles from Highway 3. Cabins can be rented for a week at a time during the months of July and August. All meals are provided. For more information, call 530-462-4677, or visit www.mountainmeadowresort.com.

Ripple Creek Cabins, on the Eagle Creek Loop north of Coffee Creek, is an all-year facility with seven housekeeping cabins, renting by the week during the summer and per night during the rest of the year. For more information, call 530-266-3505, or visit www.ripplecreekcabins.com.

Camp Unalayee is a private kid's summer camp on an inholding within the northeastern corner of Trinity Alps Wilderness. Beginning operations on the present site in 1960, the camp was grandfathered in when the area became a federally designated wilderness in 1985. For more information, call 650-969-6313, or visit www.unalayee.org.

Situated along the banks of the Klamath River about a mile from the town of Orleans, Sandy Bar Ranch is a green-friendly resort offering four rustic redwood cabins for rent, each with full bath and kitchen. Activities include rafting, fishing, and swimming in the Klamath River, and hiking in the nearby western Alps. For more information, call 530-627-3379, or visit www.sandybar.com.

Resorts near Russian Wilderness

More remote and much smaller than the Trinity Alps, the lands surrounding Russian Wilderness offer travelers little in the way of lodging options. JH Ranch is a private Christian-based resort on the west side of the Russian Wilderness, geared primarily toward junior high and high school students. For more information, visit www.jhranch.com.

Resorts near Castle Crags

Near the town of Castella along Clear Creek, Best in the West Resort is a small, all-year facility with eight housekeeping cabins and an RV park. For more information, call 530-235-2603, or visit www.eggerbestwest.com.

Cave Springs Resort, along the upper Sacramento River near Dunsmuir, rents cabins and motel rooms on a daily or weekly basis in a secluded setting. For more information, call 888-235-2721, or visit www.cavesprings.com.

Near the shore of Lake Siskiyou and southwest of City of Mt. Shasta, Mount Shasta Resort offers fully equipped chalets for rent. The resort has a golf course, day spa, restaurant (open Thursday–Sunday), and lounge. For more information, call 800-958-3363, or check out their website at www.mountshastaresort.com.

Open Memorial Day weekend to Labor Day weekend, Lake Siskiyou Camp-Resort has cabin rentals, campsites, a general store, a marina, and a swimming beach. For more information, call 888-926-2618, or visit www.lakesis.com.

Bed-and-Breakfasts near Trinity Alps

Fully restored in 1989, The Old Lewiston Inn, overlooking the Trinity River in the small community of Lewiston, offers seven guest rooms. For more information, call 877-778-3385, or visit www.theoldlewistoninn.com. The three-room Whitmore Inn occupies a restored Victorian home in the historic district of downtown Weaverville. For more information, call 503-623-2509, or visit www.whitmoreinn.com. Trinity River Bed & Breakfast is near the Trinity River in Hawkins Bar, about an hour west of Weaverville. For more information, call 530-629-1659, or visit www.trinityriverbb.com. The historic and elegant Carrville Inn, 6 miles north of Trinity Center on Carrville Loop Road immediately off Highway 3, is a spacious three-story inn offering six guest rooms and a two-bedroom cottage nearby. For more information, call the owners at 530-266-3000, or visit www.carrvilleinn.com.

Bed-and-Breakfasts near Russian Wilderness

Alderbrook Manor in Etna occupies a fully restored Victorian home on well-manicured grounds, offering four guest rooms, two with private baths. Of great interest to hikers and backpackers is the Hikers Hut, a six-bed hostel-type cabin equipped with a bathroom, microwave, toaster, coffee pot, barbecue, and computer with Wi-Fi. A washer and dryer are also available. The good news is that the rate for a night's stay was only $25 in 2009. For more information, call 530-467-3917, or visit www.alderbrookmanor.com.

Bed-and-Breakfasts near Castle Crags

The City of Mt. Shasta offers a couple of bed-and-breakfasts. Dream Inn is comprised of two neighboring houses, one Victorian and the other Spanish. For more information, call 877-375-4744, or visit www.dreaminnmtshastacity.com.

Packers, Outfitters, and Guides

A number of outfitters hold permits to operate guided trips into the Trinity Alps and Russian Wilderness, using llamas, horses, or mules as the beasts of burden. For more information, contact the Shasta Cascade Wonderland Association (see page 24).

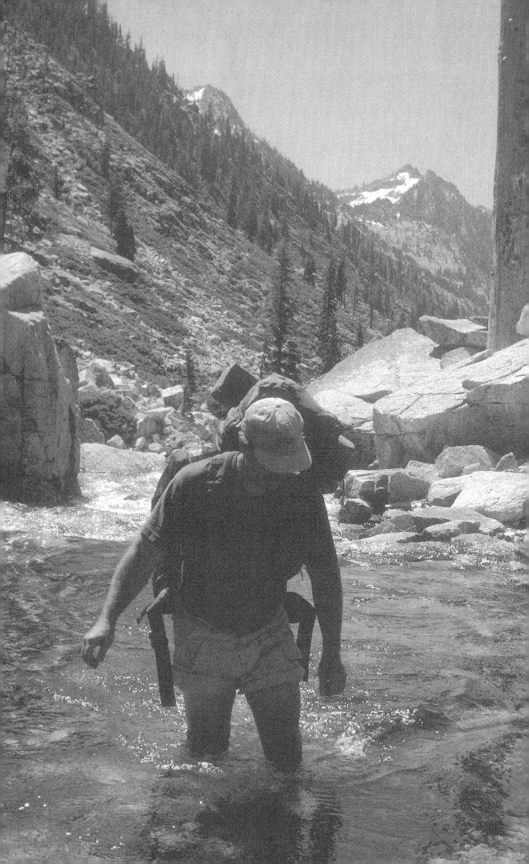

CHAPTER 3

Hiking and Backpacking Basics

This guide should provide you with all the information you need to hike, backpack, or ride horseback on the more than 500 miles of trails in the Trinity Alps Wilderness, Russian Wilderness, Whiskeytown National Recreation Area, and Castle Crags area. The well-researched information in the trip descriptions will assist you in planning trips and anticipating the pleasures of any particular area. This guide will help you choose the right trips, and inform you about when to go, what to expect, and what to carry with you. If you happen to be fortunate enough to eventually walk or ride all of the trips described in this book, you won't regret the time or effort involved.

A basic knowledge of how to read topographic maps and how to use a compass and a GPS unit are expected skills for anyone headed into the areas covered in this guide. Consequently, the book does not go into minute details about the trails. If you would like to learn more about backcountry navigation, Brian Beffort's *Joy of Backpacking* (also published by Wilderness Press) is a very helpful resource.

When and Where to Go

The relatively low elevations in Whiskeytown NRA and Castle Crags State Park provide fine early and late season hiking opportunities. In fact, many of those trails could be hiked year-round, depending on weather conditions. Most trails in the Trinity Alps and Russian Wilderness are open by late June in all years except those of inordinately heavy snowfall, and usually remain open until

Left: Fording outlet of upper lake, Canyon Creek Trail (Trip 32)

sometime in October or early November. At the beginning of each trip description is a "Season" listing, which may be slightly different from this generalization; there are usually good reasons for any discrepancies. For instance, some high-elevation passes and north-facing slopes shed their snow later than lower passes and south-facing slopes. Fords of swollen streams may not be safe at the same time every year as well. Since no two years are alike, you should always exercise good judgment and acquire all the relevant information about an area when planning your visit.

If You Want to Fish

Fishing is generally good—even fantastic at times!—in the areas covered by this guide. Almost all of the lakes in this region have been stocked with fish in the past, but stocking has been curtailed by court ruling in many of the more remote lakes in an attempt to restore the native fish populations. Reducing stocking is also a cost-cutting measure for a state government badly strapped for cash. A list of bodies of water in the state that will and will not be stocked by the Department of Fish and Game is generally available at www.dfg.ca.gov. The only lakes not stocked in the past were too small and remote, or too high and too shallow that they froze solid during the winter, killing the fish. Most of the trout in the backcountry lakes are eastern brook trout, as this species can reproduce without the aid of running water. However, a few lakes do have a good population of rainbow trout that spawn successfully in the running water of inlets or outlets. Some other lakes also contain large rainbow and brown trout that were stocked several years ago, such as Upper Canyon Creek Lake, which boasts a healthy population of good size fish of all three species.

Fishing in the Klamath River system, including streams that empty directly into the Trinity River below Lewiston Dam, and all the tributaries of these streams, is influenced by steelhead and salmon runs. You may see a few adult steelhead resting in the deep pools of these streams in the summer during spawning runs. If you're particularly fortunate, you may even see a salmon or two, but they are becoming scarce. In an effort to sustain these fisheries, salmon and steelhead runs in the anadromous waters of the Klamath and Trinity rivers is reviewed and regulated by the California Department of Fish and Game every year. Check with them for current quotas and regulations.

Of course, none of the streams that empty into Trinity Lake or the Trinity River above the lake have steelhead or salmon runs any longer. However, all

Fly-fishing in the Trinity River

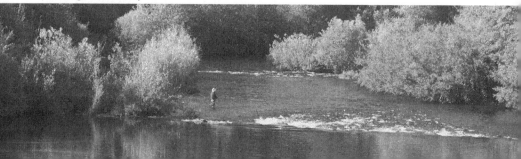

of these streams of any consequence harbor some native rainbow trout, and some of the higher tributaries have eastern brook trout. The lower, more easily reached stretches of these streams are badly overfished. Stuart Fork, Swift Creek, and Coffee Creek have been hit particularly hard.

Some of the best fishing in the state occurs in the upper Sacramento River near Castle Crags. Fishing season on this stretch of the river, and nearby Castle Creek, runs from the last Saturday in April to November 15, and is restricted to artificial lures and barbless hooks.

A few streams and lakes have been stocked with golden trout and, if so, are noted in the trip descriptions. Almost all the fishing information in the descriptions was based on the personal experience of this guide's former author, Luther Linkhart, and is biased toward dry fly-fishing. Of course, a valid California fishing license and compliance with California fishing regulations are required. Good luck!

Hunting Season

If you prefer not to hike in the backcountry during general deer hunting season, avoid scheduling trips during the last week of September and the first three weeks of October. Bow hunting usually precedes the opening of rifle season by about a month, but there's little chance that a bow hunter at close range would mistake you for a deer. The beginning of bear hunting season usually corresponds to the beginning of general deer hunting season, but either extends through the last Sunday in December, or until the yearly quota is taken. Check with the Department of Fish and Game for the actual dates of each season, as they tend to vary somewhat from year to year and district to district.

Hiking in the Trinity Alps, Russian, and Castle Crags wilderness areas during hunting season without experiencing any difficulties is quite possible. The number of hunters you encounter seems to diminish with the amount of distance you're willing to put between yourself and the nearest road. Besides, most hunters you come across in the wilderness are typically competent and respectful backcountry users. In many ways, fall is the best season for hiking the trails in theses areas and should be enjoyed by all.

To Ski or Not to Ski

Currently, there are no downhill ski areas operating near the Trinity Alps, Russian, or Castle Crags wilderness areas, and there are no plans to build any in the future. The closest developed ski area is on Mt. Shasta. Designated or groomed cross-country ski trails are also absent from this part of Northern California. Scott and Carter summits are about the only areas high enough for cross-country skiing or snowshoeing and reachable by car. Otherwise, you should expect to walk many wet miles in order to reach a sufficient amount of snow on which to practice these pursuits. Much of the backcountry is potentially avalanche prone as well.

The Trails

Factors Determining Trail Difficulty

The difficulty level of a trip is somewhat subjective and depends greatly on the weather, your physical condition, and your expectations. Of those three factors, the only one this guide can help influence is what you expect to find. For many of the same reasons, the number of days suggested for each trip is subjective as well. The fewer number of days listed is the minimum you should schedule in order to fully enjoy a trip. The greater number of days obviously includes a layover day or two when you can settle into a camp and do some nearby day-hikes, or simply enjoy a rest day. Campsites and places to acquire water will be mentioned in order to help you plan your routes efficiently.

Finding the Trailheads

All of the trailheads listed in this guide should be accessible to the average sedan. However, that sedan might be very dusty or mud-caked by the time you reach a particular trailhead. Some roads are narrow and winding, requiring a speed no faster than 15 miles per hour at times.

Directions to the trailheads should be explicit enough to get you safely there without belaboring them too much. Due to inadequate funding, the U.S. Forest Service has had to curtail much of their road maintenance, so checking on the current conditions at a ranger station may go a long way toward preventing any prospective difficulties in accessing the trails. Keep a watchful eye whenever you drive roads near active logging operations, as the typical sedan won't fare very well in a battle with a logging truck. Try to allow more time to get to a trailhead than you consider necessary, as many of the "highways" in the area can't be driven at freeway speeds. The gravel and dirt roads beyond the highways will require even slower speeds.

Some of the road and trailhead signs in this area have a habit of routinely disappearing (the TANGLE BLUE LAKE sign is a classic example), which can create obvious problems. Therefore, keep track of your odometer readings and have an up-to-date map handy in case you reach an unsigned junction.

While the safety of your vehicle when parked at a trailhead is always a legitimate concern, the chance of a break-in or other form of vandalism is quite remote in this area. Nevertheless, don't leave valuables in your vehicle, and place any unused gear or extraneous objects out of sight in your trunk—what you may consider of little value a vandal might find worth stealing.

Watching Grass Grow

Many miles of trail in the northwestern Trinity Alps are not covered in this guide for the not-so-simple reason that this area has long been inhabited by illegal farmers cultivating marijuana. During the 1970s and 1980s, pot growers virtually took over a vast area of territory that included East Fork New River,

Pony Creek, Slide Creek, Eagle Creek, and Mary Blaine Meadow. Forest Service personnel did not patrol or maintain any of these trails, advising recreational enthusiasts to avoid the area altogether. In the course of events, two guard stations were burned down, shots were fired at or near Forest Service personnel, and numerous vehicles were vandalized and burned while parked at trailheads. In 1982 the district ranger stationed at Big Bar said, "Large areas in my district are not under our control."

In the mid-80s a major law enforcement effort was carried out in this area by armed forest rangers, state and federal narcotics agents, and Trinity County deputy sheriffs. Marijuana plantations were destroyed, illegal structures torn down, and large amounts of trash packed out. Maintenance crews restored some of the trails, and they were subsequently declared safe for outdoor enthusiasts to use again. However, before you decide to travel in this area, check with the Big Bar Ranger Station or the Denny Forest Service Guard Station about current conditions.

Marijuana cultivation may be attempted in remote areas with an adequate water supply once again thanks to declining government budgets for both maintenance and patrols, as well as the passage of recent laws allowing individuals to grow and possess small amounts of the plant for medicinal purposes. Since selling, transporting, and growing larger amounts of marijuana is still illegal, some pot growers may arm themselves and may not appreciate your presence should you happen to stumble upon their illegal plantation. You should beat a hasty retreat if you come across any suspicious activity.

Signs of illegal pot-growing activity include water lines, PVC pipes, generators, or water pumps—anything out of place in a wilderness setting, for that matter. If you happen to see marijuana plants growing, stop immediately and leave the area. Do not look for more plants, take samples, or conduct your own investigation—leave these duties for trained law enforcement personnel. If you have a GPS unit, you could record the coordinates, while making a mental note of the surroundings and your route.

Staying Safe

Hiking in the Trinity Alps and the other areas covered in this guide should pose no special problems that you wouldn't encounter in any other wilderness or backcountry area in the West. However, some precautions and pre-trip planning can certainly save you some discomfort. Foolhardiness or panic can easily get you into trouble here, as is the case in any outdoor area. For instance, during the very hot and dry summer of 1981, a youth group led by two adults started up the notoriously steep and exposed trail from Portuguese Camp to the crest of Sawtooth Ridge late in the morning one hot summer day. Two-thirds of the way up to the ridge, one boy became ill with "flu-like symptoms," and was unable to continue. The unfortunate boy was left alone in the hot sun while his companions, who were in only slightly better shape, climbed over the ridge to seek help. By the time they were finally able to secure help and climb back over the ridge, the boy was dead.

Apparently no single mistake led to this boy's death, but rather a series of poor decisions, compounded by a lack of precautions, did. First, the group should not have attempted to climb up this trail without carrying a lot of water. Second, basic first-aid training would have enabled at least someone in the group to recognize the symptoms of heat exhaustion and prompted them to find some shade for the stricken boy, loosen his clothes, lower his head, fan him, and above all stay with him. In retrospect, only two people should have gone for help and the rest of the group should have tried to carry the boy to shade and water.

One of the most important considerations in the backcountry is to avoid traveling alone—help could be a long time coming in remote areas. Here's a brief summary of additional hazards.

Altitude Sickness

A cursory examination of topographic maps reveals that altitude sickness should not be much of a problem in the areas covered in this guide. Very few of the trips exceed an elevation of 7500 feet, with many of the trailheads in the Trinity Alps and Russian wildernesses below 3000 feet. Consequently, your first day on the trail should not overtly tax your body, at least from an elevation standpoint. Elevations in Whiskeytown NRA and Castle Crags State Park are even lower. Increase in altitude does aggravate distress caused by heat and dehydration, so take it easy on the trail and drink plenty of fluids, especially on the first day of a trip.

Hypothermia

Although experiencing subfreezing temperatures in this area is highly unlikely during the summer, the possibility of developing hypothermia is quite real when you're unprepared for wet conditions and/or chilly temperatures. The combination of wet clothing and windchill is enough to cause hypothermia at temperatures well above freezing. You can become wet and chilled not only from precipitation, but also by falling into a stream or lake, or even from excessive perspiration.

Hypothermia is a condition where core body temperature lowers due to loss of heat through the skin at a rate faster than the body's ability to produce heat. A drop of one degree in core body temperature is enough to produce shivering, which is the body's defense mechanism to try and raise core temperature through exertion, as well as slurred speech and loss of judgment. A two-degree drop in temperature leads to loss of coordination, loss of memory, and further loss of judgment and initiative. If your core body temperature decreases by three degrees, you will be unable to walk, will experience debilitating lassitude, and, without help, will eventually die.

Hypothermia is an insidious ailment, as the victim fails to realize his or her deteriorating condition, due to the loss of judgment brought on by the initial stages. When wet and cold conditions are encountered, every member of a group should watch each other closely for any developing signs of hypothermia. At the first signs of hypothermia in anyone, the group as a whole should seek shelter, build a fire where possible, and take every step to get the victim warm and dry.

If a person reaches the second or third stages of hypothermia, they must be helped immediately. Abandoning a victim in this situation is a death sentence. With utmost haste, the victim should be placed in a shelter, stripped of all wet clothing, and placed in a dry sleeping bag with another unaffected person, stripped of clothing as well—skin-to-skin transfer of heat is the best remedy. If warm, *nonalcoholic* beverages are available, they will also help the victim.

As with many backcountry maladies, prevention is the best cure for hypothermia. You should always bring waterproof and breathable clothing made from modern synthetics, such as Gore-Tex or its equivalent, whether you're on a dayhike or multiday expedition. At the first sign of wet and/or chilly conditions, put on a shell parka and pants and wear them until conditions improve. Base layers worn next to the skin should be made of polypropylene, or natural fibers like silk or wool—fabrics that will keep you warm and transfer perspiration to the outer layers of your clothing. Mid-layers of synthetics, such as fleece, or wool serve a similar function. Cotton clothing, while very comfortable, is the worst possible fabric for wet and chilly conditions. When wet, either from the elements or perspiration, cotton loses all ability to insulate and thereby keep you warm. A well-constructed tent with a rain fly (or waterproof tent) is an excellent investment for backpackers camping in wet weather (it also provides a haven from mosquitoes).

Sun Exposure

Dehydration is a common but easily preventable condition brought on in the backcountry by strenuous exertion. Dehydration occurs when your body loses too much fluid and you're not drinking enough to sufficiently replace that lost fluid. Symptoms can include muscle cramps and lightheadedness. Not properly rehydrating can lead to severe dehydration, which will eventually become a life-threatening condition. While on the trail, make sure you're drinking plenty of fluids and you shouldn't have to worry about becoming dehydrated.

Heat exhaustion and heatstroke (sunstroke) are not uncommon afflictions in the backcountry of sunny Northern California. Heat exhaustion is when the rate of perspiration is insufficient to cool the body. This condition occurs when a person exercises strenuously in hot weather and does not drink enough fluids to replace those lost through perspiration. Symptoms include flushed skin, rapid breathing, and possible fainting. Drinking plenty of water or electrolyte

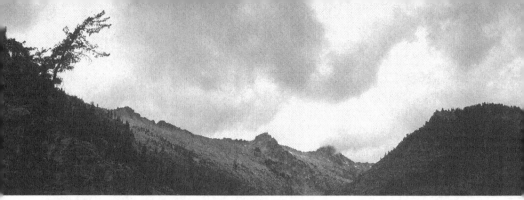

Threatening weather, Upper Canyon Creek (Trip 31)

replacement beverages, such as Gatorade, will prevent heat exhaustion. Moderate to severe heat exhaustion can lead to heatstroke, when the body is unable to regulate core temperature and that temperature continues to rise—simply put, the body produces more heat than it can lose. Symptoms include pale but hot skin, rapid heart rate, mental confusion, convulsion, and unconsciousness. Heatstroke is a serious malady requiring emergency medical intervention. Victims of both heat exhaustion and heatstroke should be removed from the sun and cooled off by sponging the skin with cool water. The treatment for someone who faints is to place their head lower than the rest of their body. Never give an unconscious or semiconscious person anything to drink.

Obviously, people with sensitive eyes should wear sunglasses while in the backcountry, especially when they're on granite- or snow-covered slopes.

Lightning

Occasional thunderstorms sporadically roll through this area during the summer months, which was made abundantly clear by the high number of lightning strikes that triggered numerous fires in June 2008. For further evidence, all you need to do is look around when you cross one of the high crests and see numerous old snags split, shattered, and seared by bolts of lightning.

The safest place during a lightning storm (other than safely tucked into your bed at home) is in the middle of a wide valley in an extensive stand of trees. In addition, you should be at least 100 feet away from metal objects, including your pack. Avoid tall, isolated trees, and high, open areas. Report any fires you see as soon as possible to the nearest Forest Service facility. Do not attempt to put out any forest fire of substantial size without help.

Drinking Water

All drinking water should be treated in the backcountry. This does not mean that all water in the backcountry is contaminated, only that since microscopic organisms are impossible to see with the naked eye, treating all drinking water is the best plan for guarding your health. Giardiasis, a severe intestinal disorder caused by the organism, *Giardia lamblia*, is common enough in the backcountry to cause concern. High coliform (including such bacteria as *E. coli*) counts are fairly common as well.

Dangerous Animals

This subject is covered to some extent in the natural history section (see page 10). In brief, don't attempt to feed or pet any wild animal, which includes carelessly leaving food lying around within easy access for any mildly resourceful critter, such as bears, deer, and rodents.

Bear encounters are few and infrequent. However, carrying your food and scented items in a bear canister, or adequately bear-bagging at the very least, is essential for the well-being of both you and the bears. The following guidelines should help campers and backpackers reduce the possibility of a bear encounter.

At the campground:
- Store all food and scented items out of sight in a bear locker or the locked trunk of your vehicle.
- Dispose of all trash in bear-proof garbage cans or dumpsters.
- Never leave food out and unattended.

In the backcountry:
- Don't leave your pack unattended on the trail.
- At your campsite, empty your pack and open flaps and pockets.
- Keep all food, scented items, and trash in a bear canister, or effectively counterbalanced from a high tree limb.
- Pack out all of your trash.

Everywhere:
- If possible, don't allow a bear to approach your food—throw rocks, make loud noises, and wave your arms. Be bold while maintaining good judgment from a safe distance.
- If a bear gets into your food, you are responsible for cleaning up the mess.
- Never attempt to retrieve food from a bear.
- Report any bear-related incidents to the appropriate government agency.

The most likely spot to encounter a rattlesnake is near or under the end of a footlog at a stream crossing. Rodents cross streams over footlogs too, and rattlesnakes oftentimes wait there for dinner to come to them. The relationship between rattlesnakes and rodents is discussed earlier (see page 11). The only incident of a rattlesnake bite in the Trinity Alps that I've heard of involved a dog owner trying to get a snake off of his dog. Separating the participants in a dog-bear encounter may prove just as unfortunate. Both bears and rattlesnakes will avoid you if they can, so always allow them a route of escape. Refrain from killing a rattlesnake simply because you happen to see it; they are an important part of the ecosystem and were here long before people.

As treatment of rattlesnake bites is somewhat controversial, influenced by numerous old wives' tales, any recommendation for treatment is offered hesitantly. A human being in reasonable condition should be able to survive a rattlesnake bite without immediate treatment, provided he or she stays reasonably calm. Fortunately, rattlesnakes do not always inject venom when they strike and, if they do, bites are very rarely fatal. Of course, a victim should be taken to a hospital or urgent care as soon as possible, but they should ride or be carried out of the backcountry, as opposed to walking out under their own power. To treat a rattlesnake bite, wash the area with soap and water. If you happen to be carrying an extractor, apply suction and use the device to pull venom from the wound, but do not incise the wound. While a tight tourniquet should not be used, application of a constricting band tight enough to slow circulation but not stop pulses will help to slow the spread of venom. Keep the affected limb immobile and below the heart.

Insects

Insect pests are covered rather thoroughly earlier (see page 13). However, although the overwhelming majority of bites cause no problems, one of California's 49 species of ticks, the western black-legged tick, may carry Lyme disease. If possible, treatments for tick bites are influenced by even more erroneous folklore than rattlesnake bites. If bitten by a tick, carefully grab the body of the insect with a pair of tweezers as close to its mouth as possible. Applying gentle traction, pull the tick straight out of the affected flesh without twisting, which can separate the head from the body. Once removed, place the tick in a container for later identification if necessary and then wash the wound thoroughly with soap and water, as well as your hands. If the bite becomes infected, you can apply an antibiotic ointment and cover with a bandage. If the wound starts to itch, swell, or develop redness, an antihistamine, such as Benadryl, may help alleviate those symptoms. Consult a physician if the wound develops a round, red rash and/or you experience flulike symptoms, which can occur anytime after three days or up to a month after being bitten.

Ford of the Stuart Fork (Trip 5)

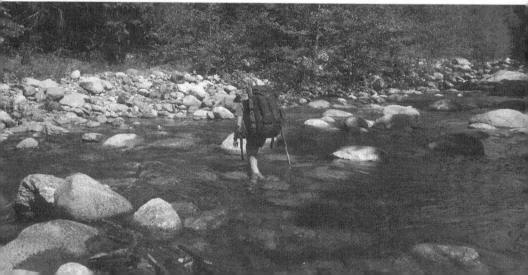

Stream Crossings

A number of stream crossings that would otherwise be dangerous early in the summer have been bridged. Some potentially problematic stream crossings without bridges are specifically mentioned in the trip descriptions. A few streams to be wary of during high water include Virgin Creek, North Fork Trinity River, Grizzly Creek, Rattlesnake Creek, Canyon Creek, Swift Creek, and Stuart Fork. For information on roped stream crossings, consult *Joy of Backpacking* by Brian Beffort. In order to rope safely across a stream of any size, you will need a 150-foot lightweight climbing rope.

Wilderness Patrols

A wilderness trail crew is comprised of some of the hardest-working, most dedicated public servants you'll ever meet. Unfortunately, there's simply not enough money to fund enough personnel to do all the things that need to be done. Most of the small force of workers in this area is made up of volunteers—if they do get paid they don't receive a ton of money. If you happen to meet a Forest, State Park, or National Park Service ranger on patrol, he or she will likely be carrying a radio, first-aid kit, shovel, axe, and some plastic bags for picking up garbage left behind by the thoughtless few who abuse the privilege of being in the backcountry. Rangers have plenty to do in directing visitors, educating the masses, overseeing trail maintenance, and conducting rescues when necessary. Rangers can and will issue citations for flagrant violations of Forest Service, National Park, or State Park regulations.

What You'll Need

Maps

The maps at the beginning of each chapter of trail descriptions provide a general idea of where trips are located. Individual trips are shown in greater detail on maps sprinkled throughout the pertinent chapters. Familiarity with topographic maps and orienteering with map and compass are skills essential to successfully following any off-trail routes described in this guide, and are highly recommended for on-trail travel as well. Some conservation and hiking associations, as well as some community colleges, offer classes in these skills.

The topographic maps listed in the heading at the beginning of each trip are for USGS 7.5-minute maps. These topographic maps are available directly from the federal government at http://store.usgs.gov, or from visitor centers, ranger stations, and some outdoor retailers. Also, software programs for making topographic maps on your home computer are available for purchase, or you can use them to make a map at kiosks in stores of some major outdoor retailers, such as REI.

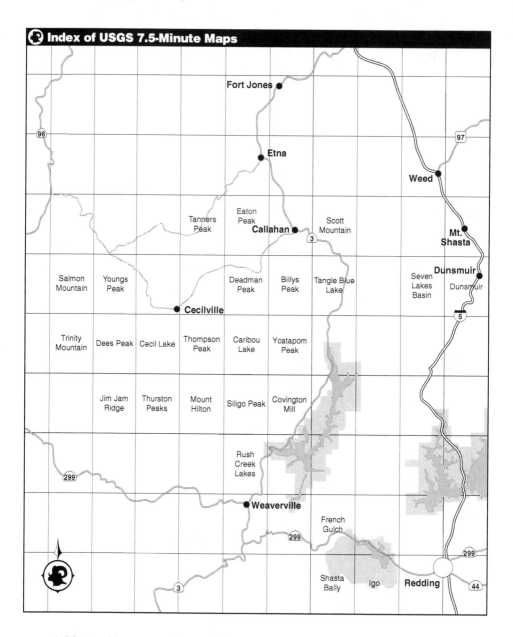

Index of USGS 7.5-Minute Maps

Fort Jones

96

97

Etna

Weed

Tanners
Peak

Eaton
Peak

Scott
Mountain

Mt.
Shasta

Callahan

3

Dunsmuir

Salmon
Mountain

Youngs
Peak

Deadman
Peak

Billys
Peak

Tangle Blue
Lake

Seven
Lakes
Basin

Dunsmuir

Cecilville

5

Trinity
Mountain

Dees Peak

Cecil Lake

Thompson
Peak

Caribou
Lake

Ycatapom
Peak

Jim Jam
Ridge

Thurston
Peaks

Mount
Hilton

Siligo Peak

Covington
Mill

Rush
Creek
Lakes

299

Weaverville

French
Gulch

299

299

Shasta
Bally

Igo

Redding

44

3

Additional listings in the heading are for useful topographic maps printed on waterproof paper and published by the Forest Service for Trinity Alps, Russian, and Castle Crags wilderness areas. *A Guide to the Trinity Alps Wilderness* (2004) is a two-sided map (scale is an inch equals a mile) printed on waterproof paper that covers the entire wilderness and is quite handy for longer trips. The same is true for *A Guide to the Marble Mountain Wilderness and Russian Wilderness* (2004), with the Marble Mountains shown on one side and the Russian Wilderness on the other. At a scale of 2 inches equals 1 mile, *A Guide to the Mt. Shasta Wilderness and Castle Crags Wilderness* (2001) is printed on waterproof paper and also has the two areas shown on opposite sides. California State Parks publishes a waterproof, topographic map at a scale of 3.75 inches equals 1 mile for Castle Crags State Park, which is available from the park's visitor center.

Not mentioned in the headings but useful for trip planning and for finding directions to campgrounds, picnic areas, trailheads, and other features, the Forest Service also publishes smaller-scale maps covering an entire national forest for Klamath (2007), Shasta-Trinity (2007), and Six Rivers (2005) national forests. All of these Forest Service maps can be purchased at ranger stations and information stations, or online at the National Forest Store at www.fs.fed.us/recreation/nationalforeststore.

Index of USGS 7.5-Minute Topographic Maps

NAME	PUBLICATION DATE	TRIPS
Billys Peak	1998	14, 20, 23, 24
Caribou Lake	2001	5, 10, 11, 15, 17, 18, 19
Cecil Lake	1998	33, 34, 35
Covington Mill	1998	7, 8, 9, 10, 11
Deadman Peak	2001	14, 16, 23, 25, 26
Dees Peak	1998	37, 38
Dunsmuir	1998	44, 45, 46, 47, 48
Eaton Peak	2001	39, 40, 41, 42, 43
French Gulch	1979	3, 4
Igo	1998	1, 2
Jim Jam Ridge	1998	36, 37, 38
Mount Hilton	1998	5, 31, 32, 34
Rush Creek Lakes	1998	5, 6, 7, 30
Salmon Mountain	1997	28, 29, 38
Scott Mountain	2001	23
Seven Lakes Basin	1998	48
Shasta Bally	1978	4
Siligo Peak	1998	5, 6, 7, 9, 10, 19
Tangle Blue Lake	1998	20, 21, 22, 23
Tanners Peak	2001	39
Thompson Peak	2001	5, 27, 33, 34
Thurston Peaks	1998	33, 34, 35, 36
Trinity Mountain	1997	38
Ycatapom Peak	1998	10, 11, 12, 13, 14, 19
Youngs Peak	2001	28, 38

Tools

Few tools are required for a trip into the wilderness. One important tool many hikers and backpackers like to carry is a shovel, not the big, cumbersome, or heavy type that you would use in your garden, but a short one with a sturdy blade and a strong handle. This kind of shovel serves three purposes—to scrape out a place for a fire, to put the fire out, and to dig a hole for disposing of human waste.

A fire can only be fully extinguished by drowning it out with water, stirring, and repeating the whole process over again. Simply covering a fire with dirt is usually insufficient enough to put out a campfire. Don't attempt to put out a fire simply by dumping some dirt on it and covering it with rocks.

Human waste should be disposed of in a 6- to 8-inch hole in mineral soil a minimum of 200 feet from a campsite or water source. If you must dig a hole in sod, remove and replace an intact piece, which requires a shovel, as opposed to a stick. Please don't bury garbage—buried garbage will be dug up by some critter. Only cook as much food as you can eat.

Modern backpacking tents have done away with the need for ditching. Digging out a level place to pitch a tent is also unnecessary. Such scars remain for a long time.

The second important tool is a good pocketknife or multi-tool, which is invaluable for a number of purposes: making repairs or cleaning fish, for instance. A pocketknife or multi-tool with a pair of pliers can be particularly useful.

Waterdog Lake in the Russian Wilderness (Trip 39)

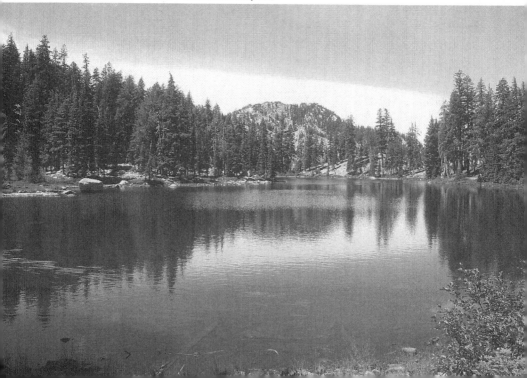

Permits and Practices in the Wilderness

Wilderness Permits

Although regulations are prone to change, a wilderness permit is likely to be a continued requirement for any overnight stay in the Trinity Alps Wilderness. Free wilderness permits are available by self-registration at any ranger station around the Trinity Alps. Currently, wilderness permits are not required for the Russian Wilderness or Castle Crags Wilderness. However, if you are planning to backpack and have a campfire in the national forests covered in this guide, you will have to procure a campfire permit, which is free and available from any Forest Service ranger station or information center. Whether or not wilderness permits are required for overnight visits, you should still inform a responsible party about your plans and itinerary, providing them with information about what agency to contact if you fail to return on time.

Visitor and information centers and ranger stations administered by Forest Service, Park Service, and State Parks personnel can usually provide good information on the current status of trails and conditions of the backcountry. For more information, contact the following facilities:

Whiskeytown National Recreation Area

Whiskeytown NRA
P.O. Box 188
Whiskeytown, CA 96095
530-242-3400
530-246-1225 (visitor information)
www.nps.gov/whis

Trinity Alps

Shasta-Trinity National Forest
3544 Avtech Parkway
Redding, CA 96002
530-226-2500
www.fs.fed.us/r5/shastatrinity

> **Big Bar Ranger District**
> Star Route 1, Box 10
> Big Bar, CA 96010
> 530-623-6106

> **Weaverville Ranger District**
> 210 Main Street, Highway 299
> Weaverville, CA 96093
> 530-623-2121

Klamath National Forest
1312 Fairlane Road
Yreka, CA 96097
530-812-6131
www.fs.fed.us/r5/klamath

Salmon River Ranger District
11263 North Highway 3
Fort Jones, CA 96032
530-468-5351

Russian Wilderness

Klamath National Forest
1312 Fairlane Road
Yreka, CA 96097
530-812-6131
www.fs.fed.us/r5/klamath

Scott River Ranger District
11263 North Highway 3
Fort Jones, CA 96032
530-468-5351

Castle Crags

Shasta-Trinity National Forest
3544 Avtech Parkway
Redding, CA 96002
530-226-2500
www.fs.fed.us/r5/shastatrinity

Mt. Shasta Ranger District
204 West Alma Street
Mt. Shasta, CA 96067
530-926-4511

California State Parks
1416 9th Street
Sacramento, CA 95814
800-777-0369 or 916-653-6995
www.parks.ca.gov

Castle Crags State Park
P.O. Box 80
Castella, CA 96017
530-235-2684

Camping Rules and Etiquette

Campsites should be at least 200 feet from streams and lakes where possible. Only dead wood lying on the ground may be used for firewood. Don't cut green foliage or upright trees for any purpose. The use of motorized equipment within wilderness areas is strictly forbidden, except where specifically authorized on existing mining claims. Equestrians should check with the U.S. Forest Service about forage and tie regulations for saddle and pack animals. A maximum group size of 10 persons is in effect for all wilderness areas covered in this guide.

Campfires and Fire Rings

Most recreational enthusiasts appreciate a fire at their campsite as a marvelous, cheery accessory to their wilderness experience. However, wise use of the firewood supply today will allow future wilderness visitors to enjoy the same experience. Nowadays, some of the most heavily used areas lack an adequate supply of firewood, and as a result campfire bans have been instituted at a handful of the more popular locations. In other areas, please consider whether or not a campfire is appropriate and, if so, keep it small.

Fire rings can be eyesores, particularly the high, built-up variety, which tend to collect trash that is hard to remove from between the rocks. They also make fully extinguishing a fire much more difficult, as coals continue to smolder in the chinks between the rocks. Start a campfire only in existing fire rings—never construct a new fire ring, and don't cook over an open fire—backpacking stoves are much more efficient.

Trail Courtesy

Cutting switchbacks causes erosion and could possibly dislodge a rock onto an unsuspecting hiker below—don't do it. When meeting others on the trail, downhill hikers should yield the right-of-way to uphill hikers. Saddle and pack animals have the right-of-way: When encountering stock, quietly step well off the trail on the downhill side, as they may become nervous when crowded or frightened by unexpected noises or movements, which ultimately could result in potential injury to both hikers and riders.

Any form of trash is an affront to a wilderness experience. Don't litter! Be a good Samaritan and pick up any trash you may encounter at camp or on the trail.

How to Use This Book

Trips are numbered and labeled to show start and finish locales. At the beginning of each trip description, the following bits of information are provided.

Trip Type
This entry describes whether the trip is an out-and-back (retracing your steps to the same trailhead), a point-to-point (beginning and ending at two different trailheads and requiring two vehicles or shuttle), or a loop. A range of days necessary to enjoy the features of the entire trip is also listed.

Distance
This figure gives the total distance in miles from the trailhead to the end point of your journey.

Elevation Change
This figure reveals how much elevation gain and loss hikers will experience from the trailhead to the ultimate destination for out-and-back trips (which should be doubled for the entire distance), and the total elevation gain and loss for point-to-point and loop trips.

Difficulty
The overall difficulty of a trip is measured as easy, moderate, or difficult. This rating is somewhat subjective, as your level of fitness, experience, and knowledge of the backcountry will influence your particular rating of a trip's difficulty. The ratings listed here should be fairly accurate for the average hiker or backpacker.

Season
This entry suggests the best times of the year to fully enjoy the attributes of a particular trip, including the average times of snow-free trails. The season may vary some from year to year based upon the previous winter's snowpack and how quickly the snowpack melts in the spring and early summer.

Maps
The USGS 7.5-minute topographic maps for each trip are listed here, along with any recommended Forest Service or State Parks maps.

Nearest Campground
This listing is for visitors who may wish to camp in a developed campground before or after a trip. In addition to the main trip description, many additional side trips, cross-country routes, or alternative routes are described and are easily identifiable so as not to be confused with the main trip description.

The Trips

Each trip description begins with some general information about the condition of the trail and the features of the area you should expect to experience. Within the trip highlights are any special considerations or necessary cautions that are important for effectively planning your trip. Also, the general information includes an idea of the amount of traffic you should expect to encounter along the trail and at destinations. Each trip also includes a map and an elevation profile. For out-and-back trips, the profile shows data for the trip from the trailhead and to your destination but not your return journey retracing your steps.

Starting Point

This section provides you with detailed driving directions and distances to each trailhead, as well as information about the road surfaces and conditions. Any trailhead facilities are also noted. Nearby campgrounds are listed in the trip summary information and are sometimes described in this section based upon level of use, scenery, privacy, protection from the elements, unique natural features, proximity to fishing, swimming potential, and the availability of possible side trips.

Map Legend

Symbol	Description	Symbol	Description
▪▪▪▪▪	Featured Trail	▲	Mountain
-----	Other Trails	■	Structure or Point of Interest
··········	Cross-Country Route	‖	Waterfall
1	Trip Number	●—●	Gate
T	Trailhead	—	Dam
P	Parking	⅊	Swamp/Wetland
A	Campground	⑤	U.S. Interstate
↑	Ranger Station	95	U.S. Highway
?	Information	③	California State Highway
$	Fee Collection Gate	421	California County Highway
⊞	Picnic Area	93	Forest Service Road

Caring for the Backcountry

Whiskeytown, Shasta, and Trinity are three separate islands of national recreation area surrounding giant reservoirs of the same names, which were set aside in 1965 and are currently managed by the National Park Service. Centered around Whiskeytown Lake, the Whiskeytown Unit consists of around 42,000 acres of land. The area has 24 different trails, many of which are favorites of dayhikers and mountain bikers.

The wilderness areas described in this guide are relatively new to the wilderness system; they were set aside two decades after the original wilderness bill was passed in 1964. The Trinity Alps, Russian, and Castle Crags wilderness areas were all created as part of the California Wilderness Act in September 1984.

The Trinity Alps Wilderness consists of approximately 518,000 acres, with boundaries close to what several conservation organizations and Trinity County lobbied for over the years prior to wilderness designation. Such a designation was a triumph for wilderness proponents and nonmechanized recreational enthusiasts. The act also required that previously existing private lands within the designated wilderness boundary would be exchanged or eventually purchased. Until such buy-outs are completed, any private inholdings will be nominally managed as wilderness. With more than 500 miles of trail, the Trinity Alps are a backpacker's paradise.

The Russian Wilderness is much smaller than the Trinity Alps, with only 12,000 acres of land set astride the apex of a divide separating the Scott and Salmon rivers. The area has a buffer of national forest land on all but the east side, land which is mostly held in private hands. With more than 30 miles of trail within the wilderness and surrounding national forest, this area is well suited for dayhikers, as well as for weekend backpackers.

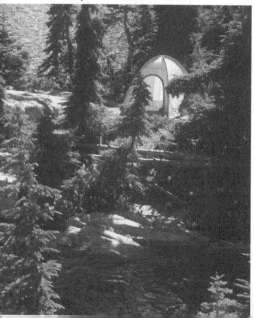

This campsite is too close to water.

Castle Crags Wilderness is even smaller than the Russian Wilderness, with only about 10,500 acres of protected wilderness. This small pocket of backcountry is bordered by Castle Crags State Park to the southeast and national forest land to the northwest, but the remaining land around the wilderness is a checkerboard of private and public holdings. There are nearly 30 miles of maintained trail within the wilderness. Castle Crags State Park adds another 4,000 acres to the Castle Crags complex, and another 30 miles of hiking trails. Due to the compact size, the Castle Crags area is best suited to dayhikers.

Owners of mining claims within the designated wilderness areas may continue to explore and mine their claims, and must be allowed reasonable access to do so. Fortunately, no new claims may be filed without an act of Congress. The Forest Service was validating all existing claims in the development of the Wilderness Operation Plan, which was to establish strict environmental regulation of all mining activities.

What these marvelous areas will look like in the future depends on how we treat them today. Since major population centers are hundreds of miles away, these areas have not been prone to the heavy recreational use that is prevalent in the Sierra Nevada. Far more people were here 150 years or so ago than now, when preservation of the wilderness was not on the minds of the early miners and settlers who ravaged the land for their own economic gain. The area has recovered quite nicely from the debacle of the mining days, thanks to a scarcity of human beings in the nearly century and a half that followed. Recreational use of the wilderness has been declining in modern times, a boon to solitude seekers, but perhaps not so great for the wilderness itself. Without enough friends of the wilderness who appreciate the numerous blessings the natural world has to offer, who knows what fate will ultimately befall this wonderful area.

Hikers can follow several guidelines for the preservation and health of the backcountry. A simple list of widely accepted wilderness practices follows:

- Don't leave any food or scented items in your vehicle. Bears have been known to break into vehicles searching for food.
- Pack out all trash, and any other trash you find, including aluminum foil packaging, which does not burn completely.
- Only have a campfire in an existing fire ring. Keep fires small and use only downed wood. Make sure fires are completely out before leaving the area.
- Wash dishes and bathe well away from lakes and streams, at least 200 feet from any water source. Use only biodegradable soap.
- Use only existing campsites whenever possible. If you must develop a new site, establish camps at inconspicuous sites away from the trail and remove all traces of your presence upon leaving. Camp only on mineral soil not vegetation. Don't build improvements such as fireplaces, rock walls, ditches, etc. Camp at least 200 feet from water.
- Filter, boil, or purify all drinking water.
- Don't cut switchbacks and avoid walking on meadows and wet areas when possible. Stay on the trail.
- Preserve the serenity of the backcountry. Avoid making loud noises.
- Keep group size to a minimum: 10 is the limit in the Trinity Alps and Castle Crags, 25 in the Russian Wilderness.
- Yield the right-of-way to equestrians. Step well off the trail on the downhill side. Yield the right-of-way to uphill hikers.
- Leave the wilderness as you found it, or better if possible.

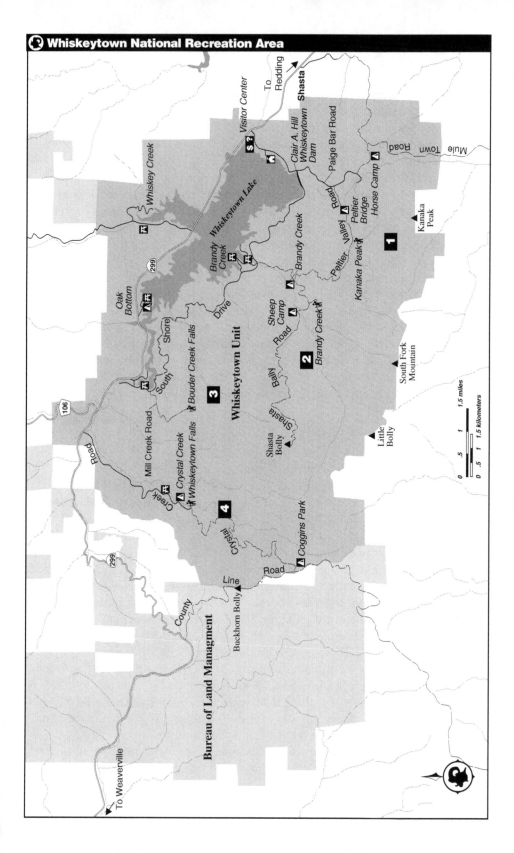

Whiskeytown National Recreation Area

CHAPTER 4

Trips in Whiskeytown National Recreation Area

A lthough the Whiskeytown Unit of Whiskeytown-Shasta-Trinity National Recreation Area is best known for holding a good-sized artificial lake where Sacramento Valley residents can beat the scorching summer heat, the area offers fine hiking, especially in spring when wildflowers cover the slopes, streams are full, and a trio of scenic waterfalls peaks. This chapter has four dayhikes: a splendid 6.5-mile loop trip to the summit of view-packed, 2616-foot-high Kanaka Peak, and three short out-and-back romps to waterfalls. While spring is best for the falls and beautiful flowers, hiking here in the fall, when daytime temperatures have abated and autumn colors reach their peak, can be pleasant as well. Summer visitors should hike in the morning or in the evening, when the temperatures are more tolerable.

The NRA status of Whiskeytown requires hikers to purchase permits to park at trailheads; they can be obtained at the visitor center near Whiskeytown Dam, on Kennedy Memorial Drive off Highway 299. America the Beautiful pass holders may park in Whiskeytown at no additional charge.

In addition to hiking and water sports, the Whiskeytown Unit offers activities well suited to recreationists of all ages. Picnic areas at Brandy Creek, Oak Bottom, Whiskey Creek, and Crystal Creek Falls are fine spots to share a meal. Three sandy beaches on Whiskeytown Lake offer swimming and sunbathing. Developed campgrounds include Oak Bottom Campground and Brandy Creek RV Campground, and there are a few primitive campgrounds above the reservoir. With a valid California license, anglers can ply the waters of Whiskeytown Lake year-round and the surrounding streams from the end of April to mid-November for a half dozen varieties of fish. Visitors can even pan for gold as a ranger-led activity.

TRIP 1

Kanaka Peak Loop

Kanaka Peak offers splendid views from Mt. Shasta all the way to the Yolla Bollys.

Trip Type:	Dayhike
Distance:	6.5 miles, loop
Elevation Change:	3600 feet, average 544 per mile
Difficulty:	Moderate to difficult
Season:	All year, best from April to early June and late September to November
Map:	USGS *Igo*
Nearest Campground:	Peltier Bridge

The splendid views from the summit of 2616-foot Kanaka Peak are well worth the physical effort. Make sure you're clad in the proper footwear and have a set of trekking poles for the steep, ankle-twisting, knee-wrenching descent off the top of the mountain. The 6.5-mile Kanaka Peak Loop passes through a mixture of black oak woodland and mixed conifer forest, with small pockets of lush riparian foliage lining the banks of Paige Boulder Creek and its tributaries. The dense vegetation clears enough on top of Kanaka Peak to allow the wide-ranging vistas that span from Mt. Shasta in the north down the Sacramento Valley to the south. If possible, pick a day right after a storm for the best views, when cleansing rains have cleared the air of dust and pollutants.

The elevations within Whiskeytown National Recreation Area are low enough to allow for year-round hiking, although snow may blanket the area for brief periods in the winter. Swollen creeks may cause more of a problem on this route for hikers then, as the Kanaka Peak Loop fords Paige Boulder Creek three times during the circuit—check with park officials for current conditions. In summer those low elevations usually produce scorching afternoon temperatures, generally more than 100 degrees, when Whiskeytown Lake is littered with water-loving recreational enthusiasts attempting to beat the heat. Spring is perhaps the best time for a visit, as the temperatures are usually mild, the creeks are flowing, and colorful wildflowers line the trail. Fall can also be a fine time to experience the area, with pleasant temperatures as well and deciduous plants and trees offering a touch of autumn color. Be watchful for poison oak along the loop, particularly on the upper ridge of the peak, where the trail is nearly overgrown with encroaching vegetation.

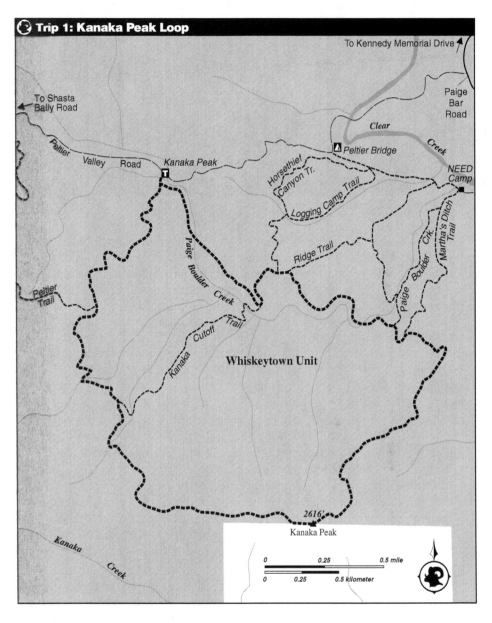

Trip 1: Kanaka Peak Loop

To Kennedy Memorial Drive

To Shasta Bally Road

Paige Bar Road

Peltier Valley Road

Clear Creek

Kanaka Peak

Peltier Bridge

NEED Camp

Horsethief Canyon Tr.

Logging Camp Trail

Ridge Trail

Paige Boulder Creek

Peltier Trail

Martha's Ditch Trail

Paige Boulder Crk.

Kanaka Cutoff Trail

Whiskeytown Unit

2616' Kanaka Peak

Kanaka Creek

Kanaka Peak

| 0 | 0.25 | 0.5 mile |
| 0 | 0.25 | 0.5 kilometer |

Starting Point

Head west from Redding on Highway 299 for 8 miles and then turn left (southwest) onto Kennedy Memorial Drive. The Visitor Center immediately on the right is the place to obtain current information and purchase a daily, weekly, or annual pass that is required to park at any NRA trailheads. With pass in hand, drive away from the Visitor Center toward Whiskeytown Dam. Do not follow Kennedy Memorial Drive across the dam, rather turn right at Paige Bar Road. After 1.1 miles turn right across from the Mt. Shasta Mine parking lot onto the

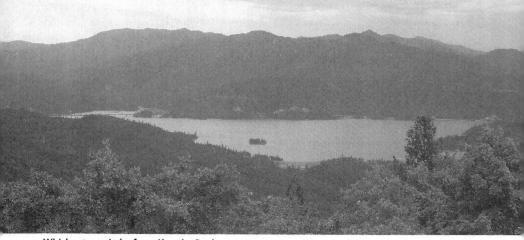

Whiskeytown Lake from Kanaka Peak

dirt surface of Peltier Valley Road, reaching Peltier Bridge Campground after 0.7 mile. The road past the campground becomes rough and steep for the next 1.1 miles on the way to a small parking area near the trailhead. This section of the road is subject to winter closure; if the gate happens to be closed, hikers must park at the campground and walk the road to the trailhead.

Description

The Kanaka Peak Loop begins by dropping immediately to a crossing of Paige Boulder Creek, and then climbing about 30 yards to an obscure, unmarked junction with a single-track path on the left heading southeast along the stream bank (this trail will be the return leg of the loop). Proceed ahead on the old road, climbing stiffly through the dappled shade of a mixed forest. Keen eyes should spy poison oak lining the side of the road, offering a reminder to avoid these plants by keeping to the roadbed. After a 0.75-mile climb, you reach a signed junction with Peltier Trail on the right.

Pleasantly graded trail leads away from the junction, around the fold of a hill, and then down to a crossing of a seasonal stream that, when flowing, picturesquely spills down a grassy and rocky nook bordered by lush plants. Shortly past the crossing is a three-way junction with the Kanaka Cutoff on the left, offering a short return to the trailhead for those looking for an early escape route.

Remaining on the loop trail, a moderate climb leads to the crossing of a usually dry seasonal stream. Beyond there, the roadbed dwindles to a single-track trail and begins a stiffer, switchbacking climb through Douglas firs, tanoaks, and Pacific madrones on the way toward the ridgecrest above. Tree-filtered views of Whiskeytown Lake along the way offer a hint of the much more extensive views that start to unfold upon gaining the top of the ridge west of Kanaka Peak. Following a fence line delineating the recreation area boundary from private property to the south, you drop steeply into a narrow saddle and then climb just as steeply toward the top of Kanaka Peak. Nearing the 2616-foot-high summit, the forest parts enough to allow stunning views from the grass-covered ridgecrest in every direction. Snowcapped Mt. Shasta is the dominant Cascade volcano to the north, while much-lower Lassen Peak and its immediate neighbors lie to the east. The range of peaks to the south is the Yolla Bolly Mountains, while the broad plain of the Sacramento River stretches away into the distance. Nearer at hand, Whiskeytown Lake lies at your feet and 6199-foot Shasta Bally, with a panoply of communication towers littering the summit, seems a stone's throw away to the west-northwest.

Once you've fully admired the view from Kanaka Peak, prepare yourself for the knee-wrenching descent down the mountain's northeast ridge, with Whiskeytown Lake in nearly constant view. Park officials have recently shown interest in realigning this section of trail to follow a less severe grade, but private property nearby limits their alternatives. After a mile or so of steep descent, the trail bends northwest and continues the sharp drop until easing just before a junction with the closed Martha's Ditch Trail on the right. A short distance farther you reach another junction with the Paige Boulder Trail, also closed to public use.

Gently graded trail leads away from the junction, crossing a usually dry drainage and then dropping down to a boulder hop of Paige Boulder Creek. From the crossing, a steady ascent leads well above the creek through open forest and continues upstream through the canyon. Where the path moves a good distance away from the creek, you come to a pair of junctions, the first with the unmarked Ridge Trail and the second with the Logging Camp Trail to Peltier Bridge Campground. Now heading southwest, the trail ascends back toward the creek, reaching the north junction of the Kanaka Cutoff Trail on the way. The sound of the creek returns shortly after the junction, as the trail proceeds upstream beneath the welcome shade from the riparian vegetation lining the banks to an easy boulder hop. Once across the creek, continue along the south bank, soon passing around a closed steel gate and then closing the loop at the junction with the old roadbed. From there, retrace your steps back across Paige Boulder Creek and shortly to the trailhead.

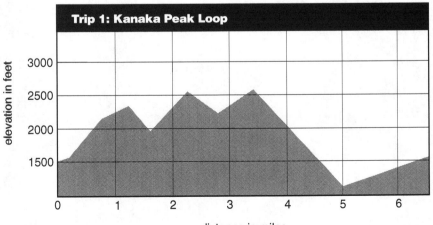

TRIP 2

Brandy Creek Falls

Two spectacular falls in a lushly foliaged canyon

Trip Type:	Dayhike
Distance:	3 miles round-trip, out-and-back
Elevation Change:	700 feet, average 467 per mile
Difficulty:	Moderate
Season:	All year, best from April to early June and late September to November
Map:	USGS *Igo*
Nearest Campground:	Sheep Camp

Lower Brandy Creek and Upper Brandy Creek falls will thrill you in the spring, when peak flows swell the creek and create a show of watery splendor. The moderate climb is a bit strenuous, but the overall distance is relatively short and the effort is easily forgotten once the dramatic scenery captivates you at the falls. Photographers will find the best light at midday.

Upper Brandy Creek Falls

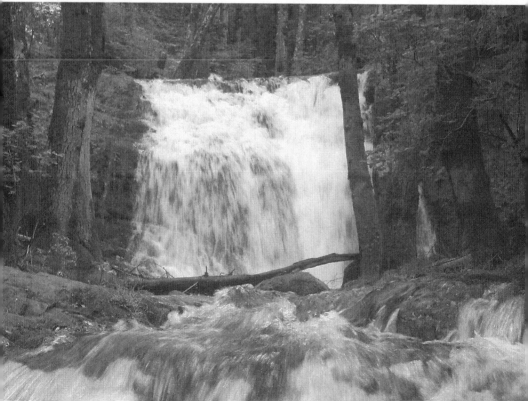

Trip 2: Brandy Creek Falls

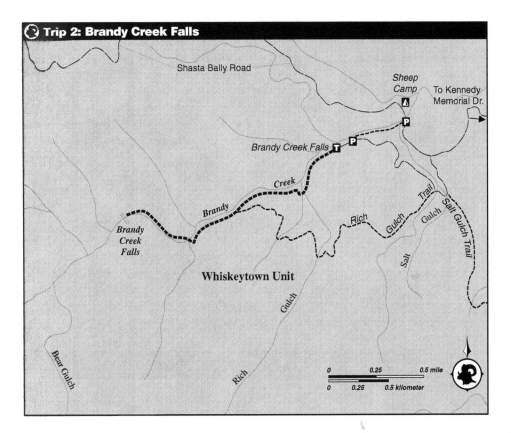

Starting Point

Head west from Redding on Highway 299 for 8 miles and then turn left (south-west) onto Kennedy Memorial Drive. The Visitor Center immediately on the right is the place to obtain current information and purchase a daily, weekly, or annual pass that is required to park at any NRA trailheads. With pass in hand, head south on Kennedy Memorial Drive toward Whiskeytown Dam, drive across the dam, and wind around above the shoreline to the Brandy Creek Beach Area. Here, immediately past a service road, turn left onto Shasta Bally Road and make a steep, winding climb on dirt road 1.3 miles to a junction and proceed ahead toward Sheep Camp and Shasta Bally.

Continue snaking up the road, avoiding the tendency to stop at two separate pullouts signed BRANDY CREEK TRAIL, to another junction, 2.2 miles from Brandy Creek Beach Area. Turn left at the junction and drive another 0.75 mile to where large boulders block the road, passing pullouts for Salt Gulch and Rich Gulch trails along the way. A small parking area with a bearproof trashcan is nearby.

Description

Walk up the continuation of the road past the boulders a short distance to where an old roadbed veers uphill on your left next to a sign reading BRANDY CREEK FALLS 1.5. Climb along this old logging road through a shady, mixed forest of black oaks, canyon live oaks, tanoaks, bigleaf maples, ponderosa pines, Douglas firs, and incense cedars, with the reverberating sound of Brandy Creek tumbling down the canyon below. A healthy understory includes a variety of ferns, as well as snowberry and dogwood. The grade momentarily eases at the bridged crossing of a tributary, followed shortly by an easy hop across a smaller rivulet cascading through large boulders, which were deposited here during a slide in the winter of 1997. Beyond the rivulet, the moderate climb resumes beneath forest cover until a very brief descent drops to a junction with the Rich Gulch Trail on your left.

A short, gently graded stretch of trail from the junction leads to a boulder hop of a thin stream, after which the trail climbs again through a narrower section of the canyon. Soon you reach a viewpoint of Lower Brandy Creek Falls, with a park bench nearby from which to rest and enjoy the view. As a sign indicates that the upper falls is still a quarter mile away, you continue upstream through the slender canyon, passing directly alongside the lower falls and the cascading creek above, aided at times by the presence of some iron handrails. Cross the creek on a twin-plank bridge and then climb along the north bank past another cascade and an inviting pool before crossing back over the creek and scrambling up to a dramatic, cathedral-like view of the upper falls.

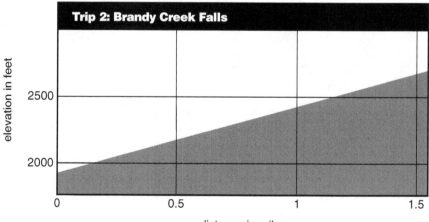

TRIP 3

Boulder Creek Falls

A short, gentle trail leads to a beautiful 81-foot-high waterfall in a cool grotto.

Trip Type:	Dayhike
Distance:	2.4 miles round-trip, out-and-back
Elevation Change:	400 feet, average 334 per mile
Difficulty:	Easy
Season:	All year, best from April to early June and late September to November
Map:	USGS *French Gulch*
Nearest Campground:	Oak Bottom

Two different trails lead to scenic Boulder Creek Falls, a dramatic 81-foot-high waterfall tucked into a narrow and shady canyon. The 2.75-mile-long trail featured by the Park Service follows the creek most of the way from a conveniently accessed trailhead just off South Shore Drive. However, following this route necessitates crossing the creek three times, and during spring, when the falls are at peak glory, you're almost guaranteed to come away with wet footwear. The alternate trail described below is considerably shorter and avoids all three fords, but does require a slightly longer drive to reach the trailhead.

Starting Point
Head west from Redding on Highway 299 for 8 miles and then turn left (southwest) onto Kennedy Memorial Drive. The Visitor Center immediately on the right is the place to obtain current information and purchase a daily, weekly, or annual pass that is required to park at any NRA

Boulder Creek Falls

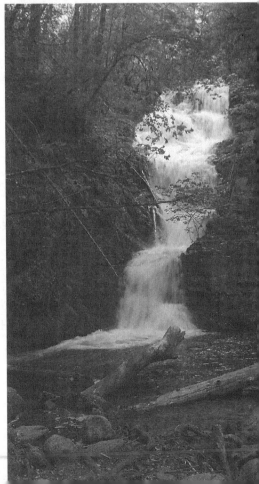

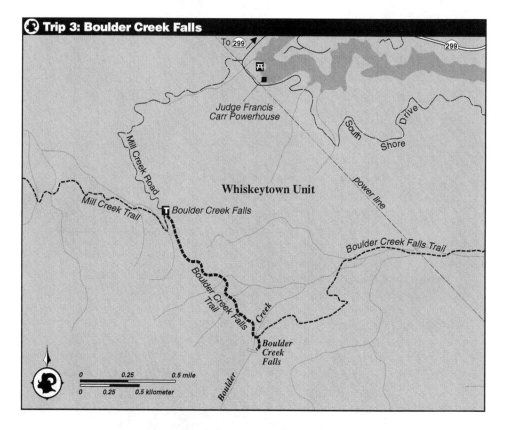

Trip 3: Boulder Creek Falls

trailhead. With pass in hand, return to Highway 299, turn left, and continue westbound 7 miles along the north shore of Whiskeytown Lake to a left-hand turn onto Carr Powerhouse Road. Cross a bridge over Clear Creek and proceed 0.5 mile to a junction with Mill Creek Road. Turn right and follow the dirt surface of Mill Creek Road for 0.4 mile to a junction and bear right. Proceed for another 1.4 miles, where the road splits again and steel chains block further vehicular progress. Park your car as space allows along the shoulder. The upper road is your route, signed BOULDER CREEK FALLS.

Description

From the gate, follow the continuation of the road on a steep and exposed climb through manzanita and widely scattered pines and oaks. Fortunately, both the steep ascent and exposure to the sun are short-lived, as the grade soon eases and a dense forest of incense cedars, ponderosa pines, Douglas firs, canyon live oaks, black oaks, and tanoaks provides some welcome shade. Springtime provides the added bonus of flowering dogwoods. Poison oak is quite prevalent along the way, but the width of the old roadbed is plenty wide enough to avoid any potential contact. Gently descending tread leads farther into the forest and across a couple of seasonal tributaries of Boulder Creek.

As you begin to hear the roar of the creek ahead, the trail curves around toward Boulder Creek, where you will soon notice an appreciable drop in the temperature in the cool and moist environment of the canyon. Cross the creek on a wood-plank bridge and immediately turn upstream, forsaking the old road for a narrow, single-track trail. Ascend steeply up the canyon, aided by wood-beam steps, and soon spy the falls through the trees. Continue climbing to the base of the falls, with a trail register and park bench nearby.

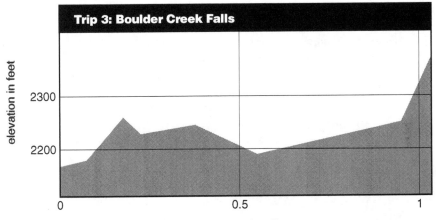

TRIP 4

Whiskeytown Falls

A rediscovered gem has become the waterfall to see at Whiskeytown National Recreation Area.

Trip Type:	Dayhike
Distance:	3.4 miles round-trip, out-and-back
Elevation Change:	1040 feet, average 612 per mile
Difficulty:	Moderate to difficult
Season:	All year, best from April to early June and late September to November
Map:	USGS *French Gulch* and *Shasta Bally*
Nearest Campground:	Oak Bottom

Whiskeytown Falls

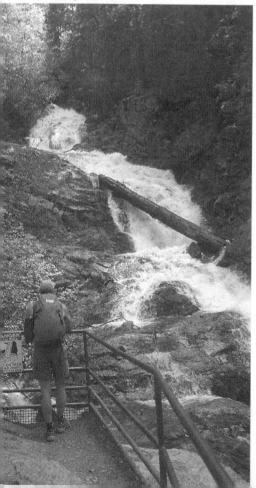

In this day and age, "losing" a significant waterfall is hard to imagine, but that's exactly what occurred with Whiskeytown Falls. In 2004 park biologist Russ Weatherbee rediscovered the falls, not as he stumbled across the dramatic cascade in the field but as he was examining some aerial photos in his office. Subsequently, Weatherbee and a fellow National Park Service geologist, Brian Rasmussen, hiked to the falls and confirmed what had been seen on the photos.

Although the distance is fairly short at 1.7 miles, after the short stretch down to the crossing of the west fork of Crystal Creek, the well-used James K. Carr Trail to Whiskeytown Falls climbs quite steeply. The stiff climb passes through a forest that was selectively logged in the 1950s, succeeded by a mixed, second-growth forest of oaks and evergreens. During weekends in spring, when the waterfall puts on a most dramatic display, you may notice a high number of tourists lumbering up the trail or catching

Trip 4: Whiskeytown Falls

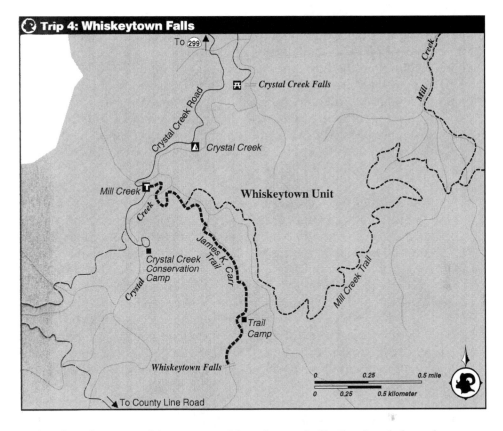

To 299

Crystal Creek Falls

Crystal Creek

Mill Creek

Whiskeytown Unit

Crystal Creek Road

James K Carr Trail

Crystal Creek Conservation Camp

Mill Creek Trail

Trail Camp

Whiskeytown Falls

0   0.25   0.5 mile
0   0.25   0.5 kilometer

To County Line Road

their breath on one of the many park benches periodically placed along the way. Nearing the falls, the trail enters a narrow canyon and climbs closely along the creek for the final quarter mile. The labor of the stiff ascent is well rewarded once the base of the falls is reached, where you'll be treated to a fine view of Whiskeytown Fall's watery splendor. A stone stairway lined with handrails leads alongside the falls for an even closer view.

Starting Point

Head west from Redding on Highway 299 for 8 miles and then turn left (southwest) onto Kennedy Memorial Drive. The Visitor Center immediately on the right is the place to obtain current information and purchase a daily, weekly, or annual pass that is required to park at any NRA trailhead. With pass in hand, return to Highway 299, turn left, and continue westbound 8 more miles to a left-hand turn onto Crystal Creek Road, which is about 0.25 mile past the turnoff for Tower House Historic District. Drive up Crystal Creek Road past junctions to the Crystal Creek Picnic Area and Crystal Creek Campground to a gravel parking area, 3.75 miles from Highway 299. The trailhead is equipped with portable toilets and trash and recycling bins. On the way back you may want to stop at Crystal Creek Picnic Area for the superb view of Crystal Creek Falls.

Description

The trail begins by following alongside a split-rail fence on a moderate descent across a mostly open slope that eventually leads into a mixed evergreen and deciduous forest on the way down to a crossing of the west fork of Crystal Creek via some well-placed beams. A short, steep climb heads away from the creek and up to the top of a rise, where the grade momentarily eases. Nearby, the first of many park benches along the way offers winded tourists the opportunity to sit down and catch their breath. From the rise, a more moderate climb leads to a junction with the much fainter tread of the Mill Creek Trail on your left.

The Story Behind the Missing Waterfall

So how does one lose such a significant physical feature as a waterfall? Prior to the creation of the 42,000-acre Whiskeytown National Recreation Area, the land was in private hands and the location of the falls was known only to a small number of loggers. Rangers became aware of the waterfall in 1967, but the National Park Service lacked the funds in those days to build a trail and pay for staffing. As time wore on, rangers with knowledge of the falls either passed away or were reassigned to other locations. Park biologist Russ Weatherbee's rediscovery quickly led to the renovation of an old logging road into the James K. Carr Trail, named for the Undersecretary of the Interior who championed national park status for the Whiskeytown area. The falls have become one of the area's most popular attractions.

Veer right at the junction and make a moderately steep to very steep climb away from the east fork of Crystal Creek up Steep Ravine, a steep, dry, and dusty gully that fortunately is well shaded by the canopy of a mixed forest. Old roads periodically fork away from the trail, but your well-traveled route is obvious at each junction. At the top of the ravine, the trail swings around a hillside

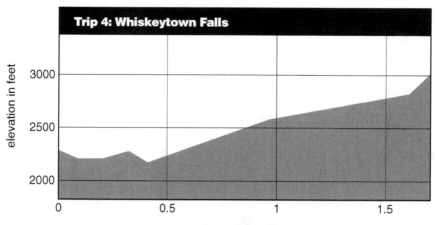

and draws closer to the creek, which noisily tumbles in the canyon below. A more moderate ascent leads to Trail Camp, complete with picnic tables, a bear box, and a tent platform.

Above the camp, you cross over the creek on a wood bridge and then climb more steeply again, headed up the narrowing canyon toward the base of Whiskeytown Falls, where another well-placed bench provides a fine place from which to watch the falls tumble into a shallow pool. To reach the upper viewpoint, clamber up a series of rock steps bordered by a steel handrail a short distance to where the multiple upper cascades of the upper falls are strikingly visible. According to the NPS "Trail Guide," the first vista point is known as Photographer's Ledge and the upper vista point is known as Artist's Ledge. Whether you're a photographer, an artist, or simply an average hiker, you are likely to be very impressed with the scenic display put on by Whiskeytown Falls.

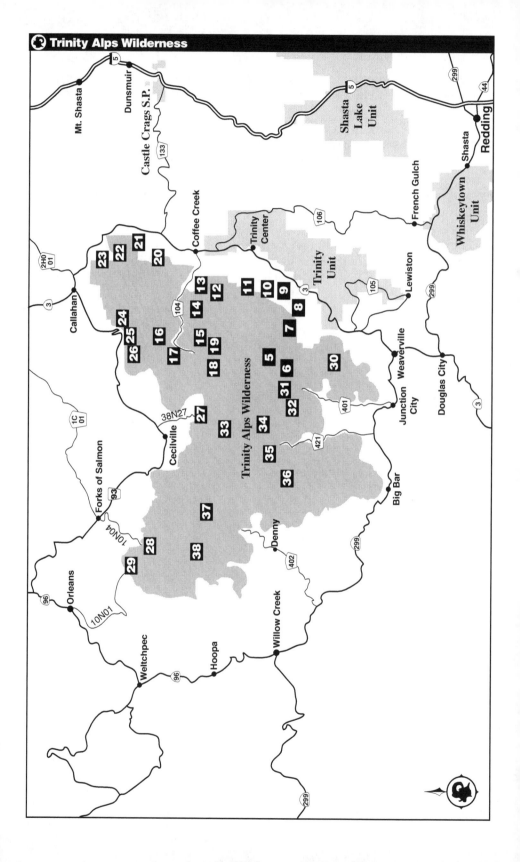

Trinity Alps Wilderness

CHAPTER 5

Trips in Trinity Alps Wilderness

The Trinity Alps region of the Klamath Mountains boasts some of the most diverse topography in California, ranging from coastal forests below 2000 feet to glacier-clad, 9002-foot Thompson Peak. One of the largest roadless tracts in the state, the area includes the headwaters of two of Northern California's most prominent rivers, the Salmon and Trinity. Far away from any major population centers, the 515,000-acre Trinity Alps Wilderness also offers recreational enthusiasts the opportunity for plenty of solitude. While some of the lower elevation trails make for excellent fall and spring hiking, most of the wilderness is best visited during the summer months.

With more than 500 miles of trails, the Trinity Alps Wilderness is a hikers' and backpackers' bonanza. Trips in this chapter run the gamut from forested walks to alpine heights and everything in between. With 34 described trips, the Trinity Alps makes up the bulk of this guide, including a fine sampling of both dayhikes and multiday backpacks.

Backpackers are required to obtain a wilderness permit for any overnight stays within the Trinity Alps Wilderness, available by self-registration at ranger stations. In addition to hiking and backpacking, the vast area of federal land around the Trinity Alps Wilderness offers numerous activities. The Trinity River is a notable fishery for anglers in search of salmon and steelhead. River runners also covet the river, which offers up to Class IV and V rapids in Burnt Ranch Gorge. Plenty of developed national recreation area and Forest Service campgrounds around the Alps' perimeter provide excellent camping opportunities, while several resorts and inns offer more luxurious overnight accommodations.

TRIP 5

Stuart Fork to Emerald, Sapphire, and Mirror Lakes

Set in glaciated granite at the head of rushing Stuart Fork, Emerald, Sapphire, and Mirror lakes are the area's crown jewels.

Trip Type:	Backpack, 4–7 days
Distance:	29 miles round-trip, out-and-back to Sapphire Lake (plus 2.6 miles round-trip cross-country to Mirror Lake)
Elevation Change:	4240 feet, average 292 feet per mile
Difficulty:	Moderate
Season:	Mid-June to mid-October
Maps:	USGS *Rush Creek Lakes, Siligo Peak, Mount Hilton, Caribou Lake,* and *Thompson Peak*; USFS *A Guide to the Trinity Alps Wilderness*
Nearest Campground:	Bridge

The long canyon of Stuart Fork and the three lakes at the head are breathtakingly beautiful in spite of a long history of human use and abuse. The hike to the lakes is delightful, although not exactly a wilderness experience. Don't expect solitude—Stuart Fork is one of the most heavily used trails in the Trinity Alps. However, overcrowding is only a problem if you insist on camping at Emerald or Sapphire lakes. Farther down the valley, Portuguese Camp, Morris Meadow, Oak Flat, and other campsites can accommodate large numbers of campers without feeling crowded.

Dense, mixed forest carpets the sides of the lower valley, and the river flows swiftly through a rocky channel with occasional wide gravel bars studded with cottonwoods and bigleaf maples. Both flowers and wildlife are abundant along the trail throughout the summer, especially in and around Morris Meadow. Since the only significant bear trouble I've experienced in the Alps occurred near Sapphire Lake, bear canisters are highly recommended. Fishing is good in Stuart Fork for rainbow trout to 10 inches and fair for eastern brook trout in Emerald and Sapphire lakes. Mirror Lake has both rainbows and brooks up to 10–12 inches. Autumn hikers will no doubt encounter deer hunters near Morris Meadow.

The amble through cool and shady forest on the way to Morris Meadow is one of the fine aspects of this trip, offering easy travel for the first day or two of hiking. Above the meadow, steeper tread matches the terrain of the canyon, passing through groves of stately red firs. Nearing the head of the canyon, sparse weeping spruces, mountain hemlocks, and whitebark pines cling to the

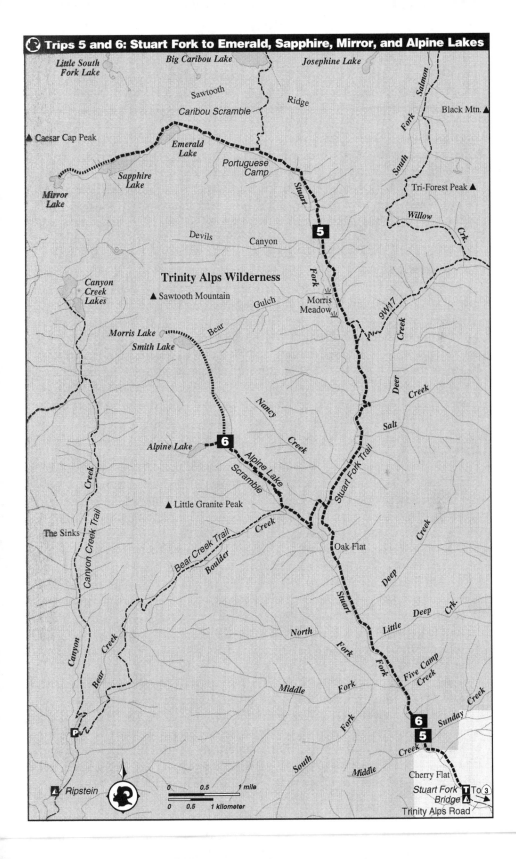

Trips 5 and 6: Stuart Fork to Emerald, Sapphire, Mirror, and Alpine Lakes

Little South Fork Lake

Big Caribou Lake

Josephine Lake

Sawtooth

Caribou Scramble

Ridge

South Fork Salmon

Black Mtn. ▲

▲ Caesar Cap Peak

Emerald Lake

Portuguese Camp

Tri-Forest Peak ▲

Sapphire Lake

Stuart

Willow Crk.

Mirror Lake

5

Devils Canyon

Fork

Trinity Alps Wilderness

▲ Sawtooth Mountain

Canyon Creek Lakes

Gulch

Morris Meadow

9W17

Deer Creek

Bear

Morris Lake

Smith Lake

Nancy Creek

Salt

Alpine Lake

6

Alpine Lake Scramble

Stuart Fork Trail

▲ Little Granite Peak

Creek

Canyon Creek Trail

The Sinks

Bear Creek Trail

Boulder

Creek

Oak Flat

Creek

Stuart

Deep

Deep Crk.

North

Little

Fork

Fork

Fork

Five Camp Creek

Middle

Fork

Creek

6

Sunday

Canyon

Bear

Creek

5

South

Fork

Middle

Creek

Cherry Flat

▲ Ripstein

Stuart Fork Bridge

To 3

Trinity Alps Road

0   0.5   1 mile

0   0.5   1 kilometer

walls of a giant, granite cirque. This subalpine environment also supports thick mats of ceanothus and huckleberry oak, as well as varieties of willow and alder in the wetter areas.

Starting Point

Approximately 13 miles north of Weaverville, Highway 3 turns northwest out of the lower end of Slate Creek canyon and runs along the shoreline of Trinity Lake past Tan Bark Picnic Area and a U.S. Forest Service information center, before crossing a bridge over the Stuart Fork arm of the lake. At the north end of the bridge, Trinity Alps Road turns west from the highway and soon leads to Trinity Alps Resort. The store, when open, is a good place to pick up last-minute supplies, and the dining room offers quite palatable meals, albeit on a limited schedule.

Beyond a row of cabins alongside the river the road switches to dirt and gravel and heads up past the resort's stable and corrals. Drive carefully through the resort and be on the alert for children and animals crossing the road. A quarter mile past the corrals you'll see the Elk Gulch trailhead on the right with room for one or two cars. Continue another couple of miles to a locked gate blocking the road. The trailhead parking area is on the left, just beyond Bridge Campground and 3.5 miles from Highway 3. Although conveniently located near the trailhead, the campground is cramped and dusty; campgrounds around Trinity Lake offer more aesthetically pleasing alternatives.

Description

Stuart Fork valley offers a cross-section of much of the natural history of the Alps. Below Oak Flat the river has cut through jumbled sedimentary and metasedimentary rock strata and glacial till. Several thousand years ago, receding glaciers left extensive terminal moraines above Oak Flat, damming a large lake that eventually filled in and dried out to become present-day Morris Meadow. At the head of the valley, Emerald, Sapphire, and Mirror lakes shimmer in their solid rock basins much as the glaciers left them.

The first mile of the Stuart Fork Trail follows the continuation of the road across private land, as signs direct you to respect the rights of the property owners by remaining on the road. Veer right at a well-signed fork immediately beyond the gate (the left-hand road leads to a mining camp near the river) and continue to the end of the road at the wilderness boundary, just past a cabin at Cherry Flat.

From the boundary, well-defined, single-track trail goes about 200 yards to a crossing of Sunday Creek, the first readily accessible water source. Above the creek you climb away from the river into dense forest of primarily Douglas fir, with occasional incense cedars, ponderosa pines, and sugar pines. Drop down to a flat beside the Stuart Fork, climb moderately up the side of the canyon, down to another flat with excellent campsites, and then up and down again to a crossing of Little Deep Creek, close to its confluence with the river. Pass another excellent campsite, climb over a mound of glacial till (the first on the way up the valley), and come to a steel girder bridge spanning Deep Creek.

After climbing moderately over another small hump above Deep Creek, you descend to yet another flat, where water from a spring runs across the trail and a number of fine campsites lie between the trail and the river. Four miles into the journey, you're probably now far enough away from the trailhead to ensure good fishing in the river. By August the water may be warm enough for swimming as well. A gentle ascent leads to the lower end of Oak Flat, a wide, gently sloping shelf, 200 to 300 yards away from the river, and heavily forested with large Douglas firs, ponderosa pines, and black oaks. About 1 mile from Deep Creek, water from a fine spring spills across the trail and, about 150 yards farther, you reach the junction of Bear Creek and Alpine Lake trails. The path on the left branches west to drop over a high bank to a forested flat and a large gravel bar beside the river. Excellent campsites, with an adequate supply of firewood, can be found on both the flat and the bar, above and below the ford. This crossing is potentially dangerous during high-water conditions. Fishing for pan-sized rainbows should be excellent.

From the junction, continue ahead on the Stuart Fork Trail, traversing a half mile of dense forest before breaking out into more open terrain well above the river on the east side of the canyon. The trail runs along the embankment of the old La Grange Ditch through here, the first place you'll notice much evidence of the mining efforts along the Stuart Fork. From this vantage point, you'll also have your first look at the high Alps at the head of the valley. Some more first-rate campsites lie in a flat between the ditch and the river. The trail soon climbs away from the ditch on the brushy east slope, and then levels off before dropping through some terminal moraines on the way to a crossing of Salt Creek. The fern- and wildflower-lined stream runs swift, clear, and cold. The remnants of an old log cabin are slowly moldering back into the soil, and some poor to fair campsites are nearby.

Other Backpacking Options in the Area

If you would prefer not to retrace your steps all the way back to the Stuart Fork trailhead and you have the luxury of two vehicles, a strenuous 30-mile, point-to-point trip over Sawtooth Ridge and through scenic Caribou Basin to Big Flat is one possibility. Another possibility is to go up Willow Creek and over the very steep divide west of Tri-Forest Peak to Big Flat, a 38-mile adventure. An even longer, 44-mile, near loop takes in the Four Lakes, Siligo Meadows, and Van Matre Meadows; crosses Stonewall Pass; passes through Red Mountain Meadows; and then descends to the Stoney Ridge trailhead. From there you must walk a mile on a dirt road and then take the Elk Gulch Trail to the trailhead on Trinity Alps Road, just above Trinity Alps Resort and 2 miles below the Stuart Fork trailhead. Additional shuttle alternatives are to go from Deer Creek to the Long Canyon trailhead, or over the divide to Granite Lake and then out to the Swift Creek trailhead.

North of Salt Creek, you climb around a shoulder of rock and ascend a series of switchbacks east up a draw before turning north again over and around more moraines. A half mile from Salt Creek, 7.5 miles from the trailhead, a steel truss bridge leads across the steep-walled, narrow canyon cut through dark sedimentary rock by the waters of Deer Creek. A pack stock bypass trail leads to a ford above a waterfall plunging into the deep pool below the bridge, which also provides access to the creek for acquiring water.

A short, steep climb heads up the north bank of Deer Creek and east into the piled-up moraines south of Morris Meadow. A half mile from the bridge, Cold Spring flows copiously across the trail and a small clearing nearby offers a few excellent campsites. You continue climbing, moderately to moderately steeply, another half mile to the south junction of the Deer Creek Trail heading east toward Four Lakes. A level stroll from there leads through open forest and patches of meadow to the north junction. Just beyond the second junction, you stroll out into the wide, lower end of expansive, lush Morris Meadow, 8.7 miles from the trailhead.

A midsummer evening at Morris Meadow can be truly memorable—an exquisite tableau of deer grazing in waist-high grass, backlit by the setting sun reflected off the multicolored backdrop of Sawtooth Ridge rising 2000 feet above the forest fringe at the north end of the meadow. The main part of the meadow is roughly a mile long by a quarter mile wide, covering the flat floor of the glacier-carved upper Stuart Fork valley. On the west side, tilted, glistening slabs of granite sweep up to remnant snowfields under the 8886-foot summit of Sawtooth Mountain. To the east, Sawtooth Ridge tapers off into a massive forested ridge separating this valley from the Willow Creek and Deer Creek drainages. Stuart Fork, hidden from view by a tangle of willows, alders, and incense cedars, meanders down the west side of the valley. White-flowering yampa dots the green expanse of meadow grass in August, and pale bog orchids hide among the sedges in marshy areas. Earlier in the summer, wide expanses of lupine and Indian paintbrush add splashes of blues and reds.

Many excellent campsites lie hidden in patches of forest interspersed with small meadows at the south end of Morris Meadow. A horse packer's camp is in a grove of incense cedars jutting into the west side of the meadow and more campsites can be found in the forest at the north end. Please refrain from camping directly in the meadow—plenty of more environmentally-friendly sites should be available along the forest fringe. Freeloading deer, too often successful, have been a problem at Morris Meadow, as are chipmunks and ground squirrels. Make sure you either hang your food effectively or use a bear canister.

To Camp or Not to Camp at the Upper Lakes

Before continuing up the valley, you should consider whether you want to haul your backpack all the way to Emerald or Sapphire lakes, or use Morris Meadow, or one of the other camps as far up as Portuguese Camp, as a base camp and then dayhike to the high lakes. The distance from the south end of Morris Meadow to Emerald Lake is a mere 5 miles, which equates to not much more than a 2-hour hike with daypacks. Campsites at Emerald and Sapphire lakes are fair at best, accommodating only about 20 people without serious overcrowding. Campfires are banned at all of the Stuart Fork lakes and only one small campsite at Emerald Lake has any trees suitable for hanging food, which are an absolute necessity if you don't have a bear canister.

Camping is possible at Mirror Lake. However, you must be in good shape and possess the requisite off-trail skills in order to carry a backpack all the way up there. Mirror Lake is seldom crowded but more than two small parties camped there will adversely impact the sense of solitude. You can check at the ranger station in Weaverville to determine if any other groups plan to camp there during your visit.

Follow the trail along the east edge of Morris Meadow to the far end and into the open red fir forest beyond. A quarter-mile stroll through grass and ferns of the floor of this beautiful mature forest leads past a few good campsites close to the now much smaller Stuart Fork. A moderately steep climb up the east side of a narrow canyon travels through patches of forest, waist-high ferns, and open, brushy slopes. Two miles past Morris Meadow, as the canyon turns west, a marvelous, cold-spring-fed rivulet gushes across the trail. Moist soil on both sides of the spring continues for some distance, as you pass through lush thickets of alders and bigleaf maples. Small openings filled with masses of flowers—larkspur, monkshood, leopard lily, bog orchid, and fireweed—crowd the trail.

Another half mile brings you into an area of small meadows and willow flats, bisected by the diminishing Stuart Fork, where a few good campsites nestle beneath groves of quaking aspen and fir. Farther on, at the head of a wide spot in the canyon and sheltered in a grove of large red firs, is Portuguese Camp, with ample room for 10–15 campers in several excellent sites. From the camp, continue along the rocky Stuart Fork Trail about 300 yards to a signed junction with the trail to Sawtooth Ridge and Caribou Lakes basin on the left.

Side Trip to Sawtooth Ridge

Opinions vary about the actual number of switchbacks on the 2200-foot climb up the very steep face of Sawtooth Ridge, varying between 89 and 98. Once you've decided to undertake the rigorous ascent, you'll have no trouble following the trail up the ridge, as there is simply no other place to walk through the thick brush and up the steep hillside of metamorphosed rock above. The distance from the junction to Big Caribou Lake is 3.6 miles; if you are carrying a backpack, you should allow a minimum of 4 hours, including some time at the crest to absorb and photograph the incredible views. Carry plenty of water, and an early morning start will help you beat some of the heat on the south-facing ascent, which can be brutally hot by noon in midsummer. A young person died on this hill in 1982, presumably of complications associated with heat exhaustion. Horses are not allowed on this section of trail.

Once you reach the crest of Sawtooth Ridge, Big Caribou Lake and the entire length of trail down to the lake is clearly visible, zigzagging down the steep slope to the south end of Caribou Lake and then following gentler terrain through the open, granite basin past Lower Caribou and Snowslide lakes. Above the far end of the basin, you have the option of following the longer but easier new trail around the northwest ridge of Caribou Mountain, or the shorter but steeper old trail directly over the ridge. The two trails reconnect at Caribou Meadows and then long-legged switchbacks, followed by a long traverse, and a shorter set of switchbacks lead to the crossing of South Fork Salmon River and the Big Flat trailhead. More complete directions from Sawtooth Ridge to Big Caribou Lake and the Big Flat trailhead can be found in reverse in Trip 19 (see page 171).

A half mile above Portuguese Camp, the Stuart Fork Trail passes a few fair campsites and draws near the tiny river for the last time before a climb up the north side of the canyon on the way to lovely Emerald Lake. The outlet cascades over ledges below to the south. Halfway along a level stretch of trail, lined with lush foliage and wildflowers, another spring-fed rivulet tumbles down a ledge and across the trail. As you steeply ascend the final quarter mile of trail to the top of a dike, the rock underfoot transitions from metamorphic to granite. The canyon walls on both sides of Emerald Lake are also granite, showing a sharp line of demarcation where the red, metamorphic strata of Sawtooth Ridge begins. You pass a terribly overused campsite in a small grove of firs at the north end of the rock dike, and then dip down almost to the lake before climbing above the north shore on the way toward Sapphire Lake.

Emerald Lake is an outstandingly beautiful 21-acre lake in a bowl gouged out of solid granite by the same glaciers that were born in the giant cirque above and were responsible for carving out the 2000-foot-deep canyon. The lake is normally warm enough by early August for comfortable swimming, with shelving rocks and a sandy slope at the northeast shore providing a convenient spot for sunbathing and for admiring the stunning scenery. Unfortunately, some ignorant people have camped here over the years; finding a worse spot to set up camp is hard to imagine—it's way too close to the water. Fishing is not spectacular here, but some small brook trout usually rise for flies toward evening. The best place to drop a line seems to be near the inlet on the southwest shore. Remember, campfires are not allowed at any of the Stuart Fork lakes.

Emerald Lake Dam

A dam of cut, fitted granite blocks was built in the 1890s to fill the notch worn by the outlet stream at the south end of the natural granite dike along the east shore. The dam raised the level of the lake more than 20 feet to store water for use at the La Grange Mine on Oregon Mountain, 29 miles to the southwest. The dam has been breached now and the lake has returned to its previous level, but the rest of the dam remains, a testament to the prodigal efforts men will exert to extract gold out of the ground.

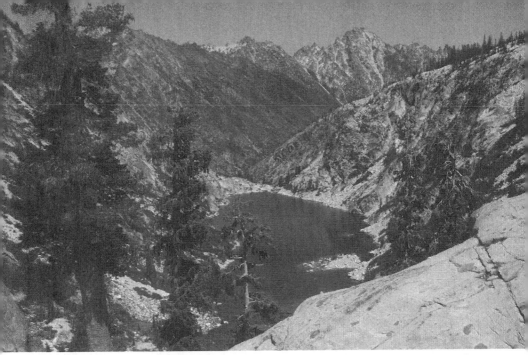

Sapphire Lake from near Mirror Lake

The trail to Sapphire Lake contours around the north shore of Emerald Lake, turning southwest through brush and across a talus slope about 100 feet above the surface. As you approach the connecting stream between the two lakes, the trail turns west to snake up over steep granite shelves on the way to the lake.

Sapphire Lake is twice the size of Emerald Lake and, with a reported depth of more than 200 feet, is the deepest lake in the Trinity Alps. The lake is spectacularly beautiful—a jewel as the name implies. From the dike at the east end of the lake, three sides of a giant granite cirque with remnant snowfields spread before your eyes. Almost directly west, a higher shelf hides Mirror Lake, hanging under the sheer upper ramparts of the canyon. Thick brush and scrub willows cover some of the lower slopes around the lake. Conifers are quite scarce, with only a few stunted weeping spruces, mountain hemlocks, red firs, and whitebark pines surviving in cracks and pockets in the granite. Fishing is no better in Sapphire Lake than in Emerald Lake, and only the hardiest swimmers will find the water warm enough for a brief, refreshing dip. A few very poor campsites have been scraped out in the rocks near the outlet, but firewood is nonexistent and there's no place to adequately hang a bag of food.

Off-Trail to Mirror Lake

To reach Mirror Lake, you'll first have to reach the west end of Sapphire Lake by heading 200 yards along a rough trail blasted and picked out of a cliff face on the north side of the lake. Beyond the cliff the tread disintegrates into several paths that cross a seep and head up through thick brush. At this point you may begin to wonder if a better route climbs over the tumbled granite blocks on the south side of the lake. Either way is difficult, but most scramblers find the north side route preferable—some of the blocks on the south side are as big as two-story houses.

On the north side of Sapphire Lake work your way up to a shelf about 100 feet or more above the surface and push through the brush almost directly west, with traces of a use trail offering some shaky assurance that you're on the right route. After about a half mile, the brush thins a tad in a slide area about 300 or 400 yards from the lake, where ducks point north toward a pair of sheer-faced granite knobs. This route is passable, crossing below a waterfall on Mirror Lake's outlet, and then scrambling around an outcrop and up a tilted ledge and a chimney to the lip of the shelf. However, a safer, although longer, route continues west to the north edge of a giant talus slope above the head of Sapphire Lake and boulder hops up to the far end of a shelf holding Mirror Lake. Either way is very strenuous, but your first glimpse of exquisite Mirror Lake beyond the ridges of glaciated granite on the shelf will make the climb seem worthwhile.

From the open east edge of the shelf a sensational panorama unfolds, including the entire upper Stuart Fork canyon. Emerald and Sapphire lakes shimmer far below, with sheer canyon walls climaxing in Sawtooth Ridge to the north and Sawtooth Mountain to the south. Sunrises seen from this lofty perch can be truly inspirational.

The heavy use that prevails around the two lower lakes is rare at Mirror Lake, and you should find the surroundings fairly pristine. Please tread lightly here and leave no remnants of your presence. A few unprotected, fair campsites lie in the hollows of rock southeast of the lake. Although more trees seem able to survive up here than down at Sapphire Lake, firewood is extremely scarce and should not be used. Shallow pockets of the lake may be warm enough for swimming by mid-August afternoons, and 10-inch rainbows cruising the drop-offs near sunset will tempt anglers. Rock climbers should find the walls of the upper cirque challenging.

Mirror Lake certainly lives up to its name; soaring walls of granite on three sides, punctuated by dwarfed weeping spruce and mountain hemlock, and a perpetual snowfield above the west shore are stunningly reflected in the usually placid water. For thousands of years, slowly moving ice ground and gouged at the resistant granite shelf, leaving behind the polished mounds and ridges and the 12- to 15-acre lake with a convoluted shoreline and four small rock islands.

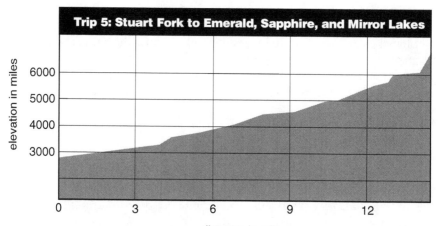

TRIP 6

Stuart Fork to Alpine Lake

Although only at an elevation of 6112 feet, Alpine Lake possesses many of the characteristics that its name suggests.

Trip Type:	Backpack, 2–4 days
Distance:	17.4 miles round-trip, out-and-back
Elevation Change:	3800 feet, average 772 feet per mile
Difficulty:	Moderate
Season:	Mid-July to late September
Maps:	USGS *Rush Creek Lakes* and *Siligo Peak*; USFS *A Guide to the Trinity Alps Wilderness*
Nearest Campground:	Bridge

see map on p. 69

Lovely, picturesque Alpine Lake covers the bottom of a glacier-carved slot on the ridge north of Little Granite Peak and west of the lower Stuart Fork valley. Little sunshine reaches the bottom of the steep-walled basin, and snowfields may linger around the lake until the end of July, resulting in an ecosystem one might expect to see at much higher altitudes. Along with the dramatic vertical scenery around the lake, the main attractions include abundant marsh-oriented wildflowers in the verdant little valley just below the lake, and the opportunity to explore, off-trail, the high ridge leading north to secluded Smith and Morris lakes immediately below rugged Sawtooth Mountain.

Since trail improvements were made in the late 1970s, adding a mile of longer switchbacks, Alpine Lake has become a more popular destination. Subsequently, the Forest Service has allowed the trail to devolve into a "scramble route," with rough and indistinct tread in places. Campfires are banned, the three small campsites around the lake are often full, and the rodent population has been problematic in the past. Fishing is only fair for small eastern brook trout in the lake and in pools in the creek below the lake. However, the view from the top of the trail back down Stuart Fork valley to Trinity Lake is still quite spectacular, and the beauty around Alpine Lake is sublime.

The 2600-foot climb from Oak Flat to the lake is arduous, with some very steep and rocky pitches. The trail is not recommended for equestrians or pack stock. If you are backpacking, plan on a four-hour climb from Oak Flat and get an early start; the last 2 miles of trail to the lake are steep and exposed. Water can be easily acquired only once along the way, at about 1.75 miles from Oak Flat, where the trail nearly reaches the outlet.

Starting Point

Approximately 13 miles north of Weaverville, Highway 3 turns northwest out of the lower end of Slate Creek canyon and runs along the shoreline of Trinity Lake past Tan Bark Picnic Area and a U.S. Forest Service information center, before crossing a bridge over the Stuart Fork arm of the lake. At the north end of the bridge, Trinity Alps Road turns west from the highway and soon leads to Trinity Alps Resort. The store, when open, is a good place to pick up last-minute supplies, and the dining room offers quite palatable meals, albeit on a limited schedule.

Beyond a row of cabins alongside the river the road switches to dirt and gravel and heads up past the resort's stable and corrals. Drive carefully through the resort and be on the alert for children and animals crossing the road. A quarter mile past the corrals you'll see the Elk Gulch trailhead on the right with room for one or two cars. Continue another couple of miles to a locked gate blocking the road. The trailhead parking area is on the left, just beyond Bridge Campground and 3.5 miles from Highway 3. Although conveniently located near the trailhead, the campground is cramped and dusty; campgrounds around Trinity Lake offer more aesthetically pleasing alternatives.

Description

The first mile of the Stuart Fork Trail follows the continuation of the road across private land, as signs direct you to respect the rights of the property owners by remaining on the road. Veer right at a well-signed fork just beyond the gate (the left-hand road leads to a mining camp near the river) and continue to the end of the road at the wilderness boundary, just past a cabin at Cherry Flat.

From the boundary, well-defined, single-track trail goes about 200 yards to a crossing of Sunday Creek, the first readily accessible water source. Above the creek you climb away from the river into dense forest of primarily Douglas fir, with occasional incense cedars, ponderosa pines, and sugar pines. Drop down to a flat beside the Stuart Fork, climb moderately up the side of the canyon, down to another flat with excellent campsites, and then up and down again to a crossing of Little Deep Creek, close to its confluence with the river. Pass another excellent campsite, climb over a mound of glacial till (the first on the way up the valley), and come to a steel girder bridge spanning Deep Creek.

After climbing moderately over another small hump above Deep Creek, you descend to yet another flat, where water from a spring runs across the trail and a number of fine campsites lie between the trail and the river. Four miles into the journey, you're probably now far enough away from the trailhead to ensure good fishing in the river. By August the water may be warm enough for swimming as well. A gentle ascent leads to the lower end of Oak Flat, a wide, gently sloping shelf, 200 to 300 yards away from the river, and heavily forested with large Douglas firs, ponderosa pines, and black oaks. About 1 mile from Deep Creek, water from a fine spring spills across the trail and, about 150 yards farther, you reach the junction of Bear Creek and Alpine Lake trails.

Turn left (west) from the junction and stroll 200 yards to where the trail drops over a steep bank to a shaded flat and a large open gravel bar beside the river. A number of excellent campsites are on the flat and beneath clumps of cottonwoods and firs on the gravel bar, where an ample supply of driftwood should provide plenty of firewood. Anglers will find the fishing better here in the Stuart Fork than above at Alpine Lake, unless the water is too high and swift, in which case you won't be able to ford it anyway. If the river is very low, you may be able to boulder hop upstream from the former site of an old diversion dam washed out by a flood, but more than likely you'll have to wade across.

Up on the west bank of the Stuart Fork the trail runs south, climbing slightly almost to Boulder Creek, then turns back to climb more steeply a little west of north before turning into the north side of Boulder Creek canyon. You soon climb higher up the side of the canyon in dense, mixed forest, amid a significant number of deadfalls, and then begin a series of moderately steep zigzags up the nose of a ridge away from Boulder Creek. As the climb eases in more open forest, about a mile from the Stuart Fork crossing, a large, dead ponderosa pine snag and a nearby cairn mark the somewhat inconspicuous junction of the Alpine Lake Trail turning steeply north.

After a short, steep start north up the Alpine Lake Trail through a field of granite boulders, you begin a series of long-legged switchbacks, climbing moderately in thick brush well east of the Alpine Lake outlet. About 0.75 mile from the junction, a switchback extends almost to the diminutive creek and to a good, but small campsite tucked under a large Jeffrey pine. A short, steep scramble down to the stream will allow you to cool your hot brow in the clear, cold water, as well as get some drinking water.

Continue up the next set of switchbacks over broken granite covered with a mat of huckleberry oak, manzanita, ceanothus, and scrubby Oregon oak. About a half mile from the water stop, you climb very steeply onto some granite knobs, from where you can hear, but not yet see, a waterfall. Another 0.3 mile through brush and over rocks leads you to the foot of the ledge from which the creek is falling, 50 yards from the trail and almost impossible to reach. Some very steep zigzags up through more rocks at the east end of the ledge lead to the top of a knob, where you can see into the cirque above Alpine Lake.

An almost level traverse across the top of the canyon takes you west through some tiny, flowery meadows to a crossing of Alpine Lake's outlet, just below a cascade over a rock dike. Instead of climbing directly up the faint track beside this cascade, look for the trail along the base of the dike and walk 50 yards south before switchbacking over the top. Beyond the dike you reach the lower end of a beautiful green valley a little less than 0.25 mile long and about half as wide. The creek meanders in a wide, still channel through lush, marshy grasses and sedges, dotted with wildflowers. Little brook trout flick a series of interlocking rings that fracture the reflections of a few huge granite boulders deposited by ancient glaciers. The trail runs up the south side of the valley for almost 300 yards, then turns and crosses the creek to continue through the grass

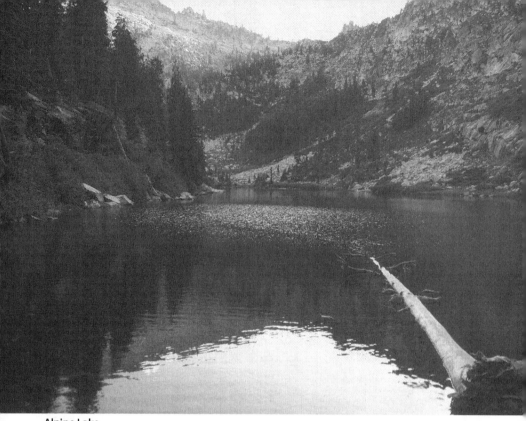

Alpine Lake

on the north side and over a low moraine to the lower end of the lake. Be sure to cross the creek, as the trail that continues up the south side of the valley leads to some vertical rock faces that block your access to the lake.

Fourteen-acre Alpine Lake fills the bottom of a deep, narrow cirque gouged out of granite and metasedimentary rock, where rows of grotesquely eroded pinnacles thrust into the sky at the top of the cliffs. Brooding, weeping spruce and firs are reflected in the dark water, while ghostly limbs of fallen snags reach from the depths near the outlet and, particularly on a cloudy day, the entire scene can be a bit somber. Camping is limited to three fair campsites in the rocks, brush, and trees at the lower end of the lake. If all these sites happen to be full, your hope for solitude will be greatly diminished, as the only items missing from the usual close quarters of the developed campground experience will be Winnebagos and boom boxes. If you're the only one camped at the lake, enjoy the magnificent blessing. Otherwise, carefully respect the desire of others for the limited amount of privacy available.

Off-Trail to Smith and Morris Lakes
Hardy cross-country enthusiasts can reap big rewards by following a strenuous route to Smith and Morris lakes. The first part of the route is by far the worst, involving steep bushwhacking on the climb out of Alpine Lake's basin. Afterward, the route becomes much more straightforward. If you are carrying a backpack, plan on at least a half day for the 2-mile off-trail climb.

From the vicinity of Alpine Lake, find a path that leads east along the north edge of the meadow just below the lake. At the east end and slightly above the meadow in a clearing is a dead snag, from which a variety of faint paths lead up into the thick brush on the hillside above. The goal is to try to locate the least offensive route through this tangle of brush to the pleasantly open slopes above. Many paths come and go all along this slope, but if you head for a spot just above or slightly below the lower set of rounded dark granitic cliffs, you should come out somewhat unscathed.

Above this demonic patch of brush, the way does indeed open up and the climbing is much more pleasant, as you ascend north through a gully over mildly sloping granite slabs interspersed with low shrubs and dotted with hemlocks and pines. While climbing to the left (west) of a small stream that drains into Alpine Lake's outlet, head for a distinctive notch at the low point in the ridge above, as increasingly spectacular scenery unfolds with each new step.

Approximately 1 mile from Alpine Lake you reach the notch in the ridge, where you're met with grand views of distant Mt. Shasta and much closer Sawtooth Mountain. In most years you'll probably encounter a snowfield on the north-facing slope below the notch. Descend this slope to the west toward a group of rocks. You'll get a glimpse of a lake from there, not Smith Lake, but the smaller and slightly higher Morris Lake (Smith Lake lies just out of view behind granite cliffs and ridges). From the rocks, make an angling descent toward a point right below the terminus of the east ridge of Sawtooth Mountain. Fixed on that point, you head over granite slabs and interlocking patches of meadow to where the outlet creek exits Smith Lake and descends through Bear Gulch.

Attempt to reach Smith Lake close to the outlet, as the slopes higher up around the lake are quite steep and difficult to descend. The outlet stream itself is wedged between granite walls 20 to 30 feet high, which makes the last part of the route down to the lake tricky: The easiest way across is right where the outlet leaves the lake, where you can scramble down some dirt ramps and hop across the stream. From there, the going is much easier.

Smith Lake is a gorgeous subalpine lake surrounded by scattered hemlocks and rugged, granite slopes leading northwest up to the dramatic summit of Sawtooth Mountain. At the far end, a stream falls picturesquely 50 feet over a sheer granite cliff before merging with the exceedingly clear, cold waters of Smith Lake. Good-sized rainbow and brook trout glide through the 24-acre lake, where fishing pressure should be minimal due to the extra time and effort necessary to get here. You should have a reasonable expectation of solitude as well. Camping is limited to benches and shelves adjacent to and above the east shore, just north of the crossing of the outlet. If you have some extra energy, even better sites may be available on the bench above the waterfall at the far (northwest) end of the lake. To get there you must climb up and over a rock knob, avoiding the steep cliffs below, and then descend slightly before traversing over to the bench. Here, wonderful campsites are nestled beneath tall hemlocks and next to tiny rivulets that dance their way over granite slabs and into delightful, little ponds.

The route to Morris Lake heads west up from the bench at the far end of Smith Lake across little brooks and up slabs to the far left of the waterfall on the outlet from Morris Lake. As you work your way up the slabs, the route draws closer to the outlet and soon

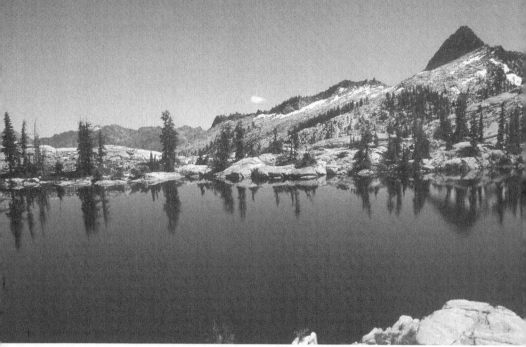

Morris Lake

follows the edge of the channel the last 200 feet into the upper basin. From there, cross over the creek and follow a use trail along the right (north) side of the outlet to the lakeshore.

Morris Lake is much smaller than Smith, but possesses its own unique charm. While Smith has much more rugged, dramatic scenery, Morris offers a more pastoral feel. The topography around Morris is not as steep as around the lower lake, consisting of rolling granite slabs softened by meadows filled with wildflowers and heather. You'll have a more intimate portrait of Sawtooth Mountain and the potential challenges posed by the possibility of an ascent. Campsites may be available above the west shore in a grove of mountain hemlocks, conveniently positioned not far from the inlet.

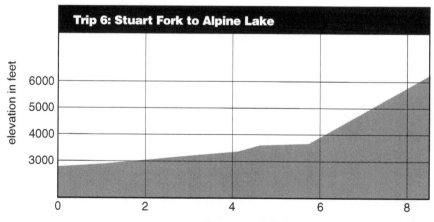

TRIP 7

Deer Creek and Four Lakes Loop to Long Canyon

Each of the four lakes is utterly delightful and unique, in character as well as size.

Trip Type:	Backpack, 5–8 days
Distance:	25 miles, point-to-point
Elevation Change:	11,545 feet, average 462 per mile
Difficulty:	Moderate
Season:	Early July to early October
Maps:	USGS *Rush Creek Lakes*, *Siligo Peak*, and *Covington Mill*; USFS *A Guide to the Trinity Alps Wilderness*
Nearest Campground:	Bridge

The Four Lakes Loop circles 8162-foot Siligo Peak, switchbacking over three spur ridges in the process and visiting Luella, Diamond, Summit, and Deer lakes. Along the way are views in all directions of the highest peaks and deepest canyons in the Trinity Alps. Sheer rock faces at the head of Deer Creek and several peaks higher than 8000 feet illustrate the mixed-up geology of this part of the Alps, offering abundant rock climbing opportunities as well. The approach up Deer Creek canyon from Morris Meadow is through a lush mix of forests, meadows, and alder and willow flats. Wide expanses of fragrant wildflowers bloom in the high basins through July and into August.

Deer Creek and the Four Lakes Loop are less crowded than the Stuart Fork, but don't expect to be alone. Deer Creek Camp and the meadows above seem to experience nearly constant use by horse packers entering the wilderness from the Long Canyon trailhead, and the trail over the ridge from Granite Lake is quite popular with backpackers as well. Stock use on the Four Lakes Loop is discouraged—the tread is steep and narrow, the area lacks good tie areas, and suitable forage is scarce.

Remote Echo Lake, Lake Anna, and Billy Be Damn Lake can be accessed via off-trail routes from the vicinity of Deer Creek Pass and Bee Tree Gap. A fine trip extension is a 44-mile loop back to the Stuart Fork trailhead (avoiding the need for two vehicles), continuing south on the Stoney Ridge Trail through Siligo Meadows and Van Matre Meadows and then over Stonewall Pass and down a section of road and the Elk Gulch Trail to Trinity Alps Resort, another 2 miles below the Stuart Fork trailhead.

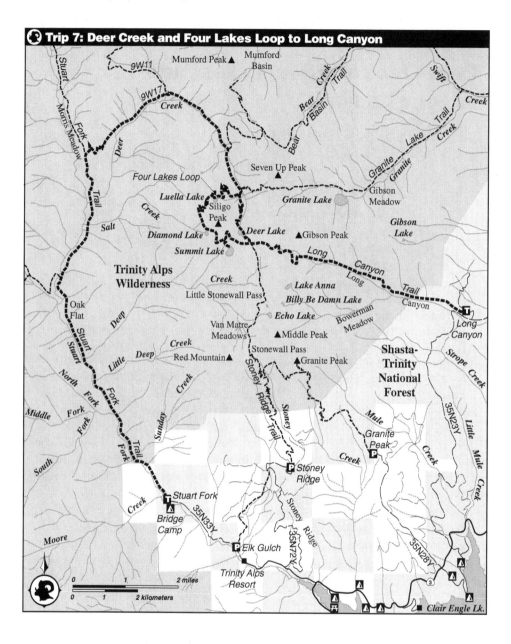

Trip 7: Deer Creek and Four Lakes Loop to Long Canyon

Starting Point

Approximately 13 miles north of Weaverville, Highway 3 turns northwest out of the lower end of Slate Creek canyon and runs along the shoreline of Trinity Lake past Tan Bark Picnic Area and a U.S. Forest Service information center, before crossing a bridge over the Stuart Fork arm of the lake. At the north end of the bridge, Trinity Alps Road turns west from the highway and soon leads to Trinity Alps Resort. The store, when open, is a good place to pick up last-minute supplies, and the dining room offers quite palatable meals, albeit on a limited schedule.

Beyond a row of cabins by the river the road switches to dirt and gravel and heads up past the resort's stable and corrals. Drive carefully through the resort and be on the alert for children and animals crossing the road. A quarter mile past the corrals you'll see the Elk Gulch trailhead on the right with room for one or two cars. Continue another couple of miles to a locked gate blocking the road. The trailhead parking area is on the left, just beyond Bridge Campground and 3.5 miles from Highway 3. Although conveniently located near the trailhead, the campground is cramped and dusty—campgrounds around Trinity Lake offer better alternatives.

Ending Point

Approximately 22.5 miles north of Weaverville, leave Highway 3 near a road sign marked LONG CANYON TRAIL 3, MULE CREEK 7 and turn left onto County Road 115. This junction is shortly beyond Guy Covington Drive on the right and immediately after a bridge over the East Fork of the Stuart Fork. Travel along paved road passing numerous turnoffs to private homes until you reach a right-hand turn onto Forest Road 35N10 at 2.6 miles, which should be signed for Long Canyon Trail. Follow this gravel road for 0.3 mile to another signed intersection, where you turn left into the ample parking area near the trailhead.

Description

The first mile of the Stuart Fork Trail follows the continuation of the road across private land, as signs direct you to respect the rights of the property owners by remaining on the road. Veer right at a well-signed fork just beyond the gate (the left-hand road leads to a mining camp near the river) and continue to the end of the road at the wilderness boundary, just past a cabin at Cherry Flat.

From the boundary, well-defined, single-track trail goes about 200 yards to a crossing of Sunday Creek, the first readily accessible water source. Above the creek you climb away from the river into dense forest of primarily Douglas fir, with occasional incense cedars, ponderosa pines, and sugar pines. Drop down to a flat beside the Stuart Fork, climb moderately up the side of the canyon, down to another flat with excellent campsites, and then up and down again to a crossing of Little Deep Creek, close to its confluence with the river. Pass another excellent campsite, climb over a mound of glacial till (the first on the way up the valley), and come to a steel girder bridge spanning Deep Creek.

After climbing moderately over another small hump above Deep Creek, you descend to yet another flat, where water from a spring runs across the trail and a number of fine campsites lie between the trail and the river. Four miles into the journey, you're probably now far enough away from the trailhead to ensure good fishing in the river. By August the water may be warm enough for swimming as well. A gentle ascent leads to the lower end of Oak Flat, a wide, gently sloping shelf, 200 to 300 yards away from the river, and heavily forested with large Douglas firs, ponderosa pines, and black oaks. About 1 mile from Deep

Creek, water from a fine spring spills across the trail and, about 150 yards farther, you reach the junction of Bear Creek and Alpine Lake. The path on the left branches west to drop over a high bank to a forested flat and a large gravel bar beside the river. Excellent campsites, with an adequate supply of firewood, can be found on both the flat and the bar, above and below the ford. This crossing is potentially dangerous during high-water conditions. Fishing for pan-sized rainbows should be excellent.

From the junction, continue ahead on the Stuart Fork Trail, traversing a half mile of dense forest before breaking out into more open terrain well above the river on the east side of the canyon. The trail runs along the embankment of the old La Grange Ditch through here, the first place you'll notice much evidence of the mining efforts along the Stuart Fork. From this vantage point, you'll also have your first look at the high Alps at the head of the valley. Some more first-rate campsites lie in a flat between the ditch and the river. The trail soon climbs away from the ditch on the brushy east slope, and then levels off before dropping through some terminal moraines on the way to a crossing of Salt Creek. The fern- and wildflower-lined stream runs swift, clear, and cold. The remnants of an old log cabin are slowly moldering back into the soil, and some poor to fair campsites are nearby.

North of Salt Creek, you climb around a shoulder of rock and ascend a series of switchbacks east up a draw before turning north again over and around more moraines. A half mile from Salt Creek, 7.5 miles from the trailhead, a steel truss bridge leads across the steep-walled, narrow canyon cut through dark sedimentary rock by the waters of Deer Creek. A pack stock bypass trail leads to a ford (a good place to acquire water) above a waterfall plunging into the deep pool below the bridge.

A short, steep climb heads up the north bank of Deer Creek and east into the piled-up moraines south of Morris Meadow. A half mile from the bridge, Cold Spring flows copiously across the trail, and a small clearing nearby offers a few excellent campsites. You continue climbing, moderately to moderately steeply, another half mile to the south junction of the Deer Creek Trail heading east toward Four Lakes. A level stroll from there leads through open forest and patches of meadow to the north junction. Just beyond the second junction, you stroll out into the wide, lower end of expansive, lush Morris Meadow, 8.7 miles from the trailhead.

Many excellent campsites lie hidden in patches of forest interspersed with small meadows at the south end of Morris Meadow. A horse packer's camp is in a grove of incense cedars jutting into the west side of the meadow, and more campsites can be found in the forest at the north end. Please refrain from camping directly in the meadow—plenty of more environmentally-friendly sites should be available along the forest fringe. Freeloading deer, too often successful, have been a problem at Morris Meadow, as are chipmunks and ground squirrels. Make sure you either hang your food effectively or use a bear canister.

Walking south out of Morris Meadows, turn southeast on the north spur of the Deer Creek Trail, meeting the south spur after 0.3 mile. Ten long-legged switchbacks lead from there to the top of the divide and an outstanding view back toward Sawtooth Mountain. From the divide, descend moderately for 0.3 mile, then level off to contour northeast along the side of Deer Creek canyon through open forest, which includes some very large ponderosa pines, sugar pines, Douglas firs, and a few incense cedars. After dipping into a small gulch containing a tiny creek, climb out onto a bench above the steep-walled gorge. Several more small rivulets cross the trail as you climb away from Deer Creek through small meadows and patches of oak brush interspersed with white fir and incense cedar on the way to a crossing of Willow Creek. The signed Willow Creek Trail junction and a good campsite await 200 yards beyond where the creek tumbles over boulders in a tangle of alders. The trail on the left heading generally northeast eventually crosses the Trinity Divide west of Tri-Forest Peak and proceeds down to the Big Flat trailhead, 7.5 miles from this junction.

Continuing east of the Deer Creek Trail, you climb gently to moderately through wide meadows and alder and willow flats. A beautiful little stream, in some dense willows, waters a splendid garden of head-high delphiniums. As the canyon bends gradually south, the trail climbs moderately on the east side over glacial till supporting sparse forest and fern-covered meadows speckled with white-flowering yampa and other flowers. After 1.5 miles from Willow Creek, you turn east to cross Deer Creek twice within a quarter mile and then climb a rocky hillside to the first campsites associated with Deer Creek Camp. The Black Basin Trail snakes up the steep east wall of the canyon from a junction about halfway through this cluster of heavily used, but still decent, campsites. Fortunately, the herds of cattle that used to graze here are long gone. However, they seem to have been replaced in part by horses and pack mules. Fishing for both eastern brook trout and rainbow trout is fair to good in the creek below camp.

From the Black Basin junction, the Deer Creek Trail descends slightly, then turns west to cross the little creek at the foot of a lush, wet meadow. You turn south again on the west side of the canyon well above a series of meadows and climb moderately for a mile to a grove of firs beside a cascade on the creek. As you turn up the side of a tree-covered hill, a well-used, unsigned trail forks steeply to the right up the hill in loose, sandy soil, which is an old trail to Luella and Diamond lakes. You can use this trail if you like, intersecting the newer Four Lakes Loop on a hill above Round Lake, but it's easier to continue south on the Deer Lakes Trail to the signed junction of the Four Lakes Loop, a short distance past the Granite Lake Trail junction. For those planning to travel to Granite Lake and exit at the Swift Creek trailhead, the 7.5-mile route climbs the steep ridge south of Seven Up Peak and then descends past the lake to the trailhead (for details on that option, see Trip 11, page 111).

Southwest of the Four Lakes Loop junction, Round Lake, more of a pond than a bona fide lake, is 200 yards west of the Deer Creek Trail, surrounded by willows in a marshy flat. Despite the lake's diminutive nature, swimming can be quite pleasant, and some anglers have taken 12-inch eastern brook trout from the lake in the past. J. W. Cow Camp, dating from the mining days, offers several excellent campsites a quarter mile farther along the trail, near the base of a hill below Luella Lake.

From the signed Four Lakes Loop junction, turn west beside a tiny tributary of Deer Creek, and climb moderately via six long-legged switchbacks to a shelf below the cirque holding Luella Lake. The big attraction at Luella Lake is staged across the upper basin of Deer Creek, as the shadow on the west ridge moves slowly up the sheer east wall across from a vantage point on the rock balcony below the lake. You may be so entranced by this wonder that you lose track of time watching the last flaming rays fade from the tops of the cliffs with the basin turning purple below—but the magnificent show is well worth the price.

Despite the snowbank that usually lingers for most of the summer above the south shore, the greenish waters of 2.5-acre Luella Lake are warm enough for hardy swimmers by mid-August. A few open gaps in the thick willows near where the trail approaches the shore may provide anglers with just enough room to cast for pan-sized brook trout. Red metamorphic rock, which extends most of the way around the lake, changes to granite on the south side and leads up to the ragged crags of Siligo Peak—a difficult climb from this side, but a walk-up from the trail near Summit Lake on the south side. One fair campsite is in the rocks above, and south of, the trail just before you dip into the little valley below the lake. From the campsite, you'll have to tunnel through thick willows to reach the outlet, or walk 250 yards to the lake to get water. Fires are not allowed around any of the Four Lakes.

From the shelf below Luella Lake most of the trail to the top of the cirque ahead is clearly visible, switchbacking across talus slides on the way up the very steep west slope. Carry plenty of water for this ascent, as there exists no dependent source between Luella and Diamond lakes. The ascent begins with a traverse north to a rim, then turns back southwest to begin a series of switchbacks that arc around the west side of the cirque. A steep, 0.7-mile climb on sometimes-rough tread is rewarded at the top of a ridge with breathtaking views west across the Stuart Fork canyon and east of Gibson and Seven Up peaks. The ridge itself is beautifully grassy under widely spaced, large foxtail pines, western white pines, and red firs.

Drop off the crest via moderate switchbacks across an open hillside carpeted with grass and adorned with myriad wildflowers, including mountain aster, mint, Indian paintbrush, and angelica. Diamond Lake, above the yawning Stuart Fork canyon, comes into view about halfway down the slope.

The shallow, 2.5-acre lake hangs on the lip of a shelf at the bottom of a U-shaped valley that funnels steeply down from a lateral ridge west of Siligo Peak. An amazing number and variety of wildflowers bloom around the grassy shoreline. The one poor, unprotected campsite at Diamond Lake is near the trail under a foxtail pine, the only large tree close to the lake—not the place to camp during a storm. Water is available from tiny streams above the lake. Perhaps the best attribute of this campsite is the view of Sawtooth Mountain and the other peaks and ridges around the head of Stuart Fork—a most breathtaking scene. Fishing in Diamond Lake is fair for eastern brook trout.

The trail from Diamond Lake to Summit Lake runs around the east side of Diamond Lake and up to a shelf, then climbs east on 10 moderately steep switchbacks through a flower garden just north of a long, red-rock-talus slide. Wild flax and stonecrop bloom profusely here among the many other species of wildflowers that carpet the hillside. Traverse the talus, and then climb another series of steeper switchbacks southwest through more flowers and rocks to a narrow crest. Summit Lake, now in full view to the southeast, is so near the top of Peak 8059 that the lake appears to be contained inside a volcanic crater. However, Peak 8059 is not volcanic—the basin was scooped out of sedimentary and metamorphosed rocks by the same glaciers that carved the rest of the local landscape. The trail climbs gradually east along the crest, then contours around the southwest flank of Siligo Peak to a junction with a lateral to Summit Lake, 1.4 miles from Diamond Lake.

From the junction, turn right and drop 0.3 mile to the north shore of Summit Lake, which is the largest (13 acres) and highest (7400 feet) of the Four Lakes. South of Siligo Peak, Summit is a lovely subalpine tarn, with the dark blue waters contrasting sharply with the stark red rocks arcing above the east shore. Without a permanent inlet or outlet, the lake itself is the only source of water. There are four or five good campsites spread among scattered foxtail and whitebark pines above the north and west shores. A base camp here allows you to explore the surrounding country on dayhikes and scrambles. Fishing is fair to good for both rainbow and brook trout to 10 inches. Only the hardiest of swimmers will stay in the chilly water for any length of time.

Return to the junction and head north toward Deer Creek Pass, climbing moderately steeply 200 yards to a notch in a solid rock ridge between Siligo Peak and Peak 8059. The terrain east of the crest lies out before you, with Deer Lake at the bottom of a giant, almost barren cirque. North of Deer Lake, a steep drop-off hides the head of Deer Creek canyon. From the notch, the trail switchbacks five times down a shoulder of Siligo Peak, and then contours just below the south lip of Deer Lake's cirque around to a junction, a quarter mile below Deer Creek Pass. An interesting botanical inversion can be witnessed on this crest: Whitebark pines, normally seen on the highest and most exposed ridges, stop short here and are replaced by wind-battered and contorted Jeffrey pines clinging to the uppermost rocks. A few upright Jeffrey pines also grow down the west side of the ridge for a short distance. You'll have plenty of time to admire the lake from several angles, as you make the long traverse around the south side of the cirque to the junction below the pass.

Off-Trail to Siligo Peak

Peakbaggers can begin a relatively easy "walk-up" climb to the top of Siligo Peak from almost any point on the trail between the Summit Lake junction and the top of the ridge above Deer Lake. A tangle of use trails heads up a steep incline of red rock, granite sand, patches of brush, and blocks of granite to the summit, a mere half mile from the trail. The summit offers a superb panorama of all the peaks and canyons of the central Trinity Alps, as well as three of the Four Lakes around the peak (Luella Lake is hidden under a ragged spur ridge to the north). Mt. Shasta, to the northeast, and Lassen Peak, farther south, punctuate the east horizon.

From the Deer Creek Pass junction, head down toward Deer Lake, which is of similar size and shape to Diamond Lake. The water appears jade green from above, contrasting vividly with the red-weathered serpentine rock around the shore. Also, as at Diamond Lake, the only usable campsite lies close to the trail above the east shore, sheltered by one large conifer. Fly-fishing on calm evenings should net anglers several pan-sized eastern brook trout.

From Deer Lake, climb back up to the junction below Deer Creek Pass and continue climbing another 0.25 mile to the pass and a junction of the Stoney Ridge Trail heading south and your trail, the Long Canyon Trail, heading east toward Bee Tree Gap. The view from the pass is somewhat hemmed in by the topography, but you overlook verdant Siligo Meadows to the south and the upper Deer Creek valley to the north.

Side Trip to Echo Lake

As long as you're this high at Deer Creek Pass, you might as well take the relatively easy 4-mile round-trip down through Siligo Meadows and up over Little Stonewall Pass to gorgeous, isolated Echo Lake. From the junction, head south on the Stoney Ridge Trail, dropping moderately steeply across a dry hillside through scattered foxtail and whitebark pines, just west of a deep ravine. Proceed across lush meadows to the bottom of the hill, pass through a belt of forest, and then start climbing toward Little Stonewall Pass in more open terrain. The lower part of Siligo Meadows, including a number of small ponds with raised grass rims, stretches away below to the northwest, where Deep Creek falls over the edge of Stuart Fork canyon. The scene is very bucolic, unfortunately including cows in some years.

Switchbacks lead up toward Little Stonewall Pass, where some different types of rock show up in slides from the cliffs to the east: slates and serpentines, as well as non-metamorphosed sandstones of various colors. The trail levels off a quarter mile south of the pass in a meadow. Look for a small pond among the erratic boulders at the east end of this meadow, walk around the pond, and continue east through a gap to where you can see Echo Lake directly below at the bottom of a deep cirque. There is no maintained trail down to the lake, but you should be able to easily follow a use trail.

Echo is a beautiful, teardrop-shaped subalpine lake of 2.5 acres. Rock slides that reach almost to the tops of some of the cirque's cliffs have leveled out and filled in around the shoreline to form exquisite little meadows and flower gardens. Water seeps and gurgles through the slides on the east and north sides of the cirque, and enough soil has formed there to support an amazing growth of flowers and ferns. A few stunted red firs, mountain hemlocks, and whitebark pines take root around the lake. The southeast shore has a poor campsite that's too close to the lake, but better sites may be available near the little pond above, or around Van Matre Meadows below. Fishing in Echo Lake is fair for small brook trout.

At least two alternatives exist to backtracking over Little Stonewall Pass and through Siligo Meadows to Deer Creek Pass or Bee Tree Gap. One is to continue south through Van Matre Meadows, over Stonewall Pass and out to Trinity Alps Resort. The other leads to Long Canyon via a strenuous cross-country route up the incline on the northwest side of the Echo Lake cirque, over the top and down past Billy Be Damn Lake to Lake Anna. From Lake Anna the way is relatively easy down to the Long Canyon Trail. Although quite rigorous, the route offers plenty of solitude and outstanding scenery.

If you plan to return to Bee Tree Gap, you need not go all the way back to Deer Creek Pass; from upper Siligo Meadows, cross the beginnings of Deep Creek and head for the hill to the east of the ravine (the one you stayed west of on the way down from the pass). Climb northeast and continue around the southeast side of a small meadow above. The well-defined tread of the trail between Deer Creek Pass and Bee Tree Gap crosses the upper edge of this meadow. Turn east on the trail and climb moderately steeply to Bee Tree Gap.

When you're ready to wind up your trip, turn east from the junction near Deer Creek Pass and make a fairly level 0.6-mile traverse to Bee Tree Gap at the head of Long Canyon. Far beyond a distant arm of Trinity Lake and a series of purple ridges, Lassen Peak thrusts above the eastern skyline, 85 miles away. Mt. Shasta hides behind the crenellated bulk of Gibson Peak, towering above the north side of the green-floored basin directly below at the head of Long Canyon. Closer up, gnarled red firs and mountain hemlocks, along with stunted lupines, pussy paws, and stonecrops, testify to the alpine character of the crest.

The Long Canyon Trail first descends north in two long-legged switchbacks, then turns back south to descend more switchbacks before rounding a spur ridge and contouring down to a delightful little meadow notched into the south wall of the canyon, 0.9 mile from the gap. An icy little stream wanders from under a

Long Canyon

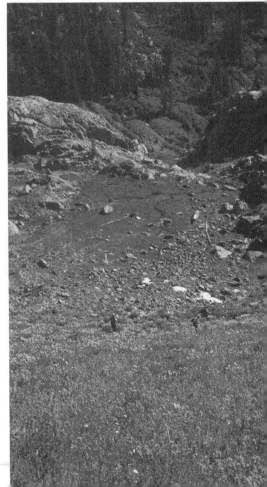

semipermanent snowbank to water the lush, green grass and refresh passersby. Two good campsites are among the boulders around the meadow. Please don't camp in the meadow or graze stock there, as the little patch of grass could be ruined by just one such transgression.

The wide, rocky slope reaching up to the base of the cliffs on the crest, west and south of the little shelf, supports the thickest and most extensive growth of wildflowers to be found in the Trinity Alps. Acres and acres of Indian paintbrush, angelica, and western pasqueflower reach almost as far as the eye can see. Under these taller flowers, an amazing number of smaller varieties flourish, including bluebell, evening primrose, and gilia.

From the little meadow hanging on the south side of the upper Long Canyon, the trail zigzags down on steep, rocky tread to cross the small creek in the bottom of the canyon, then turns east along the north slope. A series of meadows and willow flats, decorated with wildflowers in season, slopes moderately down for a mile to a narrower, wooded section of the canyon, where the trail once again drops steeply on rough, worn tread. The condition of the trail improves as the descent eases and turns away from the creek. Switchbacks lead down to a somewhat obscure junction with the trail to Bowerman Canyon, 3 miles from Bee Tree Gap. A small, poor campsite is tucked under the trees nearby, the first passable campsite since the little meadow 2 miles back.

Madrones and bigleaf maples begin to intermix with the conifers as you descend the next 0.7 mile of moderately steep trail to a crossing of a good-sized tributary stream well up the hillside above the East Fork. The trail eventually merges with an old roadbed, gradually descending another 0.4 mile to the Long Canyon trailhead.

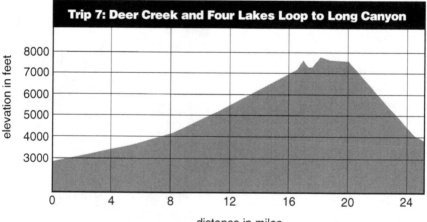

TRIP 8

Granite Peak

The brutal climb is soon forgotten after reaching the extraordinary view from the site of a former lookout.

Trip Type:	Dayhike
Distance:	10 miles round-trip, out-and-back
Elevation Change:	4450 feet, average 890 feet per mile
Difficulty:	Difficult
Season:	Early July to mid-October
Maps:	USGS *Covington Mill*; USFS *A Guide to the Trinity Alps Wilderness*
Nearest Campground:	Minersville

Five miles of steep, nearly uninterrupted climbing deter a lot of people from the 8091-foot summit of Granite Peak, one of the highest peaks in the eastern Trinity Alps, and the highest with a maintained (if unwaveringly steep) trail to the top. However, the views from the summit, which held a lookout in the bygone days of fire spotting, are outstanding and more than ample reward for the sweat equity required to get there. Thick forest blocks any sort of view for the first 3 miles and the first view is limited to part of Trinity Lake and the Trinity Mountains. The wide-ranging views of the Trinity Alps and the more distant volcanoes of Mt. Shasta and Lassen Peak, which are the true highlights, don't start to come into play until just shy of the summit.

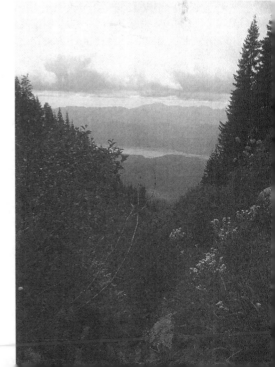

View from Granite Peak Trail

For those who don't mind an extremely rigorous climb, the trail to the summit of Granite Peak is a worthwhile endeavor. An early morning start helps hikers beat the heat; be sure to pack plenty of fluids, although water can be replenished along the way in tributaries of Stoney Creek. As the Granite Peak Trail is one of the less used trails in the eastern Alps, maintenance seems to be infrequent at best—there may be lots of deadfall across the trail.

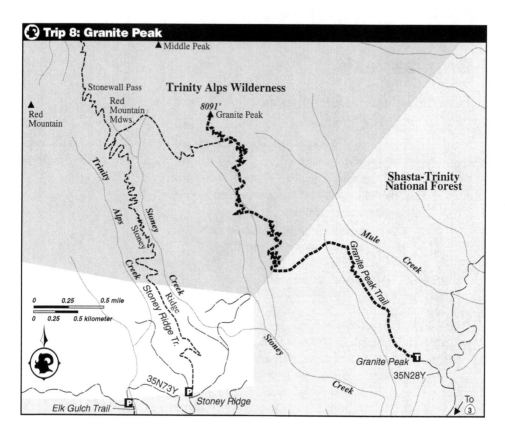

Trip 8: Granite Peak

▲ Middle Peak

Stonewall Pass   **Trinity Alps Wilderness**

Red
Mountain
Mdws.

▲
Red
Mountain

8091'
▲ Granite Peak

**Shasta-Trinity
National Forest**

Trinity

Alps

Stoney

Stoney

Creek

Mule

Creek

Creek
Ridge

Stoney Ridge Tr.

Granite Peak Trail

0   0.25   0.5 mile

0   0.25   0.5 kilometer

Stoney

Creek

35N73Y

Granite Peak

35N28Y

Elk Gulch Trail

Stoney Ridge

To
3

Starting Point

Approximately 17 miles north of Weaverville, Forest Road 35N28Y turns north from Highway 3 (this junction is opposite the road to Bushytail and Minersville campgrounds and is signed GRANITE PEAK TRAIL from the north but not the south). Follow the well-graded gravel road for a couple of miles, remaining on the obvious main road at all intersections, where lesser logging roads split off to the left and right. The road eventually narrows and the surface deteriorates a little on the way to the wide dirt turnaround at the trailhead, 2.8 miles from Highway 3. In 2008 all that marked the start of the trail was a dilapidated, empty signboard.

Description

The Granite Peak Trail starts out steeply on the course of an old road through a dense, mixed forest of primarily Douglas firs, with lesser amounts of incense cedars, ponderosa pines, canyon oaks, and sugar pines. When I hiked the trail in 2008 lots of deadfall littered the lower section of trail, making the way a tad difficult for hikers and virtually impossible for equestrians. The stiff climb continues up the rounded nose of a ridge forming the east rim of a drainage carrying the waters of the east branch of Stoney Creek. Flowering dogwoods and lupines may cheer your spirits along the grueling ascent in early summer, as the old roadbed melds into single-track trail. The grade eases as you traverse west to the crossing this alder-choked creek, 1.3 miles from the trailhead, a fine spot for taking a break and refilling your water supply for the thirst-slaking climb ahead.

From the crossing, a mildly ascending traverse heads southwest to the base of the first set of what may eventually seem like never-ending switchbacks. After the first of some 90 switchbacks on the way to the summit, you pass the signed wilderness boundary and continue zigzagging up the slope through viewless forest. Farther up the slope, you leave the deciduous trees and the Douglas firs behind as the forest transitions to include firs and western white pines. Just shy of 3 miles from the trailhead, you reach the next branch of Stoney Creek in a verdant, open swath of vegetation that allows the first views of the route, including the blue waters of Trinity Lake backdropped by the forest green Trinity Mountains.

The trail continues west for a while, almost reaching the next branch of the creek before a set of switchbacks leads back across the same stream you crossed below. Here the vegetation is even lusher, with fields of wildflowers and waist-high ferns threatening to overtake the trail. The slightly higher perch provides a minor improvement to the views of Trinity Lake and Trinity Mountains.

The views end where more switchbacks lead you back into the trees. Higher up the slope the forest eventually thins and the views expand to include more of the terrain to the south and east, precursors to the stunning vista that waits at the top of the peak. However, plenty more switchbacks must be conquered before you can begin to enjoy those views. Persistence eventually pays off as you reach a junction, 4.5 miles from the trailhead, with the mile-long trail connecting the Granite Peak Trail to the Stoney Ridge Trail to the west.

Granite Peak

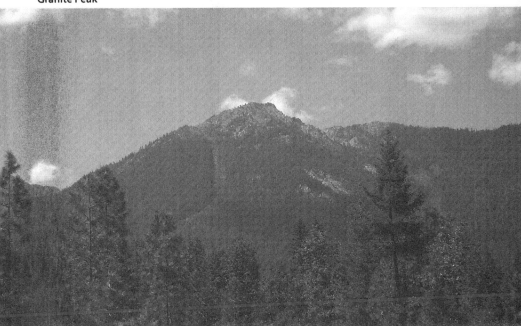

Fewer than 20 switchbacks remain, as you head away from the junction and continue to wind your way upward through mostly open terrain. The tread becomes rockier as the trail eventually swings around to the backside of the peak before climbing the last stretch to Granite Peak's 8091-foot summit, where an incredible vista unfolds. Remnants of the former fire lookout litter the summit area; it's easy to wonder about those who staffed the lookout and had this superb view to themselves. The immediate topography to the west and north is quite striking, with the rocky summits of Red Mountain, Middle Peak, Gibson Peak, and the ridges and passes between them seemingly close enough to reach out and touch. More distant landmarks include the central Trinity Alps to the northwest, Mt. Shasta to the northeast, and Lassen Peak to the southeast.

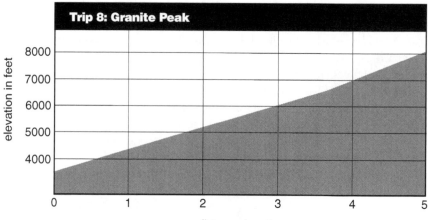

TRIP 9

Long Canyon, Lake Anna, and Billy Be Damn and Echo Lakes

Three lovely and seldom-visited lakes beckon the experienced mountain traveler who doesn't mind venturing off-trail.

Trip Type:	Backpack, 2–4 days
Distance:	12 miles, loop
Elevation Change:	9155 feet, average 763 per mile
Difficulty:	Difficult
Season:	Early July to mid-October
Maps:	USGS *Covington Mill* and *Siligo Peak*; USFS *A Guide to the Trinity Alps Wilderness*
Nearest Campground:	Alpine View

All three of these lakes are set in dramatic basins, each with its own particular charm. Combine the lakes with lush meadows, stellar wildflower displays, excellent views, rugged peaks, and the opportunity to enjoy a spectacular sunrise, and you have the necessary ingredients for a memorably spectacular Trinity Alps experience. This trip offers plenty of diverse experiences as well, with striking contrasts between the depths of forested Long and Bowerman canyons and high places such as Bee Tree Gap and Little Stonewall Pass. Solitude is almost guaranteed at the lakes, which are accessible only by off-trail travel. However, if you become too lonely at Lake Anna, Billy Be Damn Lake, or Echo Lake, you could always extend your trip by an extra day or two to include the much more popular Four Lakes Loop nearby.

This trip is not for beginning backpackers and is virtually impassable by parties traveling with stock. The route to each of the three lakes requires cross-country travel, occasionally over very steep terrain, and the ability to accurately read a map and navigate without the aid of a maintained trail. By cross-country standards, the trip is not particularly difficult, requiring a mere 2 miles of off-trail travel, but hikers must be in good physical condition and familiar enough with wilderness travel techniques to safely reach the lakes and return to the trailhead. For those up to the challenge, the rewards are well worth the extra effort.

Starting Point
Approximately 22.5 miles north of Weaverville, leave Highway 3 near a road sign marked LONG CANYON TRAIL 3, MULE CREEK 7 and turn left onto County Road 115. This junction is shortly beyond Guy Covington Drive on the right and

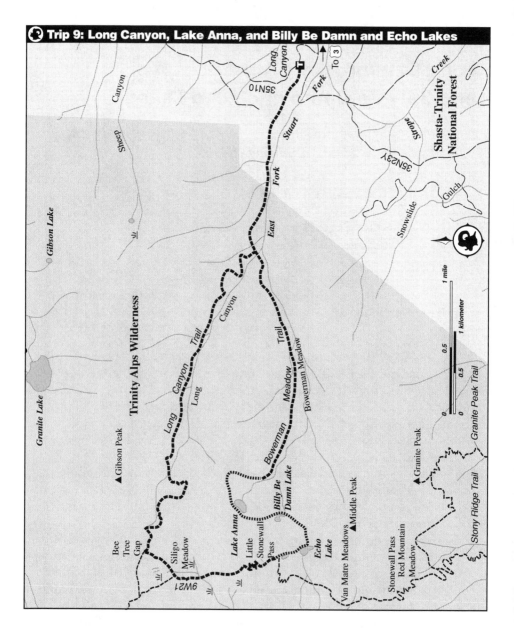

Trip 9: Long Canyon, Lake Anna, and Billy Be Damn and Echo Lakes

immediately after a bridge over the East Fork of the Stuart Fork. Travel along paved road passing numerous turnoffs to private homes until you reach a right-hand turn onto Forest Road 35N10 at 2.6 miles, which should be signed for Long Canyon Trail. Follow this gravel road for 0.3 mile to another signed intersection, where you turn left into the ample parking area near the trailhead.

Description

The trail begins by climbing moderately steeply up the continuation of an old four-wheel-drive road on red-tinted earth. The trailhead sign indicates directions and distances: LONG CANYON TRAIL, WILDERNESS BOUNDARY 3/4, BOWERMAN MEADOWS 2, DEER CREEK PASS 5, STUART FORK TRAIL 12. As you travel under a mixed, mature forest of incense cedars, Douglas firs, and Jeffrey pines, the grade moderates as you hear the roar of the creek in the canyon below. Just before reaching the signed wilderness boundary, you make a brief descent to two small rivulets that should provide a reliable source of water even in dry seasons. Continue past the boundary nearer to the creek for a while before climbing well above the water. Two switchbacks lead to a spring emerging from the ground just below the trail, followed by a longer series of switchbacks. The switchbacks end where the forest opens up a little and you reach a junction with a trail on the left to Bowerman Meadow, marked by an old wood sign nailed to a cedar, 1.9 miles from the trailhead.

Turn left and follow the trail down to a crossing of the creek, which in low water is nothing more than an easy boulder hop. When the creek is high, head 50 feet downstream to a large footlog, ax-cut on top. As you wind up and away from the creek the trail begins to climb up the ridge separating the main branch of East Fork Stuart Fork from the Long Canyon branch. Discernible tread falters a little in the tall meadow grass at the lower end of Bowerman Meadow but is soon spotted again where the trail crosses the bottom end of the meadow and briefly enters back into forest. Careful observation reveals that much of the grass in the lower meadow is being overtaken by incense cedar trees and manzanita bushes and, in areas of more moisture, alders, ferns, and bigleaf maple.

Nearing the creek, you encounter a very wet and boggy quagmire fed by a variety of seeps—watch your footing here. The trail follows alongside the creek for a stretch and then begins a switchbacking ascent beneath shady forest until leveling out near a grove of cottonwoods in the main part of Bowerman Meadow. Dramatic views of the rugged headwall and neighboring peaks dominate the eastern skyline. Your pleasant stroll through the nearly level meadow doesn't seem to last long enough, as the trail begins a steep ascent of a hillside above the creek and meadows. The trail continues up the canyon, winding up the steep hillside until leveling out again at the top of a hill carpeted with meadow grass.

Five-finger ferns

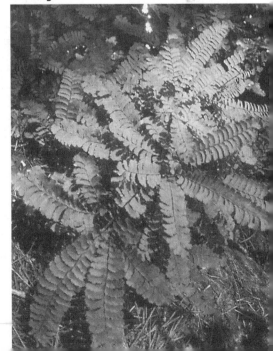

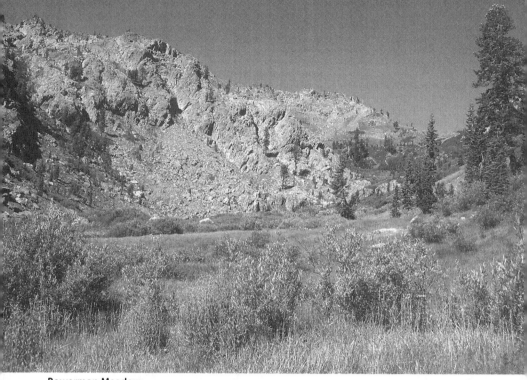

Bowerman Meadow

From the top of the hill well-defined trail leads toward a grove of alders, across a seasonal stream, and over to a large camping area. Unfortunately, this is not the trail that continues up toward the head of the canyon and the route to Lake Anna. Your route follows fainter tread straight uphill, where periodic cairns should help keep you on track. You climb steeply at first, then more moderately on the way to the top of yet another grassy hillside. From the top of the rise, keep heading uphill until you reach the upper meadow just below the headwall at the end of the canyon. Nearby, beside the creek at the edge of the trees are some good campsites, 3.5 miles from the trailhead.

Off-Trail to Lake Anna, Billy Be Damn Lake, and Echo Lake

At the head of Bowerman Meadow you begin the off-trail ascent toward Lake Anna. Although it's possible to ascend the headwall to the lake, most parties will find this nearly vertical route unfavorable. A better route, although still a rigorous climb, is to angle up to the ridgecrest and then traverse to Lake Anna around the back side: Head north from the edge of the upper meadow to the right of the cascade spilling down from the lake. Follow the line of the creek in the lower section and then diagonal over to the right, avoiding as much brush as possible in the process. A large boulder sits halfway up the slope—pass to the left and continue toward the crest of the ridge to a small saddle.

From the saddle, turn left and climb a short, steep pitch to the top, to overlook a small basin. Make a short descent into this basin, traverse the base of some cliffs, and then head up to a minor ridge on the opposite side. From the top of the minor ridge, drop down into the next small vale, as the way becomes easier on a gentle ascent over boulders and through meadows up to the top of Lake Anna's rim. The lake is a gorgeous

4-acre body of water set in a steep-sided, rockbound bowl surrounded by jagged, red cliffs. A spectacular view down Bowerman Canyon is available from the rim, as well as the possibility of some of the finest sunrises you'll see anywhere in the Alps, with the summits of Lassen Peak and Mt. Shasta tinged by the early morning light. Shasta red firs shelter a handful of campsites on the rim of the basin above the northwest shore.

Acquiring water will likely be the biggest inconvenience at Lake Anna, since the lake sits well below the rim and is the only source of water once the snow in the area has melted. If you're tempted to search for a campsite in the rocks near the outlet, don't bother—while that side of the lake offers great views, there is absolutely no place to pitch a tent. Fishing is good for eastern brook trout up to 10 inches. Lake Anna is not as infrequently visited as it once was, but you still stand a pretty good chance of having a reasonable dose of solitude and serenity during your stay.

If your plan is to visit Lake Anna only, you can make a straightforward return via the Long Canyon Trail by proceeding directly northeast from the rim of the lake down a moderately steep gully to the meadow below. Intersect the trail in the meadow and then follow the Long Canyon Trail southwest 4 miles back to the trailhead.

If few people get to Lake Anna, even fewer reach the placid waters of Billy Be Damn Lake. From the south rim of Lake Anna, ascend the slope to the top of a ridge, where you'll see the lake below. From there, descend a use trail to the northeast shore. Set in a desolate basin against a backdrop of gray, craggy spires, Billy Be Damn Lake is composed of a large oval body of water and a smaller cigar-shaped pond, the two connected by a shallow channel that dries up by late season to form two separate lakes. Campsites are scarce, but campers are scarcer still. Fishing for eastern brook trout in the shallow lake is probably fair at best. Views down Bowerman Canyon and the sunsets are even more spectacular than at Lake Anna, but the lack of both trees and smaller plants at Billy Be Damn Lake creates a much lonelier ambiance.

A use trail leaves the south end of Billy Be Damn Lake and follows an angling ascent up to a notch in the ridge southeast of the lake. Just before reaching the top of the ridge, the path disappears as the route becomes steeper. The view from the notch to the west is somewhat disappointing and Echo Lake lies out of sight, blocked by a satellite ridge. However, the view behind, including Bowerman Canyon, Trinity Lake, and Mt. Shasta, is quite spectacular. From the notch, make a winding descent down loose rock to where Echo Lake pops into view, backdropped by the rugged summits of the central Alps. As the descent continues, the route becomes both less rocky and less steep. Soon you arrive at the shore of Echo Lake.

Echo is a gorgeous, teardrop-shaped, 2.5-acre, subalpine lake located at 7250 feet. Rockslides that reach almost to the top of some of the cirque's cliffs have leveled out and filled in around the shoreline to border exquisite pocket meadows and flower gardens that contrast dramatically with the rock. Water seeps and gurgles through the slides on the east and north sides of the cirque where enough soil has accumulated in places to produce an amazing growth of flowers and ferns. A few stunted red firs, mountain hemlocks, and whitebark pines are scattered about the shoreline. One poor campsite on the southeast shore is a little too close to the lake to be legal. More acceptable sites can be found near the pond above or down in Van Matre Meadows below. Fishing is fair for small brook trout.

The distance from Echo Lake to maintained trail at Little Stonewall Pass is a mere 0.2 mile. Head directly north from the lake up and over a hill, pass by a pond, and then follow a slightly uphill traverse to the trail. More than one use trail slices through the meadow to join the main trail, but don't fret too much if you can't locate one of these paths, as the way is quite clear. If you come out at the right spot, you'll be met by a twin-trunked western white pine with an old sign marked ECHO LAKE *pointing back the way you came.*

After traveling more than 2 miles cross-country on your circuit to the three lakes, the trail up to Little Stonewall Pass seems terribly civilized. Reach the pass 5.6 miles from the trailhead and only 0.1 mile from where the cross-country route intersected the main trail. Nailed to a foxtail pine, a sign reads LITTLE STONEWALL PASS, ELEV. 7400.

From the pass you descend a series of switchbacks for 0.75 mile to the edge of Siligo Meadows, which presents a very pastoral scene with tall grasses, ponds, and meandering brooks. If cows happen to be grazing here, you may be more apt to feel like you're on the farm than in the wilderness. The trail seems to disappear in the tall grass, but large cairns should help guide you across the lower meadow to defined trail on the ascent of a low bank that divides the upper and lower meadows. If you desire to camp in the meadows, there are plenty of adequate campsites and plenty of forage for stock. At the top of the bank you come to a signed three-way junction. The trail ahead continues to Deer Pass and the Four Lakes Loop. (If you wish to add this extension to your trip, see Trip 7, page 83.)

Turn right at the junction and follow the trail around Siligo Meadows on a moderately steep, 0.4-mile climb to Bee Tree Gap. The view from the 7550-foot gap is quite impressive, as far beyond a distant arm of Trinity Lake and a series of purple ridges, Lassen Peak thrusts above the eastern skyline, 85 air miles away. Mt. Shasta hides behind the crenellated hulk of Gibson Peak, towering above the north side of the green-floored basin directly below at the head of Long Canyon. Closer up, gnarled red firs and mountain hemlocks, and stunted lupines, pussy paws, and stonecrops testify to the alpine nature of the crest.

On the Long Canyon Trail you first descend north on two short-legged switchbacks, then turn back south on more switchbacks before rounding a spur ridge and contouring down to a delightful little meadow notched into the south wall of the canyon, 0.75 mile from Bee Tree Gap. An icy little stream wanders from a semipermanent snowfield to water the lush, green grass and to refresh passersby. Two good campsites are among the boulders around the fringe of the meadow—please don't camp in the meadow or forage stock here; the little patch of grass could easily be ruined by even one such transgression. The wide, rocky slope reaching up to the base of the cliffs on the crest, west and south of the little shelf, supports the thickest and most extensive growth of wildflowers in the Alps. Acres and acres of Indian paintbrush, angelica, and western pasqueflower reach almost as far as the eye can see. Under these taller flowers are amazing numbers of smaller varieties—bluebells, evening primroses, and gilias for starters—crowding one another for spots in the sun. Another off-trail route to Lake Anna begins immediately above this little meadow, heading up the gully above directly to the lake.

The trail continues to zigzag down the canyon on steep, rocky tread to cross the small creek in the bottom of the canyon, then turns east along the north slope. A series of meadows and willow flats, decorated with wildflowers in season, slopes moderately down for a mile to a narrower, wooded section of the canyon, where the trail drops more steeply again. The descent eases as the trail turns away from the creek and then once again becomes steep on a succession of switchbacks on the way to the Bowerman Meadow junction, 3.3 miles from Bee Tree Gap.

From the junction, retrace your steps 1.9 miles to the trailhead.

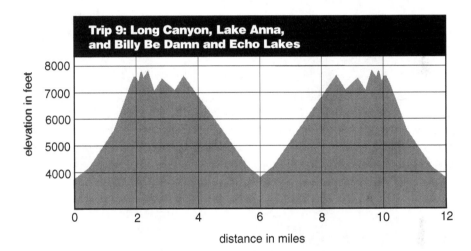

TRIP 10

Granite Lake and Bear Basin Loop

The upper part of this very pleasant and scenic loop travels all the way around 8132-foot Seven Up Peak.

Trip Type:	Backpack, 3–5 days
Distance:	17.2 miles, loop
Elevation Change:	7955 feet, average 463 per mile
Difficulty:	Moderate
Season:	Mid-July to mid-September
Maps:	USGS *Covington Mill*, *Siligo Peak*, *Caribou Lake*, and *Ycatapom Peak*; USFS *A Guide to the Trinity Alps Wilderness*
Nearest Campground:	Preacher Meadow

From the traverse of the ridge west of Deer Creek canyon you have truly magnificent views across to Siligo Peak, Luella Lake, and most of the central Trinity Alps. By adding two or three days and nearly 10 miles, you can descend a long series of switchbacks from Granite Creek summit down Deer Creek to hike the Four Lakes Loop.

Granite Lake

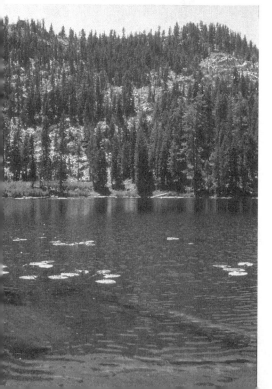

Several small lakes, including Seven Up and Gibson, hidden in the folds of massive ridges, offer off-trail goals for those who may find Granite Lake to be too overpopulated. While a large number of backpackers reach Granite Lake, and a few of those climb over the ridge to Deer Creek, far fewer end up in Bear or Black basins. However, a fair number of equestrians do reach these basins, as plenty of grass is available for stock. In spite of the heavy traffic, Granite Lake remains unique and beautiful. Catching a limit of fair-sized eastern brook trout from the evening rise is a distinct possibility. Swimming can be delightful in Granite Lake by mid-August.

Trip 10: Granite Lake and Bear Basin Loop

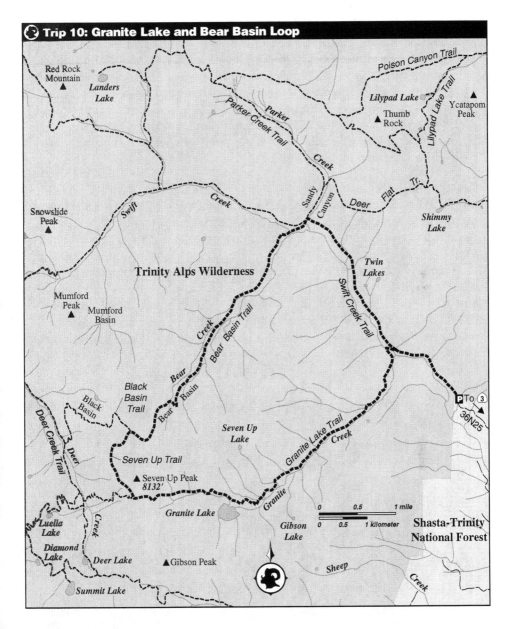

Starting Point

Highway 3 crosses Swift Creek about 29.5 miles north of Weaverville, just beyond the turnoff east to Trinity Center. The road to the Swift Creek trailhead turns west 0.25 mile north of the Swift Creek bridge and 0.25 mile south of Wyntoon Resort. The narrow pavement on the initial stretch of the Swift Creek Road ends a mile from the highway, replaced by a well-graded dirt surface wandering southwest and then west, climbing steadily well above the level of Swift Creek. You pass a number of forks along the way, including a signed junction with the road to the Lake Eleanor trailhead, but the Swift Creek Road is clearly the main thoroughfare and junctions are usually marked.

A small flat, 6.7 miles from Highway 3, offers auxiliary parking and a potential place to camp. About 200 yards farther up the road is the actual trailhead, equipped with a large parking lot, horse unloading and tie area, vault toilet, picnic table, and signboard. You would do well to ignore the camping symbol near the horse tie area, as the "camp" consists of a slanted picnic table and a fire pit on a rocky slope. A sign for stock water points the way to a beautiful large spring below the parking lot, protected by a split-rail fence.

Description

The Swift Creek Trail begins at the north end of the parking lot near a sign reading FOSTERS CABIN 5, HORSESHOE LAKE 8, GRANITE LAKE 5. You begin by descending through a dry gully and then emerging onto a bench above Swift Creek 0.5 mile from the trailhead. Rumbling through boulders, Swift Creek definitely lives up to its name here. Some excellent campsites on the bench will tempt backpackers who have gotten a late start. Rare California pitcher plant grows in clumps in a marshy area farther up the trail. Something you will more than likely notice very soon into the hike is the old California license plates periodically nailed high up some tree trunks—markers for helping personnel locate snow-survey equipment in the winter.

Gibson Meadow

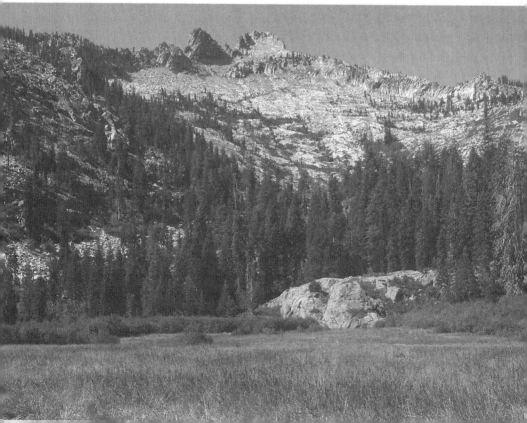

At 1.5 miles from the trailhead, you begin to climb more steeply around the north side of a deep, narrow gorge cut through solid metamorphic rock by the persistent waters of Swift Creek. You'll eventually hear the roar of two waterfalls at the upper end of the gorge, but they remain out of sight until you stroll to the overhanging outcrops along the brink. Reach a junction with the Granite Creek Trail branching southwest above the gorge, 1.9 miles from the trailhead.

Following a sign marked GRANITE LAKE, SEVEN UP PEAK, you contour almost level 200 yards to a humpbacked, steel-truss bridge over Swift Creek, climb up the south bank, and then cross a 200-yard-wide bench before switchbacking up the west side of Granite Creek canyon. The tread is steep and rocky until you cross two tributary streams. On a bench, 1.3 miles from the bridge, the trail turns closer to Granite Creek for a short stretch before climbing away again through a mature forest of Douglas firs, white firs, incense cedars, and sugar pines. After leveling out on a flat, the trail leads across another small tributary in a willow thicket, then dips into a dry draw, followed by a moderately steep climb over a moraine liberally sprinkled with erratic granite boulders. You draw close to Granite Creek again near where the creek cascades over a metamorphic rock sill, about 2 miles from the bridge. Above the cascade the trail is nearly level, following a mellow stretch of the creek through a wider part of the canyon. A half mile farther, the canyon narrows again and you climb over the toe of a red-rock talus slide past another cascade. Head-high azaleas and tall ferns line the trail in a lush dell above this cascade. Breaking out into the open at the foot of a slender meadow, you have your first unobstructed view straight up the canyon of the looming hulk of 8400-foot Gibson Peak.

After a moderate climb along the fringe of the meadow and through a belt of trees, the trail jogs northwest to climb over the end of a metasedimentary rock dike running all the way across the canyon. Turn southwest again through patches of meadow and brush on the floor of the sparse forest to an icy spring in the middle of a wide band of alders, willows, and vine maples, about 3 miles from the Swift Creek bridge. At the edge of talus falling from a glacier-carved, red-rock hump on the northwest side of the canyon, you turn south and snake up the side of another dike, only to find yet another dike ahead and a cascade above. A short climb northwest up a fern-covered side canyon leads to the top of the third dike, where you turn back south and then west to enter the lower end of Gibson Meadow.

A screen of willows hides the creek in the lower meadow and firs north of the trail shelter an excellent, large campsite, heavily used by horse packers. The trail skirts the north and northwest side of the large, wet meadow, passes two lily ponds, and then turns away from alder-choked Granite Creek up a side canyon before the final, moderately steep pitch into Granite Lake's basin. A short stroll from there leads to the east shore of the deep, 18-acre lake.

Cliffs and huge blocks of granite around the south half of the lake lead up to the magnificent bulk of Gibson Peak. Sunset colors on the peak, reflected in the lake's surface are unforgettable. Some unbelievably large incense cedars can be seen above the northwest shore, worth the effort to search out and observe—

they may be the largest cedars you'll ever see. Good campsites may be available on a ledge that the trail crosses on the way around the northwest side of the lake. Just below the lake, a use trail leads to a site beneath shady conifers, and then continues across a log over the outlet to additional sites on a hump of granite. Even if you don't plan to camp on this hump, the easy stroll to this spot offers the best view of the picturesque lake backdropped by the northeast flank of Gibson Peak. Fishing remains fair to good in Granite Lake for eastern brook trout up to 10 or 11 inches, probably because reaching the shoreline requires a trip through thick brush or over blocky talus.

The climb out of Granite Lake's basin to the crest of the ridge above Deer Creek is best accomplished in either the early morning or late afternoon, as the grade is steep and the trail is fully exposed to the sun for most of the day. The first quarter mile of trail rises moderately to steeply above some of the campsites and then crosses two small rivulets, as you continue to climb west through rocks and brush north of the inlet. Climb beside the creek, which tumbles through alders in the bottom of a gulch, the last available water on the trail until the upper end of Bear Basin, a lot of ups and downs away. A meadow carpeted with lupine, mountain aster, angelica, fireweed, corn lily, and other brilliant wildflowers, greets you above the gulch. You wander through this verdant meadow, climbing moderately west toward a gap in the ridge between the red rock of Seven Up Peak to the north and the gray granite of Gibson Peak to the south. Two steep to very steep pitches, with a brief respite between, lead to a flower-bedecked amphitheater just below the crest. A last, short, steep scramble up the west wall brings you to the crest and a junction with the Seven Up Trail branching north.

Sensational views from the crest spread out in virtually every direction. On clear days Castle Crags and Lassen Peak appear on the eastern horizon, far above the upper reaches of Trinity Lake. Seven Up Peak's ragged red cone rears up a little east of north behind skeletons of lightning-shattered foxtail and whitebark pines along the crest. The vista to the west is one of the most comprehensive views of the central Trinity Alps available in the wilderness. Luella Lake hangs in a pocket on the north flank of Siligo Peak directly across from the wide, glacier-formed chasm of upper Deer Creek canyon. Sawtooth Mountain forms the skyline behind the west wall of the canyon, leading up to the jumble of summits culminating in 9002-foot Thompson Peak, highest point on the horizon and in the Trinity Alps. The convoluted trace of the Four Lakes Loop is clearly visible across the canyon, climbing from tiny Round Lake past Luella Lake to the crest of the west ridge on the way to Diamond Lake.

Granite Lake Trail 8W14 continues west from the crest, switchbacking down the east wall to junctions with the Four Lakes Loop and Deer Creek Trail on the floor of Deer Creek canyon, 1.2 trail miles away. However, you turn north heading toward Black and Bear basins on the Seven Up Trail, which contours northwest around the flanks of Seven Up Peak, and then turns northeast around a shoulder to drop down to the divide between the two basins, 1.3 miles from the junction. Contorted Jeffrey pines and Shasta red firs add foreground interest to the views along the way. An open, vertical mineshaft is beside one of the switchbacks on the way down into Black Basin—please avoid the temptation to climb down to the shaft, throw anything down into it, or even get close to this dangerous and historic site. Farther on, a miner's collapsed cabin is beside the Black Basin Trail a short distance north of a junction at the foot of the hill.

Black Basin is a glacier-carved trough sloping northwest from the Bear Basin divide, which turns west to end as a hanging valley above Deer Creek canyon. With only one small pond and no streams to speak of, Black Basin is nonetheless a pretty valley, well worth an extra day of exploration.

The Bear Basin Trail (9W10) rises moderately north from the flat at the head of Black Basin toward a red knob, before turning east and heading down toward a small, permanent snowfield in a cirque beneath the north slope of Seven Up Peak. You descend on steep, loose dirt tread through a flower gar-den for 200 yards, and then jog north around a rock knob. Snaking down the rocky slope below the knob, you realize the reason for the jog—a 30- to 40-foot escarpment of gray, meta-morphic rock that extends from the knob across the valley. The trail turns northeast near the bottom of the hill and doesn't draw any closer than 300 yards to the inviting snowfield in the cirque. Of course, you could climb up to the snowfield if you have a craving for snow, but an icy little stream trick-les through alders 200 yards down the trail. From higher up the hill, an alder- or willow-lined pond on the east side of the upper basin is visible across the way, but the pond disap-pears from view on the descent and is difficult to locate.

Swift Creek Gorge

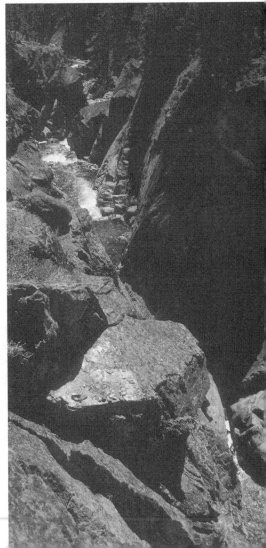

Below an outstanding grove of large red firs and western white pines, follow excellent, almost level, trail northeast above the northwest side of a wide meadow. In an airy grove of firs, 0.8 mile from the Black Basin junction, you'll find several excellent campsites with plenty of firewood nearby, the only drawback being the 200 yards you'll have to travel to acquire water from meadow-lined Bear Creek.

Below the fir grove, you drop down a little more steeply toward the middle of the valley, and then cross Bear Creek just above a cottonwood grove rising out of a tangle of alders. After climbing over a low, grassy hump on the valley floor, a moderate descent leads through a band of forest to another large, beautiful meadow. Excellent campsites abound here, some near the creek on the southeast side of the meadow, and others by springs flowing from the hill on the northwest side. Although Seven Up Peak is now out of sight, several rugged spires on the southeast rim catch the morning and evening sun above the verdant valley.

The valley narrows to a canyon below the lower meadow, and the trail becomes rough and steep in places, wandering down through open, mixed forest, with several springs and rivulets flowing across the trail. As Bear Creek drops more precipitously, you turn north on the side of the canyon, back east down to a bench, and then north again to a steel-girder bridge over Swift Creek. The Bear Creek Trail meets the Swift Creek Trail 250 yards east of the bridge, near a three-way junction above Parker Creek, and 1.3 miles from the lower meadow in Bear Basin. There's a large camping area with a spring near the junction.

From the junction, cross a heavily forested flat and begin a steady descent down Swift Creek canyon back toward the trailhead. Drop to a small meadow and follow the willow-lined stream draining the meadow to a flat. After a pair of switchbacks, you hop across an unnamed stream, cross another flat, and then proceed to a crossing of Steer Creek. Continue downstream from Steer Creek, as the trail eventually curves southeast, crosses the outlet draining Twin Lakes above, and then reaches the Granite Lake Trail junction, 1.6 miles from the previous junction above Parker Creek.

From there, retrace your steps 1.9 miles to the Swift Creek trailhead.

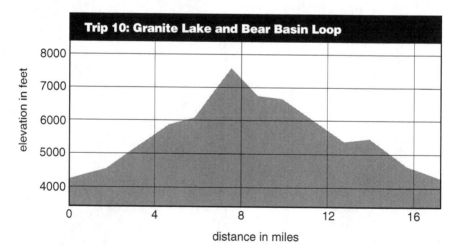

TRIP 11

Deer Flat, Thumb Rock, and Landers Creek Loop

You will see a wider variety of flora, fauna, and terrain on this trip than almost any other in the Trinity Alps.

Trip Type:	Backpack, 3–5 days
Distance:	19.7 miles, loop
Elevation Change:	11,850 feet, average 602 per mile
Difficulty:	Difficult
Season:	Mid-July to late September
Maps:	USGS *Covington Mill, Ycatapom Peak,* and *Caribou Lake;* USFS *A Guide to the Trinity Alps Wilderness*
Nearest Campground:	Preacher Meadow

This is a strenuous trip, involving almost 12,000 feet of elevation change and the crossing of four major ridge systems. Some sections of trail are steep and rough, while others are hard to find and follow. No lakes are included in the basic loop, but side trip options are easily available to Twin, Shimmy, Lilypad, and Landers lakes, and more distant Foster, Lion, and Union lakes can be added with a little more effort. You are rewarded with solitude and incomparable scenery once you get away from the thoroughfare along Swift Creek.

This trip is also one of contrasts—you probably won't be able to walk a mile along Swift Creek without the company of others, but on the traverse around Thumb Rock you may be the only one who has passed that way in weeks. Windblasted firs and Jeffrey pines have been flattened against the rocks on the 7200-foot crest above Cub Wallow, while down in Swift Creek canyon straight boles of Douglas firs and ponderosa pines soar to heights of 150 to 200 feet. The lush wet meadows at the head of Landers Creek support acres of tropical-looking California pitcher plants, a stark contrast to the near desert and sagebrush around Shimmy Lake. Deer herds graze in aptly named Deer Flat in the evenings and coyotes howl from the ridge tops, but in Mumford Meadow you're more apt to hear the radios.

Starting Point

Highway 3 crosses Swift Creek about 29.5 miles north of Weaverville, just beyond the turnoff east to Trinity Center. The road to the Swift Creek trailhead turns west 0.25 mile north of the Swift Creek bridge and 0.25 mile south of Wyntoon Resort. The narrow pavement on the initial stretch of the Swift Creek Road ends a mile from the highway, replaced by a well-graded dirt road that

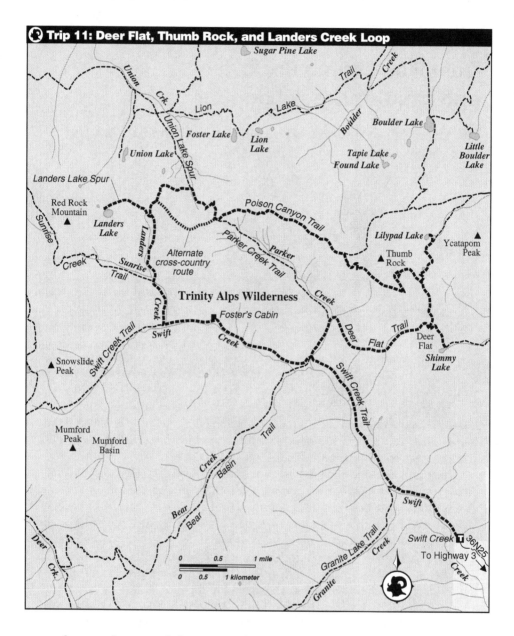

Trip 11: Deer Flat, Thumb Rock, and Landers Creek Loop

wanders southwest and then west, climbing steadily well above Swift Creek. You pass a number of forks along the way, including a junction with the road to the Lake Eleanor trailhead, but the Swift Creek Road is clearly the main thoroughfare and junctions are clearly marked.

A small flat, 6.7 miles from Highway 3, offers auxiliary parking and a potential place to camp. About 200 yards farther up the road is the trailhead, equipped with a large parking lot, horse unloading and tie area, vault toilet, picnic table, and signboard. You would do well to ignore the camping symbol near the horse tie area, as the "camp" consists of a slanted picnic table and a fire pit on a rocky slope. A sign for stock water points the way to a beautiful large spring below the parking lot, protected by a split-rail fence.

Description

The Swift Creek Trail begins at the north end of the parking lot near a sign reading FOSTERS CABIN 5, HORSESHOE LAKE 8, GRANITE LAKE 5. You begin by descending through a dry gully and then emerging onto a bench above Swift Creek 0.5 mile from the trailhead. Rumbling through boulders, Swift Creek definitely lives up to its name here. Some excellent campsites on the bench will tempt backpackers who have gotten a late start. Rare California pitcher plant grows in clumps in a marshy area farther up the trail. Something you will more than likely notice very soon into the hike is the old California license plates periodically nailed high up some tree trunks—markers for helping personnel locate snow-survey equipment in the winter.

At 1.5 miles from the trailhead, you begin to climb more steeply around the north side of a deep, narrow gorge cut through solid metamorphic rock by the persistent waters of Swift Creek. You'll eventually hear the roar of two waterfalls at the upper end of the gorge, but they remain out of sight until you stroll to the overhanging outcrops along the brink. Reach a junction with the Granite Creek Trail branching southwest above the gorge, 1.9 miles from the trailhead.

Remaining on the Swift Creek Trail, you turn northwest and climb moderately steeply up the side of the canyon. A small stream spills across the trail 0.8 mile from the junction, the outlet of Twin Lakes, two small lakes on benches above, almost entirely covered with lily pads and surrounded by azaleas and California pitcher plants. The lakes have little to offer for swimmers and anglers, but the azaleas are both fragrant and beautiful. The route up to the lakes involves some bushwhacking and a scramble up a steep and muddy hillside.

Away from the small stream, the trail gets rougher and steeper in places, as you climb moderately to the crossing of Steer Creek. From there, climb to a flat above the northwest bank, then soon drop down again to cross another small, unnamed creek. Two short-legged switchbacks lead up to another flat, where you follow a tiny, willow-lined rivulet to the source in a small meadow. The trail turns northwest away from the meadow over a low crest, and then crosses another heavily forested flat to where a bridge once crossed Parker Creek—the bridge was wiped out and the gorge filled in by a 1986 landslide. The trail crosses the creek above the former bridge site and then runs southwest for 200 yards along the brink of the gorge to a large camp area with a spring and a junction with the combination Bear Basin/Swift Creek and the Parker Creek trails.

Turn right (north-northeast) and climb up Parker Creek on steep, rocky trail, crossing a slide area and reaching a junction with the Deer Flat Trail at the foot of Sandy Canyon, 0.5 mile from the previous junction. Veer right onto the Deer Flat Trail and drop 100 yards to a stream crossing, just above the confluence of Parker Creek and the creek in Sandy Canyon. Scramble up Sandy Canyon for

50 yards and then turn south across the side of a hill. The trail contours across several small, wet meadows carpeted with wildflowers in early summer and then rises steeply northeast up a gully to begin a series of switchbacks headed generally east. About 0.5 mile from the junction of Parker and Deer creeks, you head east on a gradually sloping bench overlooking Swift Creek canyon far below. This section of trail—little-used duff tread running through open woods of ponderosa pines, Jeffrey pines, white firs, and incense cedars—is an absolute delight.

Cairns and ducks mark the way ahead, as you emerge out of the trees into a large meadow, and then pick up blazed trail climbing moderately in a belt of trees again before crossing another long strip of meadow where the tread disappears. Ducks should help guide you down to the next belt of trees and a little stream beside a large, developed campsite. Horizontal poles, wired between trees, identify this spot as a deer hunting camp. Chances are, if you're here for any length of time, you will see some deer grazing in the meadow. The trail is not clearly marked in the 10–15 acre wet meadow adjacent to this camp, but the tread should become distinct again after contouring around the edge of the meadow to the northeast side, where a rivulet flows into the clearing and a large cairn nearby signifies the resumption of trail.

A steep, zigzagging, sometimes boggy, climb of 300 yards beside the rivulet leads to a forested flat below yet another meadow. Climb moderately steeply a little east of north across this meadow and then continue climbing up the forested hill above. At the edge of the next strip of meadow, you turn east and soon come to the Deer Flat junction with the Lilypad Lake Trail, 5.8 miles from and 2700 feet higher than the Swift Creek trailhead.

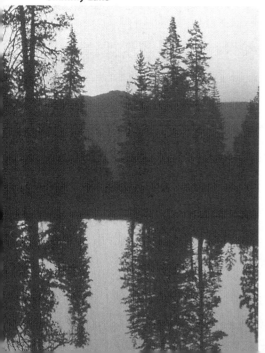

Shimmy Lake

Side Trip to Shimmy Lake

Shimmy Lake is a mere 0.5 mile southwest of the Deer Flat junction down the Eleanor Lake Trail. The vegetation thins as you descend moderately steeply, aided by a few switchbacks, on the way to the lake. Comma-shaped Shimmy Lake is lined with grasses except for a pile of broken rock that has fallen into the west end from a blood-red outcrop above. The lake has no permanent inlet or outlet and by late summer the water is brown and weedy. However, the somewhat unsavory-looking water doesn't discourage the few large and wary eastern brook trout that live in the deepest part of the lake off the rock pile. The trout make startling splashes after sundown but are very particular about what they eat. Although the basin appears level at first glance, feasible campsites are rather scarce, with one fair site next to a small meadow on the south side. The site under a large Jeffrey pine on the north side is way too close to the water.

From the Deer Flat junction, you climb north on the Lilypad Lake Trail, first through dense manzanita thickets on the crest of a ridge, and then more steeply in open forest on the east side of the crest, traveling 0.5 mile to a bare, grassy saddle. The trail becomes hard to follow, dropping down to contour around the head of a small valley beside the saddle—look for a rock cairn on the ridge northwest of the meadow at the head of the valley. A wider valley, falling away north toward Poison Canyon, lies below this second ridge.

Ycatapom Peak (supposedly "the mountain that leans" in the local Native American dialect) thrusts up ragged spires to the northeast. To the west, the granite bulk of Thumb Rock looms above lush meadows and a series of small, terraced ponds. Two signs at the crest, both with arrows pointing northwest but on opposite sides of the trail, read LILYPAD LAKE TRAIL 8W21, THUMB ROCK TRAIL, POISON CANYON TRAIL and THUMB ROCK TRAIL 8W16, POISON CANYON TRAIL, UNION CREEK TRAIL. If these two signs aren't confusing enough, the prompt disappearance of discernible tread on the hillside leading into the valley below may completely befuddle you.

Side Trip to Lilypad Lake

From the junction, without the aid of a clearly seen path, continue across the head of the valley toward the southern side of Thumb Rock. The Lilypad Lake Trail soon appears below, headed northeast across a pond-dotted terrace. Beyond the terrace the trail drops, steeply at times, eventually arriving at the northeast shore of the lake, which is set in a wide, flat basin, 1 mile from the junction. The surface of aptly named Lilypad Lake is hardly visible by midsummer, due to the profusion of lilies nearly obscuring the water. Two-thirds of the shoreline of the shallow, 2-acre lake is lined with willow thickets. All things considered, Lilypad is not the most ideal recreational lake, but the neighboring meadows and the towering peaks and ridges on all sides offer a uniquely beautiful scene. The near assurance of solitude is definitely appealing as well. Good campsites can be found in the trees near the edge of the meadows around the lake and, thanks to a general lack of visitation, firewood should be plentiful. Springs in the rocks above the lake provide a good source of water.

The Thumb Rock Trail is not easy to find. Watch for rock cairns and tree blazes that may assist your negotiation of this trailless section, which lasts for about 150 yards. The trail reappears, traversing the valley and then turning sharply uphill toward a gap in the ridgetop just southeast of Thumb Rock. Lightning-blasted red firs and foxtail pines in the gap and in the bare granite of Thumb Rock warn that this spot is not the best place to weather a thunderstorm. Splendid views of Mt. Shasta on the horizon and closer Ycatapom Peak and Poison Canyon reward your climb.

The trail becomes more evident while winding through the gap and then heading southwest down across open, grassy slopes and through scattered trees to a large meadow at the head of Sandy Canyon. The trail doesn't proceed through the meadow as you might expect, but bends slightly to the right where the path reaches the meadow and climbs uphill. A tiny stream in the meadow offers the last place to acquire water until Union Creek, 3.4 miles away. More distinct tread, marked with ducks and blazes, switchbacks moderately steeply up to the crest of a red-orange rock spur ridge west of the meadow and then contours on the back side of the ridge to a junction of the Poison Canyon Trail, 8.5 miles from the trailhead. The well-signed junction lies just below the crest of ridge running northwest from Thumb Rock, dividing the drainage of Parker Creek on the southwest from Cub Wallow and Boulder Creek on the northwest.

Bridge over Swift Creek

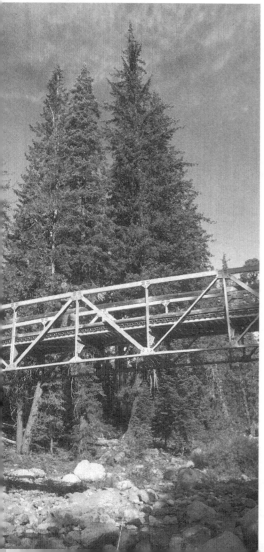

Proceed northwest on the Poison Canyon Trail, climbing to the narrow crest of the ridge and then following an undulating course along the ridge through manzanita, huckleberry oak, and ceanothus bush. Through openings in the brush, you can gaze out across the wide expanse of meadow in upper Parker Creek canyon, and catch glimpses, almost straight down, on the other side of the ridge into secluded, trackless Cub Wallow, hanging above the deep abyss of Boulder Creek canyon.

A half mile from the junction, you turn farther west and descend slightly off the crest into open fir woods. Beyond the belt of trees, you continue down around a grassy shoulder, covered with wildflowers in season, below a rounded, granite knob on the crest. Although the trail is likely to show more deer tracks than footprints or horse prints, this section of the Poison Canyon Trail is still more heavily used than the Thumb Rock Trail. Below another band of firs, the trail runs through heavy brush in places on a gradual descent toward the open saddle at the head of Parker Creek valley, which marks the divide between Parker Creek to the south and Union Creek to the north. You reach a signed three-way junction in this saddle with the Union Lake Spur and the Parker Creek Trail.

Off-Trail Route to Gap Above Landers Creek

Skilled cross-country enthusiasts can avoid the steep, dry climb from upper Union Creek to the gap in the ridge above Landers Creek, saving a half mile of hiking and 600 feet of elevation gain in the process. From the junction of Union Lake Spur and Parker Creek Trail in the saddle, traverse around the head of Union Creek to intersect the Landers Lake Trail at the gap. Following this route means forgoing the refreshing waters of Union Creek.

Proceed ahead on the Union Lake Spur, bound for the Landers Lake junction on a moderately steep, zigzagging descent down the north side of the divide. Soon a more gradual descent leads through the east side of a large meadow. You come out on a rocky dike and, as you approach the little creek draining the ponds in the meadow, you'll notice a sign on an old, dead pine beside the trail marking the Landers Lake junction, 0.8 mile from the previous junction. If you need water, get it from the little creek before starting up over the ridge to Landers Lake. If you're in need of a campsite, Union Lake is 1.8 miles down Union Creek and back up a side canyon. (From the junction follow the Union Lake Spur northwest downstream along the main branch of Union Creek to a junction with Trail 9W64A heading west. On 9W64A, travel around the nose of a ridge and soon come to a junction with the Union Lake Trail. Turn south-southwest and proceed up the canyon to Union Lake.) A number of excellent campsites may also be available along Union Creek within the first mile below the Landers Lake junction.

From the junction, head west on the Landers Lake Trail, climbing moderately across a rocky slope, then northwest up the side of a main ridge west of Union Creek valley. A short respite on a small flat brings you to the beginning of a serious climb to the crest of the ridge on a zigzagging tread of loose rock and fine dust. Reach the crest in a gap, 0.7 mile from the junction. The jagged, red cone on the skyline west of the gap is Red Rock Mountain, rising sharply behind the Landers Lake basin.

You continue moderately up the trail for 200 yards across the west side of the ridge to a small, dry meadow before descending the rocky bottom of a dry gully southwest 300 yards to a 10–12 acre meadow containing several small ponds lined with California pitcher plants. This wet meadow is the source of Landers Creek. At the lower end of the meadow, you reach the junction between the spur trail to Landers Lake and the continuation of the main trail coming up from Mumford Meadow and Swift Creek.

Side Trip to Landers Lake

Landers Lake Spur 9W09A is mucky in spots, contouring around the east side of the wet meadow at the head of Landers Creek. You ascend moderately on a rocky slope north of the meadow and then turn west into a valley with a wall of red rock across the upper end. A short, steep climb leads to a gap at the north end of this dike, from which you continue ascending moderately up a wider valley west to a final, steeper pitch over the rim of the bowl holding Landers Lake, 0.6 mile from the junction.

A large, excellent campsite is beside the trail where the path first climbs over the rim on the way to the lake. The trail continues a quarter mile to another large campsite northwest of the lake on the edge of the extensive meadows carpeting the upper part of the basin, a site apparently often used by equestrians. A small, more secluded site sheltered by trees is near the northeast shoreline. Even though the lake shrinks by late summer, the water remains cold and clear. Deer congregate in the beautiful meadows most evenings, and a constant chorus of frogs rises from two small ponds on the northwest side of the basin. Small eastern brook trout are plentiful but are difficult to catch. If you have the extra energy, a scramble to the top of the ridge on the north side of the basin affords a fine view directly down toward Union Lake and Bullards Basin 1000 feet below.

From the Landers Lake Spur junction, start down Landers Creek, snaking down the east side of the wide, glaciated upper valley through sparse forest to a dry meadow and then down through more trees to a group of fair campsites near the upper end of a large, wet meadow. The ponds in this meadow are lined and partly filled with California pitcher plants, as are the ponds in the wet meadow at the top of the valley. The trail skirts the east side of this meadow and then descends moderately through a beautiful, open forest of Douglas firs, western white pines, Jeffrey pines, and incense cedars above a grassy floor. At 1 mile from the junction, turn west down two switchbacks to cross Landers Creek and then climb moderately up the west bank to a junction with a trail branching west up Sunrise Creek canyon to Sunrise Basin and the crest above.

The trail becomes a tad rougher below the junction, descending south as the creek falls away southeast, with the last steep, quarter mile washed out and very rocky before you reach the edge of Mumford Meadow. Head south across the expansive meadow to the signed junction with the Swift Creek Trail, 1.6 miles from the Landers Lake Spur junction.

As you turn east, your feet will appreciate the nearly level, well-graded tread of the Swift Creek Trail after the previously steep and rocky section of trail. You may also discover where most of the hikers departing from the Swift Creek trailhead end up—the numerous excellent campsites near the confluence of Landers and Swift creeks at the lower end of Mumford Meadow are usually filled to overflowing. A half mile of delightfully easy descent leads to Foster's Cabin with a nearby clear, cold spring. A board-sided barn with a replacement corrugated-iron roof is the oldest building at Foster's. The original cabin has been replaced by a relatively new log structure that is open to the public. A curious, long, log-roof assembly without any shakes sits beside the trail, but there is no sign that there was ever a cabin below. There are several excellent campsites east of the cabin between the trail and Swift Creek.

Below Foster's Cabin, you stroll beside Swift Creek past additional campsites along the south edge of expansive Parker Meadow. Several seeps and one delightful little creek drain out of the east end of the meadow and run across the trail before the path turns away from Swift Creek and enters open forest. Good tread continues on a gradual descent past the Bear Basin Trail junction to the three-way junction just west of Parker Creek. From there, retrace your steps 3.5 easy miles back down Swift Creek to the Swift Creek trailhead.

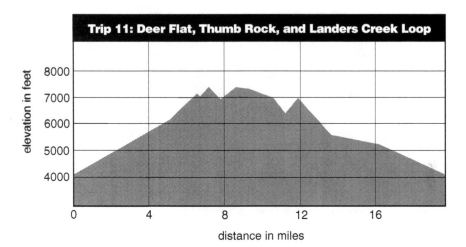

TRIP 12

Boulder Lake to Poison Canyon and Lilypad Lake

Although Poison Canyon is only a three-hour hike from the popular Boulder Lakes trailhead, it's a wild and lonely place.

Trip Type:	Backpack, 2–4 days
Distance:	9.2 miles round-trip, out-and-back
	(plus 1.5-mile off-trail side trip to Found and Tapie Lakes)
Elevation Change:	2780 feet, average 604 per mile
Difficulty:	Moderate
Season:	Mid-July to mid-October
Maps:	USGS *Ycatapom Peak*
	and USFS *A Guide to the Trinity Alps Wilderness*
Nearest Campground:	Trinity River

On this trip you'll probably hear coyotes yelping at night, see deer grazing in the meadows around sunrise or sunset, or even spot a bear. Raptors, including golden eagles and several species of hawks, soar above a wide, lush basin covered with stands of forest and pockets of meadow around Lilypad Lake, with Ycatapom Peak (which supposedly means "leaning mountain" in Wintu) as a marvelously textured backdrop and a reasonable challenge for peakbaggers. A series of terraces with flower-covered meadows and several pristine ponds lead south to Thumb Rock, a huge granite hump on the ridge above Parker Creek. You will likely see few other people around Lilypad Lake and even fewer on the terraces below Thumb Rock. Perhaps the name "Poison Canyon" discourages visitors; the climb up the steep ridge south of Boulder Lake is certainly a deterrent, as are the swarms of mosquitoes in early summer.

A short and relatively straightforward off-trail side trip over steep rock to Found and Tapie lakes is quite scenic. The best place to begin this side trip is near the top of the ridge south of Boulder Lake and, since the route rejoins maintained trail near the bottom of the ridge, you will probably prefer to do this route on your way out from Poison Canyon.

A number of alternatives continue from Poison Canyon to North Fork Swift Creek, Lake Eleanor, Swift Creek, Union Creek, and Sugar Pine Creek trailheads. Careful map research will show the way. You can attempt an interesting 21-mile loop around Thumb Rock to the Poison Canyon Trail above Cub Wallow, down to upper Union Creek, and then back to Boulder Lake via Foster and Lion lakes. (Some of this route is described in Trip 13, page 127.)

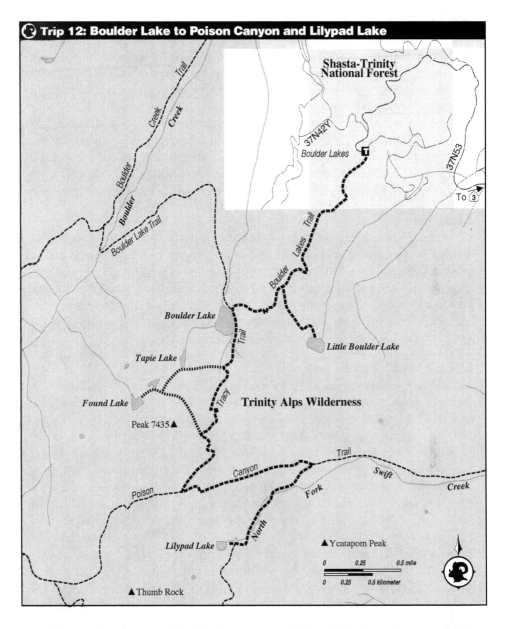

Trip 12: Boulder Lake to Poison Canyon and Lilypad Lake

Eastern brook trout inhabit the waters of Lilypad Lake and some of the ponds above, but fishing is virtually impossible due to the presence of lilies. Swimming is difficult for the same reason. Fishing in Boulder and Tapie lakes is reported to be fair to good.

Starting Point

The road to the Boulder Lakes trailhead turns off Highway 3 less than a half mile south of the junction of the Coffee Creek Road, 40 miles north of Weaverville. Increased logging activity in the area requires that you drive these roads with extreme caution. Signs would normally assist you in reaching the trailhead, but vandals seem to covet such signs in this area. Proceed on Forest Road 37N52 for 3.3 miles to a junction along a curve. Turn right here onto Forest Road 37N53 and travel another 1.1 miles to a Y-junction and bear left. From this point the main road is obvious, leading to the trailhead at the site of an old log landing on the top of a ridge between Little Boulder and Boulder creeks, 10.2 miles from Highway 3. The large landing has enough parking for a fleet of vehicles.

Description

Good tread runs southwest from the Boulder Lakes trailhead east of the top of a ridge, as you ascend moderately, with a few steeper pitches, through dense, predominantly white fir forest. Although the first 300 yards passes through a previously logged area, selective logging practices have made the logging barely noticeable. After a switchback you climb steeply back northwest, level off on the brow of the ridge, and then contour southwest to a junction with the spur to Little Boulder Lake turning east.

Side Trip to Little Boulder Lake

Little Boulder Lake is 300 feet higher than Boulder Lake, hung in a steep-sided pocket on the north side of Peak 6994. From the signed junction, climb at a moderately steep grade southeast for a quarter mile, and then straight up the nose of a ridge for 200 yards before crossing over and dropping to Little Boulder Lake, 0.4 mile from the junction.

Boulder Creek originates in the 4.5-acre lake and runs out the open north side of the basin and down into a very steep canyon below. The outlet usually dries up by midsummer. A low dam at the outlet used to raise the level of the lake, more than likely detaining water for downstream mining activities. Lush forest surrounds all but the south shore of the lake, where solid granite rises out of the water fairly steeply up to Peak 6994 above.

Although Little Boulder and Boulder lakes are only 0.6 mile apart, the smaller basin holding Little Boulder Lake has a colder microclimate, supporting a quite different range of vegetation. Lodgepole pines and red firs grow above pinemat manzanita and Labrador tea in the basin of Little Boulder, compared with white firs, sugar pines, bigleaf manzanita, and ceanothus brush around the larger lake.

Eastern brook trout to 10 inches swim lazily along the shoreline looking for something to eat. Camping is limited to a handful of poor to fair sites around the northeast shore and one fair site at the west end. Swimmers will find that the water temperature stays chilly throughout the summer.

Below the Little Boulder Lake junction, the trail switchbacks down a brushy, rock-strewn hillside, then turns west across the large basin holding Boulder Lake. At 2 miles from the trailhead, beside a large campsite near the lower end of the lake, you reach a three-way junction between the continuation of the Boulder Lakes Trail heading northwest toward Boulder Creek canyon and the Tracy Trail turning south around the east shore and then climbing over a ridge to Poison Canyon.

Boulder is a medium-sized green lake—8 acres of algae-tinted water with a ring of lily pads extending about 100 feet from a mostly grass-covered shoreline. A wet meadow borders the upper (south) end of the 27-foot-deep lake, and dense forest lines the strip of grass and willows around the rest of the shoreline. A craggy granite peak is the prominent feature of the glaciated ridge to the south.

A number of fair campsites, some quite large, nestle beneath the trees around the lower end of the lake. Other excellent sites occupy a bench 300 to 400 yards above the east shore. A pair of good sites is near where the Poison Canyon Trail crosses the inlet. Thanks to the lake's popularity, firewood is scarce. In spite of the drawbacks presented by swarms of mosquitoes in early summer and too many neighbors on weekends, Boulder Lake is a pleasant place to spend a day or two. The scenery is beautiful! Fishing is challenging around much of the tree-rimmed shoreline, but the evening rise off the logjam near the outlet may produce a fair catch of 8–9 inch eastern brook trout. Wading the muddy bottom near the inlet streams can also be fruitful, provided you don't get hung up on the lily pads; swimming off the rocks on the west side can be quite refreshing by August.

From the three-way junction near the lower end of Boulder Lake, you continue ahead (south) on the Tracy Trail around the east side of Boulder Lake just above the shoreline. Make a short climb east from the side of the wet meadow above the lake to a bench and an excellent, large campsite near the trail. In the next quarter mile, you cross two inlet streams separated by moraines. Continue climbing, steeply at times, as you wander up the second stream through open forest and small wet meadows, where a variety of wildflowers bloom through midsummer, including leopard lilies, corn lilies, shooting stars, paintbrush, mountain asters, daisies, sunflowers, and yampa.

The ascent becomes steeper up a heavily wooded slot between humps of granite before turning east to cross back over the stream, 0.7 mile from

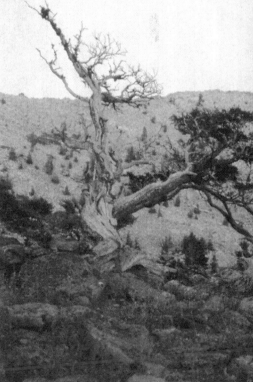

Mountain mahogany at Boulder Lake

the junction. The banks of the pretty little creek are decorated with parrot's beak, angelica, pink spiraea, and columbine. Switchbacks ease the pain of the ascent a little before you turn southwest away from the creek and scramble straight up a very steep, broken granite slope through an open forest of mountain hemlocks, red firs, and western white pines. A final, very steep zigzag brings you to the narrow crest of the ridge. By leaving the trail here and following the ridge a very short distance to the northeast, you have a fine view of the north face of Ycatapom Peak across Poison Canyon and distant Mt. Shasta.

Rather than diving straight down the side of the canyon, the trail now turns back southwest and contours a little before dropping more steeply to a bench and a junction with the Poison Canyon Trail, 1.6 mile from the junction at Boulder Lake.

Turning left at the junction, you descend three switchbacks between benches and continue the descent on a very long diagonal through open forest and thick brush. Reach a flat near the bottom of the canyon and come to a junction with the Lilypad Lake Trail, 1 mile from the previous junction. Signs and a large cairn mark the junction, which is fortunate since the trail at this particular spot is overgrown with tall grass.

Leaving the Poison Canyon Trail, you head southwest up North Fork Swift Creek canyon on pleasant, almost level tread, paralleling the creek through dense fir forest. Where the forest begins to thin, the trail crosses the creek twice before a moderate ascent on rock ledges south of the creek leads up to the wide, flat basin holding Lilypad Lake. Good campsites may be found in the trees near the edge of the meadows around the lake. You'll have to hike up to springs in the rocks above the lake to obtain running water, but firewood should be plentiful.

Lilypad Lake is aptly named—by midsummer you can barely see any water for the preponderance of lilies. Two-thirds of the shoreline around the 2-acre lake is lined with willow thickets, which makes it a less than spectacular recreational lake. However, the meadows around the lake along with the towering peaks and ridges on all sides are beautiful, and the near assurance of solitude is an attraction as well.

Faint tread continues through the meadow south of Lilypad Lake and up the steep ledges beyond to the

Mt. Shasta and Ycatapom Peak

terraces below Thumb Rock. The sky is caught here in a series of pristine little ponds set in the greenest of plush meadows. A junction above the terraces provides options of continuing over the ridge to Deer Flat, or around behind Thumb Rock and back up the Poison Canyon Trail above Cub Wallow, traveling through some of the most remote country reached by trail in the eastern Trinity Alps (see Trip 11, page 111).

Off-Trail to Found and Tapie Lakes

To explore off-trail to Found and Tapie Lake, you first have to return to the crest between Poison Canyon and Boulder Lake. From there, drop down north on the Tracy Trail about 200 yards to the top of the switchbacks, which is the best place to begin the off-trail route to Found Lake, reposing in the high, isolated basin behind the granite hulk of Peak 7435 to the west. Leaving the trail, dip down west into a delightful, flower-filled vale near the head of one of Boulder Lake's inlet streams. Cross over the stream where brush permits and then head northwest over glacier-sculpted rock to the edge of talus slopes below the vertical faces on the east side of the tor. Keep as high as feasible below the cliffs to avoid the dense brush tangles and crevices between blocks of broken rock on the slopes below.

As you traverse farther northwest around Peak 7435, Tapie Lake springs into view in a cleft above Boulder Lake. A deep gully, floored with broken rock, runs down from the north side of the peak to a pocket south of Tapie Lake. Cross this gully as close the top as feasible: The going may be rough over large talus blocks. Northwest of the top of the gulch, you enter a light forest of lodgepole pines and mountain hemlocks on the rocky floor of an open basin.

Found Lake is less than a quarter mile straight ahead, but remains out of sight until you practically step into the water, due to some intervening rock ledges. Chances are, the first lake you encounter won't be Found Lake, but a shallower, unnamed twin. Found Lake sits at the head of a basin with a rocky western shoreline that rises steeply away from the water toward the crest of the ridge above. The twin pond, 0.1 mile southwest, is shallower and is surrounded by gentler terrain.

Solitude abounds at Found Lake and the surrounding scenery is quite majestic. Swimmers and sunbathers should find the granite ledges around the lake very pleasing. Peakbaggers can scramble up Peak 7435 for additional exercise and a wide-ranging view. A quarter mile beyond Found Lake, the rocks drop away steeply, where a view opens up across the wide abyss of upper Boulder Creek canyon to the niche containing Conway and Lion lakes. Anglers will have to scramble down to Tapie Lake to fish, as Found Lake has plenty of frogs but no fish. Many excellent campsites occupy pockets of soil between the rocks and plenty of firewood should be available. Found Lake has no permanent inlet or outlet, so the lake will be the only source of water after snowmelt.

The best route down to Tapie Lake is down the nose of a spur ridge just northwest of the big gully you crossed on the way to Found Lake. Don't wander too far right (south). The scramble down is not too difficult, generally northeast back and forth over bare ledges, ending at the south shore of Tapie Lake.

Eons ago, a glacier plowed a trough through weaker rock on the steep face southwest of Boulder Lake, and Tapie Lake nowadays fills part of that trough. The lake drains

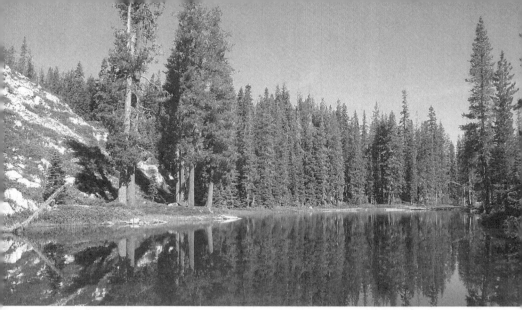

Tapie Lake

out the north end, but the south end is also open and only a few feet higher. A small lily pond in a meadow at the south end is barely separated from the lake. Thick fir forest lines the west shore, and brush covers the outlet, which makes getting all the way around the lake a little difficult. A few openings offer good spots to fish for medium-sized eastern brook trout, as well as to provide access for swimming. There is one small, fair campsite above the south shore.

A very steep and rough descent is possible from the outlet of Tapie Lake directly to the west shore of Boulder Lake. However, a better alternative leads out of the south end of the trough, east down a gully, around a shoulder of bare granite, and then south across a shelf. Remain above the tops of two brush-filled ravines on the way to the maintained tread of the Tracy Trail in a strip of trees, 0.4 mile from Tapie Lake. From there, continue the descent to Boulder Lake.

The off-trail route to Found and Tapie lakes can easily be reversed.

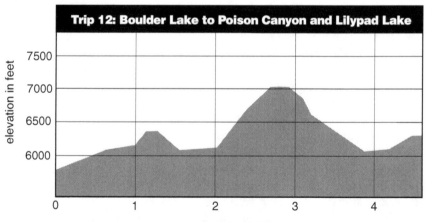

TRIP 13

Boulder, Lion, Foster, and Sugar Pine Lakes

The pass above Lion Lake offers perhaps the best view of Mt. Shasta you'll find in the Trinity Alps.

Trip Type:	Backpack, 3–5 days
Distance:	21 miles, point-to-point
	(plus 1.5-mile side trip to Little Boulder Lake)
Elevation Change:	11,200 feet, average 498 per mile
Difficulty:	Difficult
Season:	Late July to mid-September
Maps:	USGS *Ycatapom Peak*
	and USFS *A Guide to the Trinity Alps Wilderness*
Nearest Campground:	Goldfield

Anglers will love this trip—at least when they're fishing. When they're toiling up the last, brutally steep, crumbling half mile of trail to the crest above Battle Creek, however, they may feel differently. Although the trip starts high and ends low, as any ideal trip should, this excursion through the eastern Trinity Alps is quite strenuous, with hardly a flat spot in the entire 21 miles. However, the benefits include a string of four outstandingly beautiful lakes, each with their own particular charm. Adding in tiny Conway Lake and a short side trip to Boulder Lake brings the total of lakes to an even half dozen—all of them with excellent fishing.

In addition to the great fishing, you'll have a good look at most of the high country between Coffee and Swift creeks. While you're apt to see other people on this trip, the crowds drop off considerably past the Boulder Lakes—havens for both dayhikers and weekend backpackers. The basin at the upper end of Battle Creek sees few visitors, mainly cows and cowboys.

Two vehicles are necessary for this trip (unless you can find someone to pick you up and drop you off). Hitchhiking the 18 miles between the two trailheads is not practical. Of course, you could do an out-and-back trip from either trailhead, eliminating the climb to upper Battle Creek, but missing such a scenic wonder would be a real shame. If you want to shorten the trip by 7 miles and two sets of ridges, there's a 1.5-mile off-trail shortcut over the ridge between Lion and Sugar Pine lakes.

Starting Point

The road to the Boulder Lakes trailhead turns off Highway 3 less than a half mile south of the junction of the Coffee Creek Road, 40 miles north of Weaverville. Increased logging activity in the area requires that you drive these roads with

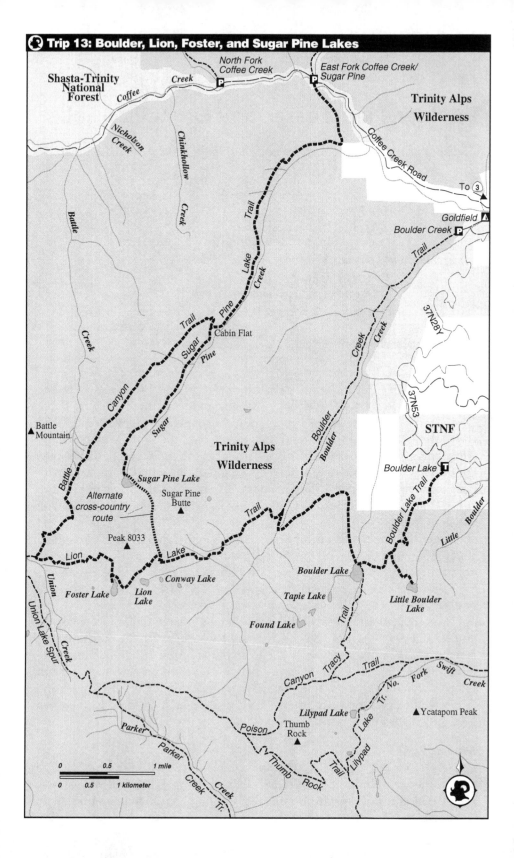

extreme caution. Signs would normally assist you in reaching the trailhead, but vandals seem to covet such signs in this area. Proceed on Forest Road 37N52 for 3.3 miles to a junction along a curve. Turn right here onto Forest Road 37N53 and travel another 1.1 miles to a Y-junction and bear left. From this point the main road is obvious, leading to the trailhead at the site of an old log landing on the top of a ridge between Little Boulder and Boulder creeks, 10.2 miles from Highway 3. The large landing has enough parking for a fleet of vehicles.

Ending Point

From Highway 3, about 40 miles north of Weaverville and immediately past the Coffee Creek bridge, turn west on Coffee Creek Road. The Coffee Creek ranger station is 300 yards down the first road to the right after you turn off the highway. Continue on well-graded road past Goldfield Campground and the Boulder Creek trailhead to the East Fork Coffee Creek/Sugar Pine trailhead on the right, 7.3 miles from Highway 3. Park your vehicle on the side of the road as space allows. Goldfield is a pleasant, no-fee campground with six sites and no running water next to Coffee Creek. The developed campgrounds around Trinity Lake and on up Trinity River have piped water and offer more refined car camping opportunities.

Description

Good tread runs southwest from the Boulder Lakes trailhead east of the top of a ridge, as you ascend moderately, with a few steeper pitches, through dense, predominantly white fir forest. Although the first 300 yards passes through a previously logged area, selective logging practices have made the logging barely noticeable. After a switchback you climb steeply back northwest, level off on the brow of the ridge, and then contour southwest to a junction with the spur to Little Boulder Lake turning east.

Side Trip to Little Boulder Lake

Little Boulder Lake is 300 feet higher than Boulder Lake, hung in a steep-sided pocket on the north side of Peak 6994. From the signed junction, climb at a moderately steep grade southeast for a quarter mile, and then straight up the nose of a ridge for 200 yards before crossing over and dropping to Little Boulder Lake, 0.4 mile from the junction.

Boulder Creek originates in the 4.5-acre lake and runs out the open north side of the basin and down into a very steep canyon below. The outlet usually dries up by midsummer. A low dam at the outlet used to raise the level of the lake, more than likely detaining water for downstream mining activities. Lush forest surrounds all but the south shore of the lake, where solid granite rises out of the water fairly steeply up to Peak 6994 above.

Although Little Boulder and Boulder lakes are only 0.6 mile apart, the smaller basin holding Little Boulder Lake has a colder microclimate, supporting a quite different range of vegetation. Lodgepole pines and red firs grow above pinemat manzanita and Labrador tea in the basin of Little Boulder, compared with white firs, sugar pines, bigleaf manzanita, and ceanothus brush around the larger lake.

Eastern brook trout to 10 inches swim lazily along the shoreline looking for something to eat. Camping is limited to a handful of poor to fair sites around the northeast shore and one fair site at the west end. Swimmers will find that the water temperature stays chilly throughout the summer.

Below the Little Boulder Lake junction, the trail switchbacks down a brushy, rock-strewn hillside, then turns west across the large basin holding Boulder Lake. At 2 miles from the trailhead, beside a large campsite near the lower end of the lake, you reach a three-way junction with a trail that turns south around the east shore and then climbs over a ridge to Poison Canyon.

Boulder is a medium-sized green lake—8 acres of algae-tinted water with a ring of lily pads extending about 100 feet from a mostly grass-covered shoreline. A wet meadow borders the upper (south) end of the 27-foot-deep lake, and dense forest lines the grass and willows around the rest of the shoreline. A craggy granite peak is the prominent feature of the glaciated ridge to the south.

A number of fair campsites, some quite large, nestle beneath the trees around the lower end of the lake. Other excellent sites occupy a bench 300 to 400 yards above the east shore. A pair of good sites is near where the Poison Canyon Trail crosses the inlet. Thanks to the lake's popularity, firewood is a bit scarce. In spite the drawbacks presented by swarms of mosquitoes in early summer and too many neighbors on weekends, Boulder Lake is a pleasant place to spend a day or two. The scenery is beautiful! Fishing is challenging around much of the tree-rimmed shoreline, but the evening rise off the logjam near the outlet may produce a fair catch of 8–9 inch eastern brook trout. Wading the muddy bottom near the inlet streams can also be fruitful, provided you don't get hung up on the lily pads; swimming off the rocks on the west side can be quite refreshing by August.

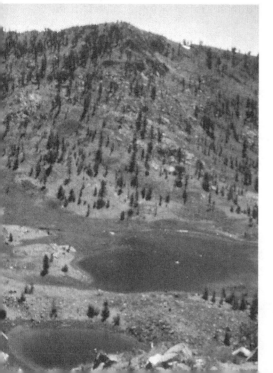

Boulder Lakes

From the three-way junction near the lower end of Boulder Lake, you follow the trail north toward Lion Lake, which is 5 miles distant and 900 vertical feet higher (you descend 800 feet into Boulder Creek canyon on the way). Sections of those 5 miles are very steep, but most of the scenery is fantastic. The trail crosses the west bank of the outlet in a gully below the lake, and then contours around the point of the ridge between Boulder Lake's outlet and the main branch of Boulder Creek. Once around the ridge you contour southwest along the wall of Boulder Creek canyon, and then start a protracted descent toward Boulder Creek. Beyond a short switchback, a break in the forest reveals the first view of the white granite wall behind Conway and Lion lakes far above. Eventually you reach the bottom of Boulder Creek canyon, 2 miles from Boulder Lake.

Traverse the floor of the canyon through a small alder thicket and across a thin strip of meadow, where 6-foot delphiniums and monkshoods bloom through midsummer. Boulder hop willow- and alder-lined Boulder Creek, which probably harbors trout but whose thick brush makes fishing virtually impossible. A use trail branching left on the west bank leads to a couple of good campsites above the creek. Continue another 0.2 mile from the creek, where the trail turns north and comes to a junction with the Lion Lake Trail on the left and the Boulder Creek Trail on the right.

Turn southwest on the Lion Lake Trail and begin a steep, zigzagging ascent on rough and washed-out tread up the side of the canyon. Beyond a small rivulet flowing across the trail, 0.5 mile from the junction, the grade eases to merely moderate along a shelf far above Boulder Creek. Directly across the canyon, a sizable amount of bare granite rises up to the basin containing Found Lake and Peak 7435 on the horizon south of the Boulder Lake basin. Farther south, Boulder Creek spills out of a basin named Cub Wallow, tucked under the crest of the divide between this drainage and Parker Creek. Climbing higher, the trail traverses a series of benches with steep pitches between them. Patches of thick forest composed of red firs, Jeffrey pines, and incense cedars alternate with pockets of flower-filled meadows and alder thickets hiding tiny creeks. Pipsissewas, twinflowers, and mahonia grow beneath the trees, while mint, phlox, wild hollyhock, angelica, paintbrush, owl's clover, and sulfur flowers carpet the meadows.

The flower gardens end around 1.5 miles from the junction, as you turn north to climb very steep zigzags, crossing a tiny creek twice within a quarter mile before turning southwest again across the side of the canyon. The ascent eventually eases a little as you pass through meadows and patches of brush. Enter a dense stand of red firs and reach a junction with a path heading south toward Conway Lake, 4.7 miles from Boulder Lake.

Side Trip to Conway Lake and Lion Lake

Leaving maintained trail to Foster Lake, turn onto the path toward Conway Lake, soon breaking out of the trees and into the upper fringe of a large, beautiful wet meadow that gracefully sweeps down to diminutive, lily pad–covered Conway Lake. The lake is tucked into a rocky shelf above the wide chasm of Boulder Creek canyon. West of the meadow and the lake, a tiny stream falls through a slot in a sloping wall cut into the glacier-sculpted granite. There are a few poor campsites in the edge of the trees at the top of the meadow, but the rocks east of Conway Lake have better sites. Firewood is extremely scarce. Small eastern brook trout hide beneath the lily pads at Conway Lake; more may be found in the small creek running through the meadow below the lake, but fishing is obviously difficult in both spots.

The easy off-trail route to Lion Lake begins across the creek at the bottom of the slot in the granite wall: Pass around the first hump on the south side, and then climb west up a gully to the top of the dike east of the lake. There is one small campsite on top of this dike, but firewood is nonexistent.

Filling a cup gouged out of solid granite by a glacier, Lion is the quintessential subalpine lake. The 3-acre lake is vaguely heart-shaped, deep blue, and quite deep (37 feet). Sheer walls of rock rise almost directly from the water's edge on three sides. Even on the lower east side the shoreline is steep, with the slot cut through the dike by the outlet as the only exception. A large slide has almost filled in the north side of the lake with broken rock. The remainder of the lake drops off very steeply from the shoreline. Only a few red firs, mountain hemlocks, and patches of low brush have found a foothold in the rock walls.

From the junction to Conway Lake, continue west a short distance to switchbacks climbing steeply north through large red firs for a quarter mile before traversing the mountain above Lion Lake. The lake is directly below, providing a good view of the mass of broken rock filling the depths almost to the surface on the north side. A generally moderate ascent southwest, with some ups and downs, leads to a final short switchback to the crest of Peak 8033's south ridge, which separates the basins of Lion and Foster lakes. Before you continue, ascend one of the large granite blocks on this crest and enjoy the view back down Boulder Creek and up and away to snow-cloaked Mt. Shasta.

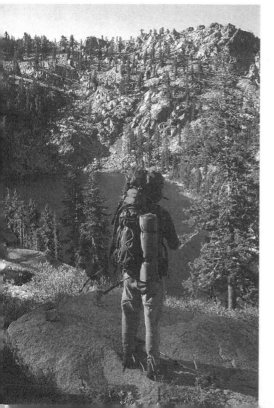

Foster Lake from the trail

Beyond a series of short-legged switchbacks, rough trail turns slightly west of north and descends moderately across granite ledges and around large blocks of talus. From a point where you can see down Union Creek to the northwest, the trail turns and drops to a junction on a shelf north of the lake. Turn left (south) at the junction and continue 200 yards, crossing the outlet on the way, to the northwest shore of Foster Lake. There are excellent campsites scattered around the outlet, one of which has an old Forest Service stove beneath a grove of mountain hemlocks. The rocks to the west hold a few more fair campsites. Firewood is not particularly plentiful.

At 7250 feet, subalpine Foster Lake is one of the higher lakes in the Trinity Alps, with snow lingering on the north-facing wall of the basin well into August in some years. On most evenings a vivid sunset floods the cliffs above the east shore—grandstand seats are on ledges beyond two exquisite seasonal ponds southwest of the outlet's camping area. Still evenings provide a double feature—one on the basin wall and the other reflected on the lake's surface. Anglers should have some success catching 8- to 9-inch eastern brook trout near the logjam by the outlet, or from drop-offs along the rocky east shore. Foster Lake's exposed perch allows the wind to blow furiously at times, the only flaw in this otherwise delightful spot.

Foster Lake or Bear Lake?

Old-time Trinity Alps hikers once referred to this 5.5-acre lake as Bear Lake, not Foster Lake. However, since the Alps already boast a Big Bear Lake and a Little Bear Lake, the name Foster *is likely the name that will stick for the foreseeable future. Besides, the Fosters were very prominent pioneers in the area.*

When your time at Foster Lake comes to an end, retrace your steps the short distance from Foster Lake to the junction on the shelf to the south of the lake.

Off-Trail Route to Sugar Pine Lake

From the junction north of Foster Lake, retrace your steps on the Lion Lake Trail to the ridge between Foster and Lion lakes and then down to the top of the first set of switchbacks above Lion Lake. Leave the maintained trail here and head north cross-country toward a gap in the ridgeline above, between Peak 8033 on the left and Sugar Pine Butte on the right. After crossing the ridge, keep to the east side of the cirque holding Sugar Pine Lake and work your way downslope to the east side of the lake. While the route is steep up to the ridge and even steeper down to the lake, the total distance is a mere 1.4 miles, compared to 8.5 miles by trail.

After pausing at the junction north of Foster Lake to admire the view across the wide, lush upper basin of Union Creek, descend a moderately steep set of switchbacks northwest through boulders and brush. Below a steep pitch straight west down the side of the canyon, you traverse northwest into a belt of firs, and then down again along the south edge of a large, beautiful meadow. Away from the meadow, the steep zigzags resume northwest through head-high ceanothus and other brush to an alder-lined dell, where a copious, ice-cold spring cascades across the trail—you'll be hard-pressed to find a finer source of pure, clear water anywhere. Beyond the spring, you soon come out onto the open floor of Union Creek valley and reach a junction with the Battle Canyon Trail 8W07, 1.5 miles from the junction near Foster Lake.

Options to Union and Landers Lakes

If you have some extra time, Union Lake is a little more than a mile away by trail: Follow the Lion Lake Trail west from the Battle Canyon Trail junction, crossing Union Creek on the way to a junction with the Union Lake Spur, and then around a shoulder of a ridge to join the Union Lake Trail, which runs up a side canyon to Union Lake. A full description of the lake can be found in Trip 15 (see page 147).

Landers Lake is almost 3 miles away by trail: From the junction with the Union Lake Spur, head southeast on the spur trail to a junction with the Landers Lake Trail, head west and south to the Landers Lake Spur, and then proceed generally west to the lake. A full description of the lake can be found in Trip 11 (see page 111). There are many excellent campsites with an adequate supply of firewood along Union Creek above and below the Lion Lake Trail crossing. Unfortunately for anglers, the creek is a little too small at this point to fish.

From the Lion Lake Trail junction, a row of ducks marks the faint tread of the Battle Canyon Trail heading north across a meadow. Beyond the meadow, you immediately start climbing east via short, steep switchbacks through an open forest of firs and incense cedars, and patches of meadow. A half mile from the junction, you turn northeast across a brushy hillside, and then east up into the lower end of a steeply sloping meadow that extends all the way up the mountain. Ducks help guide you across the bottom of the meadow and over a little stream, before the trail ascends steeply northeast along the southeast edge of the meadow beside the stream.

Farther up, you weave in and out of majestic fir forest and meadow, sometimes beside the tiny creek, where both white and purple monkshoods bloom, along with several varieties of orchids. The trail crosses the little stream, almost at the source, and then zigzags very steeply up the open face of the mountain before heading back into open forest, about a mile from the Lion Lake Trail junction. The trail soon bends north across the upper end of the long meadow. Midway along this traverse, you gaze straight down a gully and rockslide all the way to Union Creek. A switchback on an open slope north of the top of the meadow leads to a saddle at the crest, 1.5 miles from the Lion Lake Trail junction.

A wide panorama to the south and west rewards your climb to the crest. Caribou Mountain looms on the western skyline, along with the high Alps above the head of Stuart Fork, including the Alp's highest summit, Thompson Peak. Ragged ridges farther south lead up to Siligo, Seven Up, and Gibson peaks. In the middle distance, beyond the wide upper basin of Union Creek, Red Rock Mountain stands out above the basin holding Landers Lake. On the opposite side of the crest is the verdant basin at the head of Battle Creek, where a row of rugged knobs and pinnacles runs along the east side of the divide separating Battle and Sugar Pine creeks.

From the saddle, the trail drops very steeply down the canyon's headwall, then turns north to contour along the east slope below the knobs and pinnacles. About one-third mile from the saddle, a spring waters a garden filled with angelica, delphinium, monkshood, corn lily, sneezeweed, lupine, yarrow, yampa, paintbrush, and other flowers. Below the trail the hillside is covered with wild onion. Beyond another, larger spring bursting forth from the hillside above the trail, you traverse a steep slope aromatic with angelica, mint, and lupine. Farther on the tread becomes indistinct—look for ducks pointing the way east uphill. You snake very steeply up to what appears to be the crest, only to find you're on a spur of the main ridge, which requires you to traverse north on a moderate climb before a final steep rise leads to a saddle on the top of the ridge, a mile from the Union Creek crest.

Gnarled foxtail pines cling to cracks in the rugged rocks along this summit, adding foreground interest, while the more distant views are quite fantastic. On the west side you look down Battle Creek canyon to Coffee Creek, and then up to the Scott Mountain crest. On the Sugar Pine Creek side, Mount Shasta crowns the horizon beyond a series of ridges, and jagged Sugar Pine Buttes face you across the canyon.

After a short, steep drop from the crest, the trail makes a long traverse a little east of north along the side of the canyon. This section of trail is not for acrophobes—the slope is so steep that you look nearly straight down to the floor of the canyon, where the Sugar Pine Lake Trail runs across a small, deep green meadow. Beyond a switchback, about 0.6 mile from the crest, the descent becomes steeper, passing through patches of manzanita. In a grove of firs, you turn back southeast and descend to a bench. Headed northeast again, cross a delightful creek on the bench, a mile from the crest. You continue the moderate descent northeast for another mile through meadows and groves of conifers, and then begin a series of moderately steep switchbacks east down to the floor of the canyon. The trail becomes embedded in a network of cattle tracks, as you cross the wide meadow named Cabin Flat on the way to a junction with the more clearly defined Sugar Pine Lake Trail. Signs attached to the stub of a large snag provide directions at this indistinct junction.

Although your next destination is obviously upstream to the southwest, the Sugar Pine Lake Trail is hard to follow as you enter forest south of Cabin Flat. The trail runs well away from the creek, near the west side of the canyon. If you happen to find yourself on an old trail, confused by a maze of cattle tracks and piles or rocks, you'll have a tough time negotiating deadfalls and washouts. On the other side of a strip of trees, you cross another wide meadow, enter forest again, and draw near to alder-choked Sugar Pine Creek, 1 mile from the Battle Canyon Trail junction in Cabin Flat.

A gradual to moderate climb through more forest leads to the little meadow you previously looked straight down at from the top of the west ridge above. A quarter mile of gently graded tread winds through large red firs south of the little meadow, before a moderate climb through jumbled granite boulders and over a moraine leads to Sugar Pine Lake, 1.8 miles from the junction in Cabin Flat.

Jagged pinnacles cap the high walls around the lake's cirque. Except for a talus slide running into the water on the southwest side, trees line the shoreline of the 8-acre lake. However, only a few of those conifers happen to be sugar pines, belying the lake's name. Several good campsites occupy a relatively flat area east of the outlet. Since Sugar Pine Lake sees few visitors and trees surround the lake, firewood should be readily available. Fishing is good for small eastern brook trout.

When your visit to Sugar Pine Lake comes to an end, retrace your steps 1.8 miles to the junction with the Battle Canyon Trail at Cabin Flat. From there, head northwest down the canyon along the Sugar Pine Lake Trail, descending gradually to the lower edge of the meadow, and then more steeply on zigzagging tread down a rocky hillside in open forest. After 0.6 mile, you skirt the edge of a steep-sided ravine with Sugar Pine Creek at the bottom and, 0.2 mile farther, drop down a steep, gullied pitch to a small tributary flowing from the west side of the canyon.

The trail crosses a bench on a moderate descent, and then drops more steeply on better tread through dense, lush forest. Some tall sugar pines line the trail here before you begin another steep descent to an alder-tangled tributary. You traverse far up the side of a V-cut canyon, and then cross a trio of side streams before a steeper descent leads down the side of the canyon through a thicket of willows, dogwoods, alders, vine maples, and bigleaf maples. Beyond one more tributary crossing, you pass through a gate in a drift fence, remembering to close the gate behind you, and then contour back into a ravine, crossing yet another tributary along the way.

The trail remains well up the side of the canyon away from the creek, descending at mostly a moderate grade. Black oaks and ponderosa pines join the mixed forest below a lone switchback, with madrones and blue-flowering ceanothus present for the final mile. You finally near Sugar Pine Creek again, just before reaching the East Fork Coffee Creek/Sugar Pine trailhead, 4.2 miles from the junction at Cabin Flat.

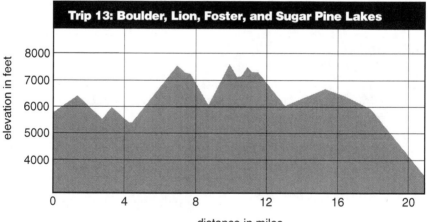

TRIP 14

North Fork to East Fork Coffee Creek Loop

And the lakes—oh, what lakes!

Trip Type:	Backpack, 3–7 days
Distance:	27.5 miles, loop (1 mile between trailheads, plus side trip to South Fork Lakes)
Elevation Change:	12,035 feet, average 438 per mile
Difficulty:	Moderate
Season:	Mid-July to mid-October
Maps:	USGS *Ycatapom Peak*, *Billys Peak*, and *Deadman Peak*; USFS *A Guide to the Trinity Alps Wilderness*
Nearest Campgrounds:	Goldfield and Big Flat

From busy, dusty Coffee Creek Road to a seldom-used 2.6-mile sample of the Pacific Crest Trail on the Scott River Divide, this trip offers a series of contrasts. Several miles of steep, badly worn trail are balanced by pleasant, level strolls through idyllic meadows. Brushy hillsides and mixed low-elevation forest near Coffee Creek give way to subalpine vistas alternating with forests of giant red firs along the ridge between Granite and Doe lakes. However, the lakes are the real draw on this trip, ranging from large, heavily used Stoddard (at 5900 feet the destination of trail rides from Coffee Creek Ranch), to tiny, remote Section Line in a 7000-foot-plus cirque, where you might not see another party for a whole week or two.

This trip doesn't pass through the highest and most rugged part of the Trinity Alps, nonetheless the countryside is both very pleasant and quite interesting. The journey includes a fair cross-section of the country north of Coffee Creek up to the Scott River Divide, where fishing is good to excellent most of the way, including angling for golden trout in Salmon Creek and the upper reaches of the North Fork. Some of the trail is heavily used, but there remains plenty of opportunity for solitude in the higher part of the loop. Mining relics are common in much of the area and miners still work a few of the claims. Until the mid-1930s, a small town endured along the North Fork between Lick and Granite creeks. Fortunately, the Forest Service has acquired a private inholding at Hodges Cabin, and now all of the area is part of the Trinity Alps Wilderness.

Starting Point
From Highway 3, about 40 miles north of Weaverville and immediately past the Coffee Creek bridge, turn west on Coffee Creek Road. The Coffee Creek ranger station is 300 yards down the first road to the right after you turn off the

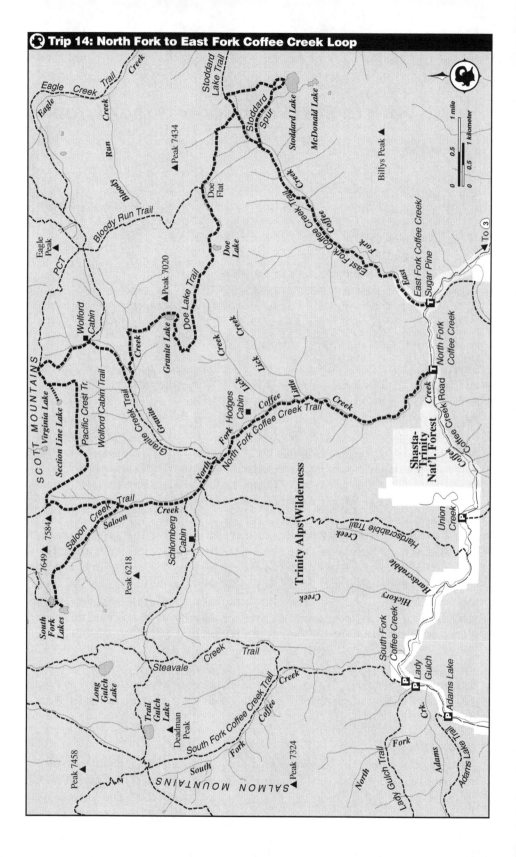

highway. Continue on well-graded road past Goldfield Campground and the Boulder Creek trailhead to the East Fork Coffee Creek/Sugar Pine trailhead on the right, 7.3 miles from Highway 3. The North Fork trailhead is another mile up the Coffee Creek Road, just before the North Fork bridge. Park your vehicle on the side of the road as space allows at both trailheads. Unless you have a vehicle at both trailheads, or have arranged for pick-up and drop-off, you will have to walk along Coffee Creek Road the last mile between trailheads.

Goldfield is a pleasant, no-fee campground with six sites and no running water next to Coffee Creek. The Big Flat campground is small, primitive, and usually overcrowded on summer weekends. The developed campgrounds around Trinity Lake and on up Trinity River have piped water and offer more refined car camping opportunities.

Description

While both Coffee Creek and the North Fork look as though they should have an abundance of trout in their waters near the trailhead, anglers will have to work hard for a few small rainbows. Fishing should be much better a few miles up the North Fork.

You climb moderately to moderately steeply northwest on good tread for the first mile, well up the side of the steep and narrow North Fork canyon. The next half mile of trail contours almost level past an old cabin site and some fine campsites perched on ledges and benches, and then dips down to cross the North Fork on a steel-truss bridge. Just above the bridge, a large, excellent campsite is on a flat beside the creek, immediately beyond a tributary cascading down the west side of the canyon.

A marvelous, wide valley, wooded with Douglas firs, ponderosa pines, and incense cedars, extends 1.7 miles from the bridge to Hodges Cabin. The stretch of creek alongside the trail is a fly-fishing angler's dream—a positively beautiful stream, flowing swiftly over a wide, open bed of gravel and rocks, with long riffles, deep pools, and plenty of room for casting. More importantly, the creek has trout—nice, fat rainbows, plus a few golden trout and some hybrids.

On excellent tread, you ascend gradually, not very far up the west slope, except for one stretch where the trail switchbacks to climb over a rock shoulder. At 3.2 miles from the trailhead, you stand across the creek from Hodges Cabin.

Hodges Cabin

Hodges Cabin is a large, two-story rustic structure built in the 1920s. The U.S. Forest Service acquired the property, including the cabin, horse barn, corral, and outbuildings, in 1987. The site once boasted a hydroelectric plant and an extensive water system. Jockey Billy Pearson (1920–2002), who rode during the '40s and '50s, and was a famous quiz show contestant, art dealer, and bit-part actor, owned the complex at one time. The cabin has been proposed as a future wilderness hostel.

The trail continues rising gradually away from Hodges Cabin, on the west side of a wide, flat valley, which shows abundant evidence of past mining activity. Fortunately, no current claims are active along this stretch of the North Fork. A little over a mile from the cabin, and 4.5 miles from the trailhead, the trail bends to cross another steel-truss bridge over the North Fork to the northeast side, a short distance above the confluence of Granite Creek. Reach a junction with the Granite Creek Trail branching right from a flat, 150 yards from the bridge. You could cut 5 to 6 miles from the trip, along with some steep ups and downs, by turning up the Granite Creek Trail to Granite Lake, but by doing so you would miss out on some marvelous scenery up on the crest. A number of excellent campsites lie between the trail and the North Fork beyond the junction.

Continue up the northeast side of the North Fork on excellent tread, climbing gradually, then a little more steeply, as the valley narrows on the way to the confluence of Saloon Creek, 0.6 mile from the junction. Boulder hop or wade across Saloon Creek near the edge of a small meadow, and then follow a rocky spit between the two creeks. As you start climbing up a spur ridge, take the time to gaze down on a sometimes-occupied miner's cabin positioned on a flat next to Saloon Creek. The narrow structure with stucco walls seems unique in the Trinity Alps backcountry. Reach a junction with the Saloon Creek Trail on a small bench, 0.3 mile from the crossing of Saloon Creek. The North Fork Coffee Creek Trail continues west to Schlomberg Cabin and then climbs to the Salmon River crest above Long Gulch.

Turning onto the Saloon Creek Trail, you rise moderately through open fir forest past an unsigned leg of the trail to Schlomberg Cabin. The moderate ascent continues for a half mile on a series of benches crisscrossed by cattle trails, before a gradual descent leads to a crossing of the creek. A fine campsite occupies a flat on the west bank just before you cross the creek on a large deadfall. Proceed a short distance to the crossing of the East Fork and a junction with the East Fork Saloon Creek Trail. An excellent campsite on a small flat between the forks of the creek will tempt overnighters. Small trout below the forks sometimes rise to flies.

Side Trip to South Fork Lakes
Lower and Upper South Fork Lakes are just over the crest beyond the head of Saloon Creek, 2.3 trail miles and a 1250-foot climb away. The South Fork Lakes represent the source of South Fork Scott River, flowing north, east of the ridge dividing the Salmon River and Scott River drainages. Little South Fork Lake, not to be confused with these lakes, is the source of Little South Fork Salmon River, and is west of Caribou Basin, 17 air miles southwest.

Along the first half mile of the East Fork Saloon Creek Trail, you rise gently on good, lightly used tread through shady, thick forest. Beyond this forested segment, you climb more steeply on rough, stony tread up a dry creek bed and over wooded benches, where a few fair campsites can be found between the trail and the creek. After a mile, reach a quarter-mile-long meadow, frequently overgrazed and trod to dust by the hooves of cat-

tle by late summer. Look for ducks leading north uphill away from the creek across the meadow before more distinct tread reappears where the trail heads back into the trees.

Patches of shorn meadow with ducks alternates with belts of trees, as the trail climbs higher to another, larger meadow, where the trail runs to the right of, then in, a small, dry stream bed headed generally northwest. At the floor of the steepest part of the ridge, ducks lead you into thick forest, where an obvious, blazed trail climbs to the north. After 0.3 mile of very steep climbing with occasional zigzags, the grade eases for a short distance, before the climb resumes west on the north side of the ridge, Pass around a hump, then descend steeply for 200 yards, before climbing again over another hump of slate and metamorphosed sandstone. The next short downhill leads out onto the floor of the valley holding the South Fork Lakes. Lower South Fork Lake is 150 yards north of where the trail branches in many directions beneath dense timber. Upper South Fork Lake is a quarter mile south through dense firs and hemlocks.

The 4.5-acre lower lake is shallow and set in a ring of lush grass backed by tall firs and hemlocks at the lower end of a hanging valley. The outlet stream falls over an escarpment a few yards from the lake and brilliant wildflowers carpet the meadows bordering the shoreline. Lower South Fork Lake offers excellent swimming and camping opportunities, with ample firewood beneath the trees beyond the south shore.

Upper South Fork Lake at 6.5 acres is set in a cirque with cliffs rimming the south and west sides. Excellent campsites above the northeast shore will surely lure backpackers to an extended stay. Small eastern brook trout rise in the evening to almost anything that touches the surface of the water. All in all, the South Fork Lakes basin is a fine place for a one- or two-day layover. Although the lakes can be accessed by 2.5 miles of trail from Carter Summit on Forest Highway 93, travel is light in this remote section of the Alps, ensuring that your visit to South Fork Lakes is relatively uncrowded.

From the East Fork Saloon Creek Trail junction, you break out of the trees and climb on a steep to very steep grade through manzanita and huckleberry oak on rough, washed-out tread. After a mile, the trail tops out momentarily on the nose of a ridge between the forks of Saloon Creek, and then continues steeply north through red-fir forest and out onto open slopes. An abundance of cattle trails may confuse the route through here—if so, stay 200 to 300 yards west of the little creek and climb toward a point just west of the lowest notch in the skyline. Near the crest, you may notice traces of an old road that lead to the gap and a junction with the much-better-defined tread of the Pacific Crest Trail. As late as the 1930s, a road led from the town of Callahan through this pass and down to the settlement around Hodges Cabin on the North Fork.

After the route up to the crest on the indistinct tread of the upper section of the Saloon Creek Trail, the PCT appears like a freeway. Turn southeast and follow the PCT through open red-fir forest and around a shoulder of Peak 7649. A mile of almost level, smooth, 3-foot-wide tread leads to the southeast side of the peak and a welcome break where an icy spring flows across the trail from the cut bank on the uphill side. From there, the trail ascends moderately past more seeps and springs, then turns to contour east well below the Scott River crest. A mile from the spring, you climb slightly around a rocky, manzanita-covered shoulder offering wide views across Granite Creek, North Fork, and Coffee Creek canyons. At 2.3 miles from the Saloon Creek junction, the trail turns east again on top of the crest. Just where you can see over the north side of the narrow crest, a rock cairn marks the spot where a use trail drops down the north slope, bound for Section Line Lake.

Off-Trail to Section Line Lake

From a cairn on the PCT, a rough use trail drops steeply northwest down the north slope and then disappears after about 200 yards, from where Section Line Lake is still 0.3 mile southwest. The way forward is a little rough and rocky through open forest and across some humps and gullies. The most direct route to the lake stays above (south of) an area of large talus blocks.

Section Line is a gorgeous little lake between 2 and 3 acres, set in a cirque right under the Scott River crest. A white granite talus slope falls directly into the south side of the lake, and red firs, mountain hemlocks, and a few western white pines surround the rest of the shoreline. By late summer the water level falls below the outlet, and the water temperature rises almost to a comfortable level for swimming. However, access to the water is somewhat difficult due to the broken rock and deadfalls around the shoreline. The only established campsite is much too close to the northwest shore, but there is plenty of room for a tent farther back from the lake. Firewood is relatively abundant.

Somewhat surprisingly, rainbow trout outnumber eastern brook trout in this lake. The rainbows vary greatly in size, indicating that they are reproducing, although they normally spawn only in running water. Perhaps they spawn during snowmelt runoff, and both fry and adults return to the lake before the streams dry up. Anglers are not apt to catch any trophy fish, but the fishing should be fun and, with a little luck, perhaps it will be enough to eat.

The 0.3 mile from the use trail to Section Line Lake and the junction of the Wolford Cabin Trail is along classic Pacific Crest Trail tread—boulders have been moved at least 3 feet to the side of a minimum 2-foot-wide path that contours continually through an 8-foot-wide swath cut through the manzanita. From the junction, Mavis Lake can be seen below, sitting in a basin north of the

Wolford Cabin

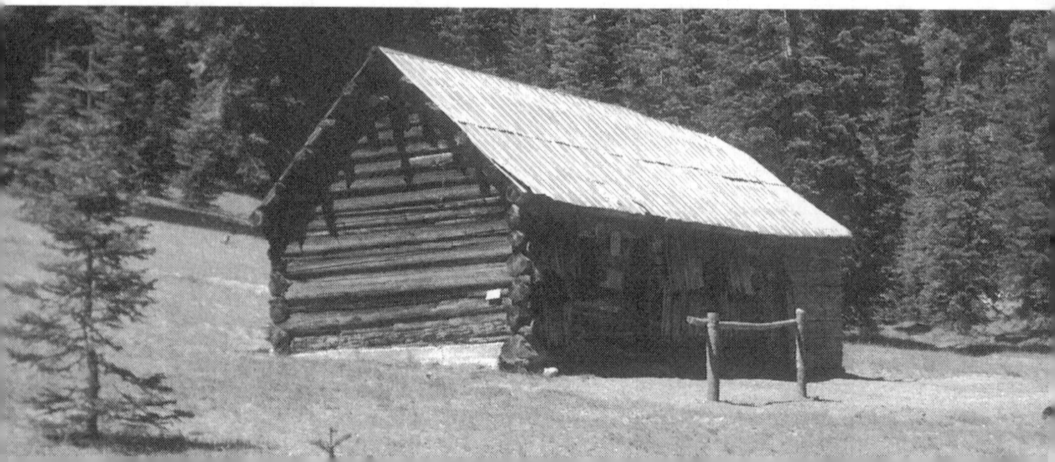

crest, while Fox Creek Lake is out of sight behind a spur ridge to the northwest. Much farther to the north is the broad expanse of Scott Valley. These two lakes and the trails to them from the Fox Creek Ridge trailhead, 4 miles away, are described in Trip 24 (see page 203).

Leaving the PCT, you turn down the Wolford Cabin Trail and drop steeply southwest out of sparse firs and hemlocks, and then zigzag down a steep, sandy, open slope partly covered with sagebrush, grasses, yellow bush daisies, and pinemat manzanita. At the upper fringe of red-fir forest, you turn southwest and, as you enter the trees, draw near a tiny creek, the first available running water since the spring near Peak 7649. As you continue southeast, a few switchbacks moderate the rate of descent. Near the bottom of Wolford Gulch, you turn a little more south, cross a small tributary, and enjoy a gradual 0.3-mile descent beside a cascading stream on the way to Wolford Cabin and a junction with the Granite Creek Trail, 1.2 miles from the PCT junction.

Wolford Cabin is a substantial log cabin in a relatively good condition with an aluminum roof. The cabin is still frequented by cattlemen and trail and snow-survey crews. Sitting in the center of a verdant forest glade, the cabin is unlocked and available for use if you are in sudden need of shelter. Please respect and preserve the historic nature of the cabin if you visit.

The section of the Granite Creek Trail heading southeast from the junction climbs 1.7 miles to the Eagle Creek divide and a junction with the Bloody Run and Eagle Creek trails (see Trip 20, page 179). Turning southwest, the Granite Creek Trail to Granite Creek and Granite Lake descends moderately to moderately steeply southwest, well up on the northwest side of Wolford Gulch, for 0.5 mile to a junction with the Doe Lake Trail.

Turning east on the Doe Lake Trail, you drop steeply into Wolford Gulch, cross the north branch of Granite Creek, and then follow a gradual ascent east above the creek. About 0.4 mile from the junction the trail veers south and crosses the main stem of Granite Creek. The first quarter mile from the crossing is nearly level through parklike forest and meadows. The rest of the mile to Granite Lake is on rough, moderately steep tread that snakes up brushy hillsides and crosses wooded benches. Rather than take a direct approach to the lake, the trail circles above the east and south shores.

This Granite Lake is sometimes referred to as "Little Granite Lake," since this body of water is not as large, or as glamorous, as the Granite Lake in the Swift Creek drainage. However, this lake has far fewer visitors than its more popular counterpart. At 6400 feet, the 6-acre, shallow lake has lily pads floating on the surface and grass growing on the ends of the water-soaked logs sticking out of the water. Thanks to the lily pads and the debris-covered bottom, swimming is less than ideal, but a good population of average-sized eastern brook trout makes for fine angling. Several fair campsites around the north and south sides seem adequate for the low number of campers who stay here overnight, but firewood is scarce.

From Granite Lake, switchbacks lead northwest to the top of a rocky spur west of the lake. Zigzag down the far side of the spur, then contour around the head of a small valley to the base of a very steep, switchbacking climb south to a saddle on a 7000-foot-plus, east-west trending ridge.

After the steep to very steep climb to the saddle, you can begin to enjoy the long traverse of the ridge. The first 300 yards rise gradually on top of the narrow crest; then you contour southeast around a granite peak. Once around the flanks of the peak, the trail continues climbing moderately east below the crest of the ridge through open red-fir forest and across slopes of granite and sand, decorated with bush daisies, sulfur flowers, and mints. A little more than a mile of gentle travel on good tread leads to a delightful dell with a sweet, clear spring, the only water on this side of the hill.

From the spring, you climb more steeply out onto a granite ledge with stupendous views across Coffee Creek canyon to the highest peaks of the Trinity Alps, including Sawtooth Mountain, Thompson Peak, and Caribou Mountain. The next half mile of trail ascends moderately at first, but ends with a 200-yard scramble up zigzags in broken granite to a saddle between two granite knobs overlooking Doe Lake basin. From here, you can now see Mt. Shasta on the northeast horizon and Castle Crags directly east. A few more steep zigzags take you down into a hanging valley; at the east and lower end of this valley you drop very steeply over a granite ledge, and then traverse east across a steep slope to the north shore of Doe Lake, 0.4 mile from the top of the ridge.

Doe Lake is a beautiful 4.5-acre subalpine lake in a steep-walled granite cirque beneath rugged Peak 7616 to the southwest. Fishing is good for eastern brook trout, but they don't seem to grow any larger than 8–9 inches. The water is warm enough for swimming in the shallower areas by mid-August. Campers should look for a few good campsites among the boulders above the northeast shore. Although the lake doesn't see a lot of traffic, firewood is scarce.

From Doe Lake you descend east down a wide valley littered with erratic granite boulders, first on the north side of the outlet stream and then crossing to the south side. At the lower end of the valley, you wander through a maze of alder thickets and meandering stream channels, where the trail is hard to follow in places until emerging into several acres of corn lilies at the upper end of half-mile-long Doe Flat. In the middle of the gently sloping flat, you pass the southern junction of the Bloody Run Trail, which runs north across a burnt-over ridge to connect with the Eagle Creek and Granite Creek trails near Eagle Peak. A mile of rough trail, steep in places, twists down a little south of east from Doe Flat to a well-signed junction with the East Fork Coffee Creek Trail. By heading northeast, you have access to the remnants of Stoddard Cabin, several excellent campsites, and a connection with the Stoddard Lake Trail to Stoddard Lake.

Side Trip to Stoddard Lake

Stoddard is a 25-acre deep blue lake that shares a wide, forested basin with much smaller McDonald Lake. Stoddard harbors a good population of small- to medium-sized eastern brook trout. A little mountaineering gets you up to delightful Little Stoddard Lake on a shelf gouged out of the side of Billys Peak. Plenty of good to excellent campsites spread throughout the basin offer options for spending a night or two.

If all this sounds idyllic, there are a few drawbacks—namely an abundance of four-legged cows and horses, two-legged humans, and winged mosquitoes. A large herd of cattle often grazes in this area most summers, and Coffee Creek Ranch runs a trail ride to the lake with some regularity. Logging roads have pushed the trailhead to within 3 miles of the lake, making this a fairly easy destination for dayhikers, anglers, and tourists. With an elevation below 6000 feet and a significant marshy area between Stoddard and McDonald lakes, conditions are prime for the production of clouds of mosquitoes through July. In spite of all these drawbacks, the basin remains a fine place to visit.

Although two trails provide access to Stoddard Lake from the East Fork Coffee Creek Trail, you'll probably prefer the northern route from Stoddard Cabin, as this trail sees much less horse traffic. From the junction near the tumbled logs of the old cabin, turn south to cross, within 200 yards, two small streams that are the beginning of the East Fork. Continue south across a lush flat, and then climb moderately through open grass-floored woods. The trail skirts some brushy patches higher up the hill and then tops out on a rim overlooking Stoddard Lake, 1 mile from the junction. A short, steep drop leads to the north shore.

Rather than retrace your steps back to Stoddard Cabin, you can intercept the East Fork Coffee Creek northwest of the lake by following a badly worn, dusty trail that heads initially north, about 250 yards east of the outlet. Starting out nearly level, the trail turns northwest to parallel the outlet creek a mile down to the East Fork. The junction with the East Fork Coffee Creek Trail is 100 yards north of the crossing.

Turn southwest on the East Fork Coffee Creek Trail and descend through an area that was burned in 1987. Openings in the forest here reveal vistas of the valley below and southeast toward Billys Peak, the high point on the massive ridge rising behind Stoddard Lake. A small tributary courses across the trail about 300 yards below a junction of the Stoddard Spur Trail. A gradual, half-mile descent leads to another small tributary, below which the creek drops away in a steeper section of the canyon and, correspondingly, the trail descends more steeply on the northwest slope through a towering forest of Douglas firs, ponderosa pines, and Jeffrey pines, with an occasional sugar pine and white fir. Just shy of 1.5 miles from the Stoddard Spur junction, the trail draws near to the creek once more.

Stoddard Lake

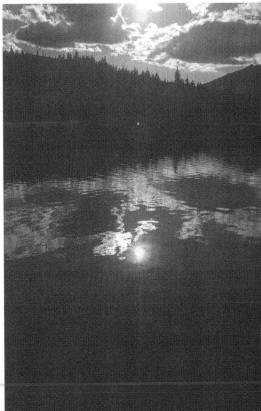

Holland Mine and the 1983 Flood

A tremendous flood and slide came down a tributary of East Fork Coffee Creek in 1983, completely inundating a flat along the East Fork with rocks, mud, and forest debris. Relics from what was the site of the Holland Mine now lie buried under all that debris, and the only mark that a mine once existed here is a sign nailed to a tree near the relocated trail.

Climb away from this area of devastation to pick up the track of an old road, then descend moderately, crossing two tributary streams before reaching a fork. Your route follows the upper, right-hand fork—the other fork leads down to the ruins of some more recent mine buildings that collapsed into the bottom of the canyon. The road soon disappears again, as you turn farther southward on a foot trail to continue down, steeply at times, above a steep rock-walled gulch cut by the creek into the bottom of the canyon. The trail becomes rougher and dustier as you round a shoulder of rock. After a steep drop aided by a few switchbacks across the remnants of an old wood flume, you may notice a sheet-metal outhouse perched on the hillside below—this incongruous sight served a miner's cabin around the corner of the canyon. A pair of long-legged switchbacks leads down to intersect the miner's road, 2.3 miles from the former site of the Holland Mine. The North Fork has cut a course far below you in a rugged canyon of gray metamorphic rock.

After 0.7 mile of moderately steep and dusty downhill along the miner's road, you stand directly uphill from the East Fork Coffee Creek trailhead, where a short stub leads down to the trailhead alongside Coffee Creek Road. However, if you're hiking the road back to the North Fork trailhead, remain on the miner's road and intersect the Coffee Creek Road farther west.

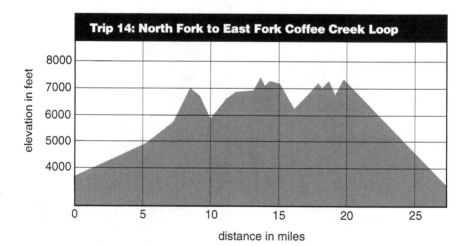

TRIP 15

Union Creek and Dorleska Mine to Big Flat

Gold was a powerful incentive, as huge piles of rock, dug and moved by hand, still testify.

Trip Type:	Backpack, 2–5 days
Distance:	10.3 miles, point-to-point (plus 2.6-mile side trip to Union Lake)
Elevation Change:	5125 feet, average 397 per mile
Difficulty:	Easy
Season:	Late June to mid-October
Maps:	USGS *Caribou Lake* and USFS *A Guide to the Trinity Alps Wilderness*
Nearest Campground:	Big Flat

Union Creek canyon is not as spectacular as some other Trinity Alps canyons, but can't be beat for being just plain nice. The hiking is easy and campsites are numerous with plentiful firewood. Fishing is excellent in Union Creek for feisty, pan-sized trout up to the confluence with the creek from Bullards Basin. Fishing is not quite as good up at Union Lake, but the side trip there provides opportunities to fish and swim, or scramble up to Landers Lake.

Although a road once ran up into Bullards Basin, most of the magnificent forest in Union Creek canyon was untouched by loggers and is still intact. However, Bullards Basin is another story: Many of the trees around Dorleska Mine were felled in the early 1900s to construct buildings, timber the mine shafts, and fire boilers to operate the equipment of the mine and mill. Mining was concentrated on the ridge between the Union Creek drainage and South Fork Salmon River to the north. The trip leads past the Yellow Rose Mine on the way down the north side of this ridge to Big Flat. The heavy machinery now rusting away at these historic mines inspires wonder as to how men and mules ever brought all that equipment in and set it up in a virtually roadless wilderness. A small amount of placer mining may still be underway on private land near the mouth of Union Creek, but the rest of the canyon remains virtually untouched. Cattle may be seen grazing along Union Creek from time to time.

Since this is a point-to-point trip, you will need a second vehicle, or someone to pick you up, at the Big Flat trailhead. However, hitchhiking the 9 miles between trailheads is not too difficult along the Coffee Creek Road, at least during peak season.

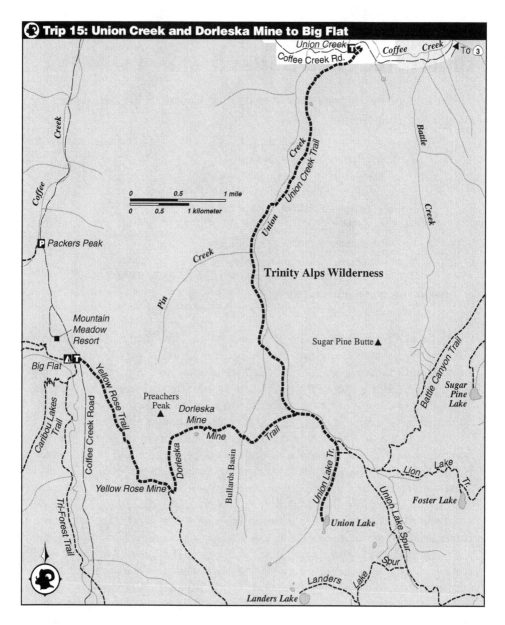

Starting Point

From Highway 3, about 40 miles north of Weaverville and immediately past the Coffee Creek bridge, turn west on Coffee Creek Road. The Coffee Creek ranger station is 300 yards down the first road to the right after you turn off the highway. Continue on well-graded road past Goldfield Campground, and the Boulder Creek, East Fork Coffee Creek/Sugar Pine, and North Fork Coffee Creek trailheads to the road up Union Creek, 11.5 miles up Coffee Creek Road and 0.5 mile east of Union Creek. Signs designating the location of the trailhead seem to regularly disappear here—if you reach the Union Creek bridge you've gone a half mile too far. The first part of the trail follows an old logging road turning south up the side of Coffee Creek canyon through broken rock. Parking is below a locked gate about 50 yards up the hill, or along the Coffee Creek Road as conditions allow. Wherever you park, don't block access to the gate.

Ending Point

The Big Flat trailhead is farther up Coffee Creek Road, 20.5 miles from Highway 3, beside Big Flat Campground.

Description

For the first 300 yards above the gate on an old road, you climb east at a moderately steep grade, then turn back southwest along the side of Coffee Creek canyon. Beyond the first mile, you look down at the tops of a fine strand of sugar pines in the canyon below, and some large specimens drop their foot-long cones along the path a little farther along. A few large ponderosa pines are also beside the road, providing a good opportunity to note the differences between these two valuable species.

At 0.8 mile the road turns south into Union Creek canyon, as you continue the moderate ascent well above the level of the creek. Where the road levels off and begins a gradual descent, about 2 miles from the trailhead, another little creek flows across, partly through an iron pipe under the roadbed. A half mile farther, you can see Union Creek flowing through a bed of boulders below, as you pass a series of slides across the road. Union Creek has washed out the road beyond these slides, as you climb along the top of a bank to a bridge across the creek's steep-sided gulch, 2.3 miles from the trailhead. Late starters will find excellent campsites on both sides of the creek near the bridge.

The route above the bridge follows a road trace that appears to be much older than the one below the bridge. You turn away from the creek near a meadow and climb moderately to a crossing of good-sized Pin Creek, a half mile from the bridge. The trail continues south, rising gradually through beautiful forest of Douglas firs, incense cedars, sugar pines, and a few ponderosa pines. A few open meadows appear between the trail and Union Creek, with excellent campsites spread about nearly everywhere. If Union Creek is not running too high, eager 7- to 8-inch rainbow trout will rise in almost every hole along the rocky bed between the bridge and the confluence with the creek draining Bullards Basin. Once in a while, a 10-incher may even surprise you.

You near and then cross the stream from Bullards Basin at 1.3 miles from the bridge, and then continue south in heavy forest, out of sight of Union Creek. In an area of seeps and springs, you leave the road trace and cross a small tributary running into a wet meadow covered with wildflowers. Turn toward Union Creek again, and skirt the bottom of a large meadow leading up to the foot of a rugged ridge separating Union Lake and Union Creek from Bullards Basin. Reach a junction in this meadow with the Dorleska Mine Trail heading west, 4.9 miles from the trailhead.

Side Trip to Union Lake

From the Dorleska Mine Trail junction, continue on the Union Lake Trail up the canyon through dense forest, within sound of Union Creek, to a crossing of the small stream flowing down from Union Lake, 0.4 mile from the junction. Turn right at a signed junction 100 feet beyond the ford, and then follow good duff tread south into a wide valley between two high spur ridges. After 0.4 mile from the previous junction, you reach another junction, this one with a trail from farther up Union Creek canyon that has run around the nose of the eastern spur ridge. Cross the creek again, 0.2 mile above the junction, and begin a steeper rise to the lake up the open top of a low ridge dividing the upper part of the valley.

Long and narrow Union Lake occupies a deep depression on the east side of the ridge, 1.3 miles from the Dorleska Mine Trail junction. A tiny creek meanders through a wet meadow carpeted with wildflowers west of the ridge. Many excellent campsites nestle beneath widely spaced firs along the top of the ridge. Despite the lake's popularity, firewood is plentiful. Lush grasses and willows line most of the irregularly shaped shoreline, and a marvelously textured rock wall, with hanging gardens and meadows, rises above the south end of the basin. Except for one deep spot in the lower end, the 3.5-acre lake is quite shallow, with logs protruding through the surface. By midsummer the water is warm enough for swimming, but the banks are quite mucky. The lake has a healthy population of good-sized eastern brook trout. Plenty of forage in the meadows to the west and north makes Union Lake very popular with equestrians. For the same reason, you're apt to see deer in your camp at night.

If you're inclined to steep, off-trail exploration, a tiny, unnamed tarn nestled under the shoulder of Red Rock Mountain to the southwest may be tempting. Also, Landers Lake basin is less than a mile away in a straight line over the south crest.

From the junction of Dorleska Mine and Union Lake trails, turn sharply right and climb moderately west above the top of a big meadow at the base of a spur ridge. At the meadow's bottom edge, you can see the Union Lake Trail that you followed earlier. A steep rise of 200 yards beyond the meadow leads to the northwest side of the ridge, where the grade eases and the forest transitions from mostly Douglas firs to mostly white firs. Beyond another short, steep rise, you cross the bottom edge of another large meadow and then turn west across the floor of Bullards Basin. The trail crosses a tiny stream in open forest and then, 1.2 miles from the Union Lake junction, crosses the rocky channel of the main creek draining the basin.

A steep climb up the west ridge begins immediately beyond the creek crossing, zigzagging on rough tread, very steeply at times, up a rocky slope through an open forest of Jeffrey pines, white firs, incense cedars, western white pines, and the stumps of some long-ago logging operation. Father up, you climb beside a little stream and a wet meadow before leveling out on a bench just below the tailings pond and one of the rock dumps belonging to the Dorleska Mine. As soon as you climb around these features, you look directly at the remnants of Dorleska's large stamp mill, 2 miles from the Union Lake junction.

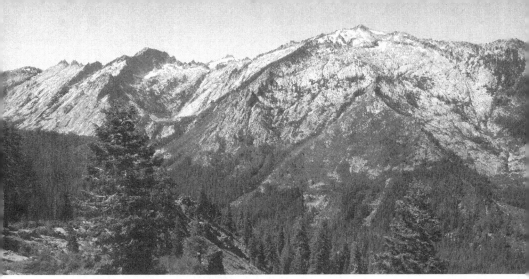

Caribou Mountain from crest above Dorleska Mine

Dorleska Mine

Eight heavy stamps in two stands pounded away at the Dorleska Mine from the turn of the 20th century to the mid-1930s, powered by steam from a wood-burning boiler. Two steam engines and the boiler remain in place among the debris of a building that once sheltered them. However, the mill stands are not in nearly as good of shape. The giant camshafts have fallen, and the stamps lean on each other like a row of drunks. Two little ore cars still sit on rusting tracks near the caved-in mouth of a drift, running into the side of the ridge at the west edge of the bench. There are no longer any buildings standing at Dorleska. One can only wonder at how in the world men and mules managed to move all of this heavy machinery to this site without benefit of a road beyond the lower end of Bullards Basin.

As you climb up to the next bench above the mill, an old sign beside the trail tells the story of the mine and the origin of its name: GOLD DISCOVERED IN 1898 BY R. D. LAWRENCE. MINE NAMED AFTER HIS WIFE DORLESKA. ALL MACHINERY AND MATERIAL HAULED IN BY MULES. LAST OPERATED ABOUT 1934. A spring behind the sign drains into a willow swamp below. Boards from miners' shacks have been recycled into a rather elaborate campsite beside the willows and beneath the only tree in the immediate area. Please refrain from burning these boards or carrying away souvenirs; they're of historic value. Between the bench and a larger flat above to the southwest, you walk an old road trace again; this stretch was used to haul ore from the upper diggings to the stamp mill. A boiler sits near a large rock dump on the upper flat, perhaps used to operate a draw works, although no evidence of a head works or shaft appears nowadays.

Rough, gravel trail snakes southwest up the steep, bare slope beyond the upper diggings to the crest of the ridge, 0.5 mile from the stamp mill. Forests on the benches and the side of the ridge have never recovered from the logging done to fire the boilers and build the mine works and shacks. However, the contorted western white pines, foxtail pines, Jeffrey pines, and mountain hemlocks on the crest were fortunately spared. From the aerie of the crest you look down into the South Fork valley south of Big Flat and northwest across to Packers Peak and southwest to Caribou Mountain. Josephine Lake hangs in a slot on the side of Caribou Mountain, and the Caribou Lakes Trail switchbacks up the brushy northwest shoulder. Preachers Peak is the high point on the rocky crest directly north.

Drop off the ridge, moderately at first, and then more steeply, bending slightly west of south across the west side of the ridge. The trail slices through two dumps from prospect holes on the way down and then, a half mile from the crest, turns straight down the side of the ridge to meet a junction of the Yellow Rose Trail.

If you turn right, a short stroll north from the junction is the Yellow Rose Mine, where, below a large rock dump, an upright boiler and the remnants of a rotary rock crusher provide historic interest. A short walk along the top of the dump will bring you to the mouth of a caved-in drift running into the hill. A small stream of water, stinky and mineralized, runs from the drift. A leaning, funny-looking, two-story shack to the south up a hill from the drift may not last many more winters.

From the Yellow Rose Mine, the level trail runs north on a flat for about 300 yards, then begins to descend moderately steeply northwest across the side of the ridge. The first mile below the mine is mostly under fir forest, with occasional open or brushy gaps. Cross several small seeps and streams, all mossy and heavily mineralized. The trees thin and the brush thickens as you continue the descent. Finally, 1.8 miles below the mine, a crystal-clear stream flows across the trail in the bottom of a steep gully.

Past a grove of Douglas firs, you see Big Blat below and Mountain Meadow Ranch across the valley. Traveling past more brush and sparse Oregon oaks, you come to a large grove of Douglas firs at Big Flat, 2.3 miles from the mine. The trailhead parking lot is across the main road before the campground.

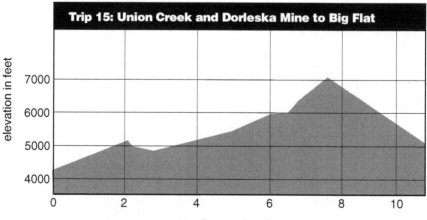

Trip 15: Union Creek and Dorleska Mine to Big Flat

TRIP 16

South Fork Coffee Creek Loop
to Trail Gulch and Long Gulch Lakes

Pleasant canyon strolls and two stunning lakes

Trip Type:	Backpack, 3–5 days
Distance:	17 miles, loop
Elevation Change:	9135 feet, average 537 per mile
Difficulty:	Easy to moderate
Season:	Mid-July to mid-September
Maps:	USGS *Deadman Peak* and USFS *A Guide to the Trinity Alps Wilderness*
Nearest Campground:	Big Flat

A very pleasant trail—not too steep, well shaded except at the upper meadows, and quite scenic—leads up the South Fork. Above the confluence of Steavale Creek the steep-sided lower canyon gives way to a wide, glaciated valley, bedecked with flower-filled meadows and backed by glistening granite ridges and peaks. Once you've climbed the last half mile to the crest of the divide, you drop into the cirque holding Long Gulch Lake.

Trail Gulch and Long Gulch lakes are both charming, subalpine lakes, 12 to 15 acres in size, and picturesquely typical of the string of lakes along the north side of the Salmon and Scott River Divide. Although a mere mile separates the two lakes, the trail between them crosses and recrosses the divide in 3.4 torturous miles. Of course, some of that climbing could be avoided by descending the trail down Long Gulch and then back up Trail Gulch, but doing so would miss a substantial amount of gorgeous scenery, as well as walking nearly 3 extra miles.

Both lakes are within easy dayhiking or riding distance from trailheads north of the divide, but the remoteness of those trailheads off the Callahan-Cecilville Road helps restrict the number of visitors. The lakes warm up for pleasant swimming by mid-August, and fishing for rainbow trout to 10 inches is reported to be fair to good. South Fork Coffee Creek supports a good-sized population of pan-sized rainbows below Steavale Creek, but you'll have to crawl down into the canyon to fish.

The return side of the loop trip across the upper basin of North Fork Coffee Creek and down through Steavale Meadow is mostly downhill through oftentimes distinctly different scenery. Cattle have been known to graze here, so you may have to consider them part of the scenery.

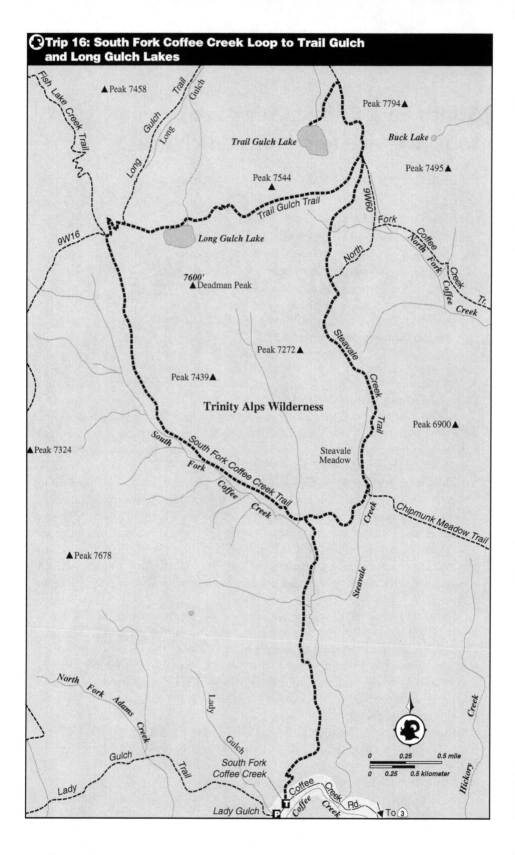

Trip 16: South Fork Coffee Creek Loop to Trail Gulch and Long Gulch Lakes

▲ Peak 7458

Peak 7794 ▲

Fish Lake Creek Trail

Long Gulch Trail

Long Gulch Trail

Trail Gulch Lake

Buck Lake ○

Peak 7495 ▲

Peak 7544 ▲

Trail Gulch Trail

9W60

North Fork Coffee Creek North Fork Coffee Creek Tr.

9W16

Long Gulch Lake

7600' ▲ Deadman Peak

North

Steavale Creek Trail

Peak 7272 ▲

Creek

Peak 7439 ▲

Trinity Alps Wilderness

Peak 6900 ▲

▲ Peak 7324

South Fork

South Fork Coffee Creek Trail

Steavale Meadow

Coffee Creek

Steavale Creek

Chipmunk Meadow Trail

▲ Peak 7678

Steavale Creek

North Fork Adams Creek

Lady Gulch

Lady Gulch Trail

South Fork Coffee Creek

Coffee Creek

Coffee Creek Rd.

To ③

Lady Gulch

T P

| 0 | 0.25 | 0.5 mile |
| 0 | 0.25 | 0.5 kilometer |

Starting Point

From Highway 3, about 40 miles north of Weaverville and immediately past the Coffee Creek bridge, turn west on Coffee Creek Road. The Coffee Creek ranger station is 300 yards down the first road to the right after you turn off the highway. Continue on well-graded road past Goldfield Campground, and the Boulder Creek, East Fork Coffee Creek/Sugar Pine, North Fork Coffee Creek, and Union Creek trailheads to the South Fork Coffee Creek trailhead, 15 miles from Highway 3 and 8.3 miles past the North Fork trailhead.

The signed turnoff for the trailhead is 0.4 mile above the road bridge over the South Fork and beside an area of former heavy dredging along Coffee Creek. Four to five vehicles could park here, provided you're careful not to block access. Don't park above the gate across the turnoff; even if the gate is open when you arrive, you may find it locked upon your return. If all the available parking space is being used, you may find enough room in the one or two turnouts within the next half mile near the Lady Gulch and Adams Lake trailheads.

Description

South Fork Coffee Creek has a misleading name—it flows from the north, well north of North Fork Coffee Creek and almost at the northernmost point of Coffee Creek's crooked course through the northern Trinity Alps. And at some point in the past the names for Trail Gulch and Long Gulch lakes were transposed, a mistake perpetuated for years in guidebooks and on maps. The mistake has been corrected on the U.S. Forest Service's 2004 *A Guide to the Trinity Alps Wilderness* map, with Trail Gulch Lake northeast of Long Gulch Lake.

A Forest Service gate, 50 yards from the Coffee Creek Road, is intended to block vehicle access to the four-wheel-drive road that marks the beginning of the South Fork Trail. The road ascends gradually north for 150 yards, before a steep climb begins northeast, first up a washed-out gully and then on switchbacks up the side of a ridge. After 0.6 mile, you round a shoulder of the ridge in thick Douglas-fir forest and then level off to contour north across the west slope of South Fork Coffee Creek canyon, still following the course of the old road. Large Douglas firs, ponderosa pines, and sugar pines shade the trail on the way to a fork, 1 mile from the trailhead. The right-hand fork disappears in the trees headed for the bottom of the canyon.

Follow the left-hand fork, signed SOUTH FORK TRAIL, and continue another 0.2 mile to the end of the road, near an old cabin site just beyond a small stream. A rusty bedspring and the remnants of an enameled kitchen range resting on a concrete slab suggest the relatively recent vintage of this cabin, but the former structure has completely disappeared. Backpackers who have gotten a late start could camp here, provided the trash in the gully below is not an aesthetic deterrent. Away from the cabin site, you climb moderately out into fern-filled meadows before turning to ford the South Fork, 2 miles from the trailhead. There are a few good campsites beyond a screen of willows on the east bank. A short, steep climb east from the crossing brings you 0.3 mile to a bench, where you level off near a junction with the Steavale Creek Trail heading east.

Continuing on the South Fork Trail, you ascend moderately northwest across forested benches and meadows to the crossing of a small tributary, 0.3 mile from the junction, and then draw near to the South Fork again. The tributary is the last easily accessible water until you climb over the divide and drop down to Long Gulch Lake, 3.5 miles away. Continue the moderate ascent through fern-filled meadows and, as the trail turns more to the north, a massive, glacier-carved, granite ridge pops into view across the valley. Steeper pitches of trail lead higher, as Shasta red firs and foxtail pines make appearances in the stands of forest between the meadows. Beyond a sandy flat, the last half mile of tread to a gap in the Salmon River divide has steep to very steep sections.

At the gap, a trail junction marks the top of the divide. Trail 9W16 branches west to cross the divide through another gap, near a junction with the Poison and Onion Meadow trails. Northwest, the Fish Lake Creek Trail cuts a dim track contouring along the side of a spur ridge and eventually crossing over and descending to Fish Lake—except for the view from the top of the spur ridge, a side trip to this oversized pond is hardly worth the effort.

Your trail to Long Gulch Lake leads northeast over the crest and the spar-kling, deep blue lake nestled into the cirque below soon springs into view. Five moderately steep switchbacks descend the north face of the divide to an unsigned junction, 0.3 mile west of the lake. From this spot, the Long Gulch Trail continues north 2.8 miles to a trailhead near Carter Meadow.

Carter Meadow summit from the crest above South Fork Lakes (Trip 14)

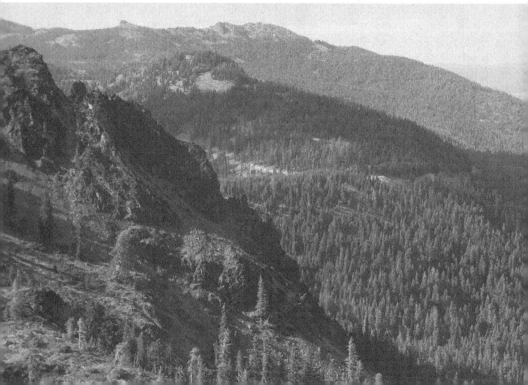

Turn right from the junction and head east through broken granite, climbing slightly over a rim before running along the north shore of Long Gulch Lake, 6 miles from the South Fork trailhead. You pass below a number of excellent campsites in an open red fir and hemlock forest on the way to the shoreline, although there's very little firewood for campfires. The 7600-foot summit of Deadman Peak towers 1100 feet directly above the south shore of the 14-acre lake, with granite cliffs surrounding more than half of the shoreline. A mammoth rockfall has formed a small island near the south shore that competent swimmers can easily access. In spite of relatively heavy fishing pressure, a limit of 10- to 11-inch rainbows is possible. All in all, Long Gulch Lake is a very nice place to spend a day or two.

After your stay at Long Gulch Lake is over, follow the trail to the outlet at the northeast shore, and then turn north along the edge of the trees past a large horse camp. About 75 yards from the lake, you'll see a small clump of blazed lodgepole pines beside a tiny meadow—the trail runs east across this meadow, crosses the outlet, and proceeds through a gap in thick alders on the far bank. Beyond the alders, the trail turns back toward the lake, then heads east again to climb past a campsite.

From there, follow ducks east up an open, cow-tracked hill. On the approach to a rock wall at the top of a moderately steep slope, ducked tread turns northeast below a thicket of alders and climbs into dense forest. Better-defined tread snakes up through mature Shasta red firs and mountain hemlocks north of the alders to a 200-yard-long stretch of very steep, gravelly, open slope, some of which is quite loose and may cause you to slip back a couple of steps for every few you climb. Fortunately, the tread improves above this obstacle. Zigzag east through younger, open forest and broken rock, very steeply at times, to the crest, just south-southwest of Peak 7544 and 0.8 mile from Long Gulch Lake's outlet. From here, you'll have marvelous views north to the Marble Mountains and west across Long Gulch.

Traverse along the south side of the crest and then drop down to a gap in the crest above Trail Gulch Lake, where you reach a junction with Trail 9W60 coming up from the south and the Steavale Creek Trail coming up from the southwest, 0.9 mile from the previous gap. From this spot at the top of the divide, Trail Gulch Lake, your next destination, springs into view to the northwest.

The trail dives steeply down the north side of the divide through a dense forest composed almost entirely of mountain hemlocks to a granite ledge, and then descends more moderately north across the west side of a ridge on the east side of Trail Gulch. After 0.3 mile, you turn west and zigzag steeply down an open slope to the lower end of a lush little meadow. Although you may be tempted by the view from above into believing that an easy approach to the lake lies up this meadow and over a spur ridge, by going this way you'd end up struggling down a rough talus slope through a tangle of thick brush. The easier route is to continue down the Trail Gulch Trail 0.25 mile to the junction and then back up the east bank of the outlet to the lakeshore.

The cirque walls around 10-acre Trail Gulch Lake are much darker granite than those around Long Gulch Lake, also containing some metamorphic rock strata. Otherwise, the two lakes and their settings are quite similar. Rainbow trout fingerlings along the shoreline and in the outlet confirm that trout are indeed successfully spawning here. However, since the lake is less than 2 miles away from a trailhead near Carter Meadow, anglers may find catching anything bigger than 6 to 7 inches difficult. A number of good campsites in a wide, wooded area above the north shore would be considered excellent except they're heavily used and lack firewood. Swimmers will find the water temperature warm enough for comfortable swimming by mid-August.

After an enjoyable stay at Trail Gulch Lake, retrace your steps 1.3 miles back to the top of the Salmon River divide and the junction with Trail 9W60 and the Steavale Creek Trail.

From the junction, follow the Steavale Creek Trail 9W61 southwest across the valley, skirting some large flats covered with alders, to a junction with the North Fork Coffee Creek Trail 9W02 at the foot of a spur ridge, 1 mile from the divide.

Away from the junction, you climb moderately southeast for 200 yards, and then turn southwest around the shoulder of a ridge to begin tracing a long contour around a wide, upper basin that drains east into North Fork Coffee Creek. This traverse offers panoramic views across the basin to the ridges east of the North Fork and the summit of Mt. Shasta on the skyline. On the other side of the basin, the trail turns southeast on the crest of the divide between Steavale Creek and North Fork drainages and descends to a saddle at the head of Steavale Meadow.

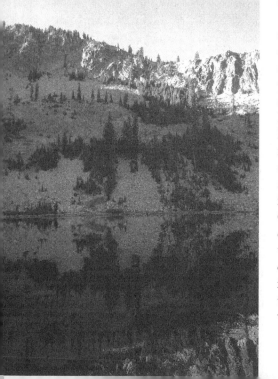

Trail Gulch Lake

Steavale Meadow slopes steeply south from the saddle in a spread of grasses and alder thickets before dropping into the steep-walled canyon below. As you start down, you can line up the distant tip of Caribou Mountain in the notch formed by the lower canyon. A half mile down the moderately steep trail on the east side of the meadow, you enter a strip of fir forest, beyond which you emerge into meadow again, with Steavale Creek burbling under a thick cover of alders—the first readily accessible water since Trail Gulch Lake. A hand-carved sign at a much-used campsite in the lower end of the meadow dubs the site CAMP SIBERIA. Perhaps the sign was carved by a lonesome cowpoke who herded cattle up Steavale Creek. A few yards below the campsite is an important, but unsigned, junction. Although it appears to be merely another cattle path, the track diving into the alders and crossing Steavale Creek to the west side is indeed your trail—the continuation of the Steavale Creek Trail. The faint, little-used trail on the east side is the Chipmunk Meadow Trail, which soon turns up a ravine and eventually climbs east to a junction of the Milk Ranch and Hardscrabble trails. A good-sized mine was once operational in the lower end of the ravine, not too far away if you're interested in a short side trip.

Steavale Creek falls away in a steep-sided canyon as the trail continues almost level above the west bank. Turn a little southwest, and then northwest around the point of a ridge between Steavale and South Fork Coffee creeks. A moderate to steep, 0.3-mile descent through dense firs brings you to a junction with the South Fork Trail, 0.9 mile from the Chipmunk Meadow Trail junction.

From there, retrace your steps 2.3 miles to the South Fork Coffee Creek trailhead.

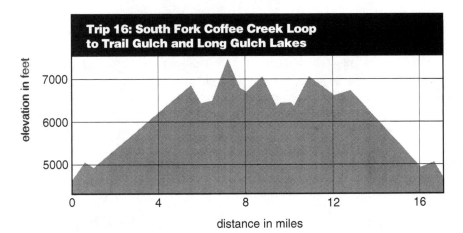

TRIP 17

Adams Lake

At 6200 feet, Adams Lake may not be alpine, or even subalpine, but what a pretty place.

Trip Type:	Dayhike or overnight backpack
Distance:	4.6 miles, out-and-back
Elevation Change:	1160 feet, average 504 per mile
Difficulty:	Moderate
Season:	Late June to early October
Maps:	USGS *Caribou Lake* and USFS *A Guide to the Trinity Alps Wilderness*
Nearest Campground:	Big Flat

Pleasant Adams Lake is only a half-hour horseback ride or an hour-plus hike from a trailhead along the Coffee Creek Road. A long time ago, off-road vehicles had access to the lake, which seems hard to believe nowadays. The 1-acre lake sits below a rugged-looking, 7500-foot granite peak and is bordered by a lush, flower-dotted meadow on the opposite side. A unique patch of cattails thrives near the outlet, wetland plants that we haven't seen anywhere else in the Alps. So close to a trailhead, fishing is only fair for pan-sized eastern brook trout. The muddy banks and bottom make the idea of swimming in the lake a trifle unappealing.

Adams Lake

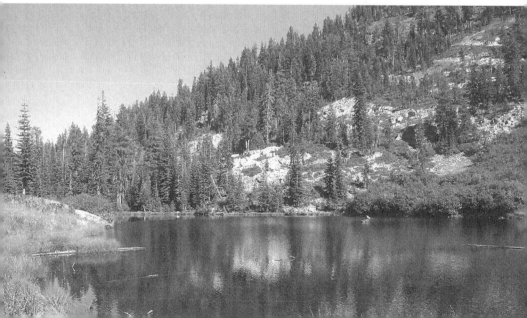

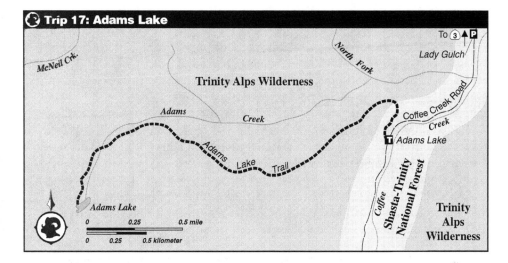

Trip 17: Adams Lake

McNeil Crk.

North Fork

To ③⚠🅿

Lady Gulch

Trinity Alps Wilderness

Adams   Creek

Coffee Creek Road

Creek

🔟 Adams Lake

Adams

Lake   Trail

Adams Lake

0   0.25   0.5 mile

0   0.25   0.5 kilometer

Coffee

Shasta-Trinity

National Forest

Trinity
Alps
Wilderness

Starting Point

From Highway 3, about 40 miles north of Weaverville and immediately past the Coffee Creek bridge, turn west on Coffee Creek Road. The Coffee Creek ranger station is 300 yards down the first road to the right after you turn off the highway. Continue on well-graded road past Goldfield Campground, and the Boulder Creek, East Fork Coffee Creek/Sugar Pine, North Fork Coffee Creek, Union Creek, Hardscrabble, South Fork Coffee Creek, and Lady Gulch trailheads to the Adams Lake trailhead, 15.8 miles from Highway 3 and 0.8 mile past the South Fork Coffee Creek trailhead.

The trailhead is not particularly obvious—the trail starts out as an old four-wheel-drive road, chopped off by a 3- to 4-foot cut on the north side of Coffee Creek Road, a half mile beyond a road bridge over Adams Creek and just as you approach the reworked area of the Upper Nash Mine. A small trailhead signboard (bearing absolutely no information in 2008) is all that marks the beginning of the trail. Minimal parking is limited to the narrow shoulder of the road.

Description

A broken-down, steel gate with a ROAD CLOSED sign lies off the trail about 100 yards up the course of the old Adams Lake Road, as you make a stiff climb that snakes north 0.3 mile to the top of a ridge dividing the drainages of Adams and Coffee creeks. The road turns a tad south of west and follows directly up the crest of the ridge through a magnificent forest composed primarily of Douglas firs and white firs, mixed with occasional sugar pines, western white pines, and incense cedars. Surprisingly, the old roadbed remains in good condition, although steep to very steep and without checks or culverts to prevent it from washing out.

At 0.8 mile from the trailhead, you turn northwest over the side of the ridge and contour above the canyon of Adams Creek. After a "zig" south up a ravine and a "zag" northwest over a minor spur ridge, the trail contours west and draws near to Adams Creek, trickling through a patch of thick alders in a steep-sided gulch. After a quarter mile of moderate climbing between the creek and a small meadow, you cross to the north bank and proceed up the glaciated valley. The trail bends south to a larger meadow and Adams Lake, which lies in a grassy cup at the meadow's upper southwest side.

While the water appears green and uninviting by late summer, the lake's surroundings are picturesquely lush. Willows border about half of the muddy shoreline from the cattails near the outlet around to talus falling into the south side from the granite peak above. A sweet little spring offers some clear-running water near built-up campsites in the trees northwest of the lake. A rope stretched between two trees near the farthest campsite from the lake provides a convenient place to hang your food. You may meet a trail-ride party from Mountain Meadow Ranch, but they seldom stay overnight.

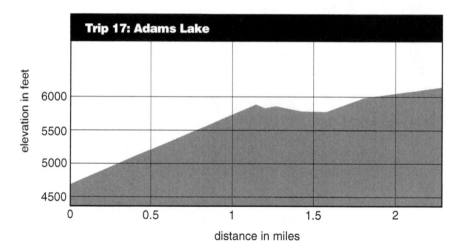

TRIP 18

Caribou Basin and Sawtooth Ridge

The moon still shines on white granite, and angelica still blooms sweetly in the meadows.

Trip Type:	Backpack, 2–5 days
Distance:	16.6 miles, out-and-back to Big Caribou Lake via New Trail; 13.6 miles, out-and-back via Old Trail (plus 0.7 mile round-trip to Little Caribou Lake)
Elevation Change:	3910 feet, average 471 per mile via New Trail; 5100 feet, average 750 per mile via Old Trail
Difficulty:	Moderate
Season:	Mid-July to late September
Maps:	USGS *Caribou Lake* and USFS *A Guide to the Trinity Alps Wilderness*
Nearest Campground:	Big Flat

Talk to any old-timer about the Trinity Alps, and you're sure to hear about a pack trip to Caribou Basin in the "good ol' days," a story likely to include prodigious numbers of trout as long as your arm, at least one marauding bear, a pack mule that nearly fell off the almost vertical trail over Caribou Mountain, and a late season snowfall with 100-mile-per-hour winds. Unfortunately, Caribou Basin is not the same pristine wilderness the old-timer remembers, but the scenery is still utterly fantastic. The deep blue lakes continue to picturesquely reflect untouched cliffs and peaks; the trout are still there but smaller these days; and the views from Sawtooth Ridge are still superlative.

The steep, 100-plus-year-old, trail over Caribou Mountain is still in place, although few people and almost no equestrians use the old path anymore—the newer trail is nearly 2 miles longer, but has only one or two short steep pitches. However, the Old Trail offers cross-country enthusiasts the opportunity to detour a short distance to remote, seldom-visited, and lovely Little Caribou Lake, as well as providing one of the most majestic views in all of the Trinity Alps from atop the northwest ridge of Caribou Mountain

Caribou Basin is one of the more heavily visited areas in the Trinity Alps but is not as crowded as other places in the wilderness. The basin is quite large, with the capacity to adequately disperse many parties. The tendency of visitors to crowd around Snowslide Lake and tiny Middle Caribou Lake creates the impression that the basin is more crowded than it is. A little thought about where and how you plan to camp will go a long way to preserve the basin. Wherever you set down temporary roots, please do so at least 200 yards or more from any body of water. Improper sanitation practices, too many pack

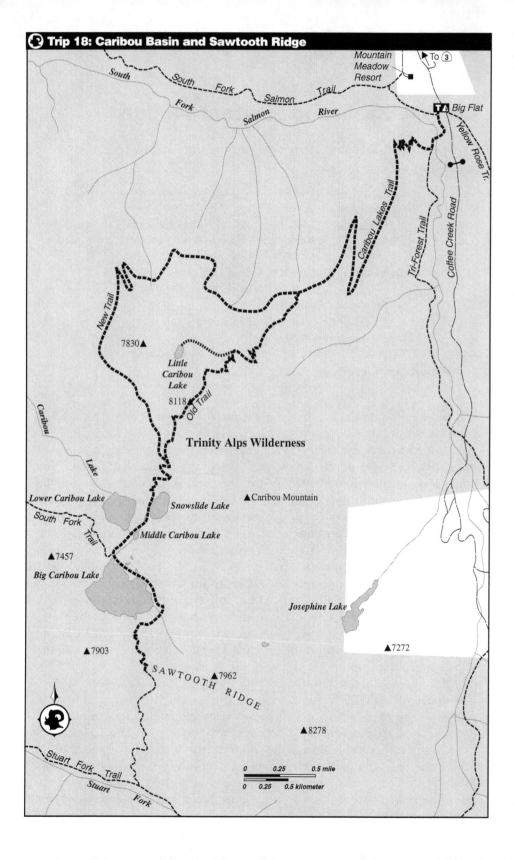

South

South Fork Salmon Trail

Fork

Salmon River

Mountain Meadow Resort

To ③

🅣🅐 Big Flat

Yellow Rose Tr.

Caribou Lakes Trail

Tri-Forest Trail

Coffee Creek Road

New Trail

7830▲

Little Caribou Lake

8118

Old Trail

Trinity Alps Wilderness

Caribou Lake

Lower Caribou Lake

South Fork Trail

Snowslide Lake

▲Caribou Mountain

Middle Caribou Lake

▲7457

Big Caribou Lake

Josephine Lake

▲7903

▲7272

S A W T O O T H   R I D G E

▲7962

▲8278

Stuart Fork Trail

Stuart Fork

0	0.25	0.5 mile
0	0.25	0.5 kilometer

animals, and the inability of solid rock to absorb wasters have all contributed to an overall decline in water quality here. Please observe all accepted wilderness ethics.

While hiking to Caribou Basin you'll likely see some of the effects of one of the many lightning-caused fires that burned in the Trinity Alps during 2008.

Starting Point

From Highway 3, about 40 miles north of Weaverville and immediately past the Coffee Creek bridge, turn west on Coffee Creek Road. The Coffee Creek ranger station is 300 yards down the first road to the right after you turn off the highway. Continue on well-graded road past Goldfield Campground, and the Boulder Creek, East Fork Coffee Creek/Sugar Pine, North Fork Coffee Creek, Union Creek, Hardscrabble, South Fork Coffee Creek, Lady Gulch, Adams Lake, and Packers Peak trailheads to the Big Flat trailhead beside Big Flat Campground, 20.5 miles from Highway 3 and 0.7 mile past the road to Mountain Meadow Ranch. If you reach a gate across the road and signs for a private subdivision, you've gone 0.3 mile past Big Flat. Parking is available for about two dozen vehicles.

While conveniently located near the trailhead, Big Flat Campground is small, primitive, and usually overcrowded—particularly on weekends. Car camping is much more pleasant in developed campgrounds near Trinity Lake.

Description

If the trail sign is missing from the parking area, you may be confused as to which direction you should head to begin the hike, as numerous roads and a half-dozen trails crisscross Big Flat. In the absence of clearer instruction, head south on a dirt road that soon narrows to single-track trail, following signs for Tri-Forest Peak and Kidd Creek. The trail soon leads to a junction just before crossing South Fork Salmon River. From this junction, proceed west to the crossing of the river, following signed directions for Caribou Lake. Early in the season South Fork Salmon River may be running high enough to be somewhat daunting, but the crossing shouldn't present any major obstacles. If the river is high, look downstream for a footlog.

Shortly beyond the crossing, you climb the hillside (passing an old, unmarked trail on the right that heads around the ridge and up Caribou Gulch), turn away from the creek, and reach another junction. The trail on the right is the Tri-Forest Trail, the western part of the Valley Loop trail toward Josephine Creek Lodge. Your trail ahead (west) should be signed CARIBOU LAKE.

A series of moderate switchbacks leads halfway up the hill, followed by a long, gradually ascending traverse south across the face of a ridge through thick manzanita and ceanothus brush. Welcome, cool shade greets you in a strip of forest across the slope. On the far side of the trees, the glistening granite slopes of Caribou Mountain briefly spring into view until you head back into forest cover and begin a long traverse north. Panoramic views of Big Flat, Mountain Meadow Ranch, and the Yellow Rose Trail slanting up the ridge across the valley open up along this traverse, which lasts for a half mile before the trail turns back southwest. Another 0.6 mile leads to Caribou Meadow in a sloping saddle on the top of the ridge, 3 miles from the trailhead.

Approximately 100 feet after entering Caribou Meadow, you reach a junction, perhaps unsigned, with the Old Trail heading over Caribou Mountain, where you're faced with a decision about which way to proceed: You can follow **Option 1** and remain on the newer trail around the northwest ridge of Caribou Mountain, or follow **Option 2** and climb steeply up and directly over the northwest ridge of Caribou Mountain on the Old Trail. While the more gently graded tread of Option 1 is less physically taxing (at the cost of nearly 2 additional miles), Option 2 offers one of the best Trinity Alps views from the top of an 8118-foot satellite peak along the ridge, as well as an off-trail side trip to Little Caribou Lake. For those with the necessary stamina, I recommend hiking in on the Old Trail and returning on the new one. A description of both options follows.

Option 1: Caribou Lake via the New Trail from Caribou Meadow

From the meadow, contour around the west side of the ridge you just climbed and soon emerge from the woods onto the solid granite, northwest face of Caribou Mountain. Rough tread, blasted directly out of the rock, climbs moderately northwest for the next half mile. Beyond a strip of sedimentary rock, you cross two small seasonal streams at the head of Caribou Gulch and then contour around a north-facing shoulder of the mountain to Brown's Meadow. The trail runs across the bottom of the large, steeply sloping meadow to dive into a thicket of alders on the west side, the dense vegetation concealing a sluggish little stream. There are a few fair campsites close to the alders and under some trees. Water is available from a spring flowing through a pipe beneath the trail 300 yards west up the hill.

Caribou Lake and Sawtooth Ridge

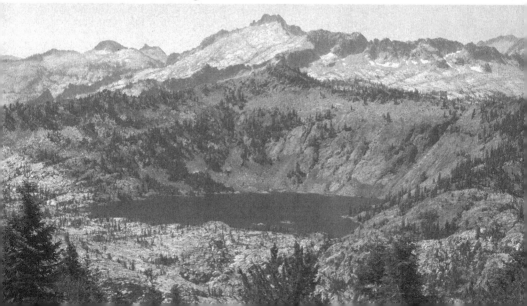

Four long, dusty switchbacks lead up the mostly forested slope of the next spur ridge. You climb directly up the crest of this spur for 100 yards, and then bend gradually southwest and south around the mountain on a moderate climb through dense forest and across old talus slopes. About 6 miles from the trailhead, head southeast across a very steep, open granite slope overlooking the dramatic chasm through which Caribou Creek drains northwest. A panorama of glacier-carved rock rises above the opposite side of the canyon, leading up to the highest summit in the Trinity Alps, 9002-foot Thompson Peak on the southwest horizon. Big Caribou Lake and Lower Caribou Lake soon appear in the giant basin above the head of the canyon, but Snowslide Lake and Middle Caribou Lake remain hidden behind folds of rock. Pinemat manzanita carpets some of the granite, and sparsely distributed red firs, mountain hemlocks, Jeffrey pines, whitebark pines, and mountain mahoganies cling to the slender cracks and narrow ledges.

Halfway along the canyon wall, the trail turns and descends into a chute gouged into the mountain. From this chute you have an unobstructed view between your feet of the canyon bottom a half mile below—not appealing for those who suffer from vertigo. Three short-legged, steep switchbacks lead up to the next point of rock, from where you continue on mostly level tread to a belt of trees. On the far side of the trees, you gaze down a brushy slope directly into Snowslide Lake, nestled into a trough between a granite dike and some cliffs on the west side of Caribou Mountain. Soon you reach the junction with the Old Trail.

Option 2: Caribou Lake via the Old Trail from Caribou Meadow

Immediately, you realize a significant difference in the grades from that of the previous section of trail to Caribou Meadow and the Old Trail heading up and over Caribou Mountain, which steeply switchbacks up the hillside above the meadow. The old-timers who constructed this path took a more direct approach than that of their modern-day counterparts. Climbing 0.4 mile on well-defined, good tread under light forest cover brings you to a little knob, from where the steep incline abates and even gives way to an all-too-short descent to an adjoining ridge. Good views of Caribou Mountain open up through gaps between the trees. Along the ridge the trail starts climbing again, this time a little more gently. Sharp eyes may notice quartz spread out all along this ridge, as a set of switchbacks heralds the trail's return to a steeper ascent. Just past the west end of the longest switchback, 1 mile from the junction, keep your eyes peeled for some ducks marking where a use trail heads off the ridge toward Little Caribou Lake.

Off-Trail Side Trip to Little Caribou Lake

Leaving the ridge and the tread of the old Caribou Lake Trail, you drop down on the use trail across rock slabs to the forest floor. Avoiding steep talus slopes above, begin a level traverse, initially over granite blocks and then over granite slabs toward the notch from which flows the seasonal outlet of Little Caribou Lake toward Caribou Gulch. Cairns may help guide you, but the route is obvious and you shouldn't have to depend on these markers to reach the lake. After reaching the canyon of the outlet, turn upstream and follow the creek to the east shore of Little Caribou Lake, 0.4 mile from the trail.

Three-acre Little Caribou Lake is a diminutive cousin of the much larger lakes ahead in Caribou Basin. Solitude is the chief advantage when compared to the more popular lakes to the south. Few backpackers and hardly any equestrians opt to climb the Old Trail to Caribou Basin, and only a small percentage of those who do take the Old Trail make the short, off-trail traverse over to Little Caribou Lake.

Little Caribou Lake is set in a cirque basin rimmed on three sides with sloping granite cliffs dotted with sporadic stands of mountain hemlock. Campsites are limited to the north shoreline, but they seem plentiful enough to handle the low number of overnighters the lake receives and, not surprisingly, plenty of firewood is available. Although the water temperature of the 7165-foot lake is icy cold until mid-August, and then merely cold afterward, swimming is good in the south end near some large rocks that offer sunny spots for sunbathing—the north half is too shallow for decent swimming.

Beyond the use trail junction, the arduous ascent resumes up steep switchbacks 0.8 mile to the summit of Peak 8118. As your heart rate slowly returns to normal, your breathing becomes less labored, and your sweat begins to dry, you begin to understand, perhaps, why the original trail crew decided to construct a trail straight up over the shoulder of Caribou Mountain: The wide-ranging view is utterly spectacular. Mt. Shasta shines as big as life to the northeast; the glistening granite peak of Caribou Mountain seems a stone's throw away; and—the most dramatic sight of all—Caribou Lake sprawls across a glacier-carved granite basin below razor sharp, serrated Sawtooth Ridge, backdropped by the snow-tinged summits of the central Trinity Alps. Mt. Thompson, Mt. Hilton, and Sawtooth Mountain are a few of the more noteworthy peaks visible in this sweeping panorama, one of the best views in the entire Alps.

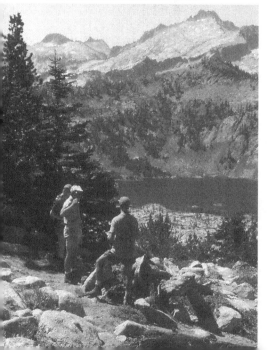

Sawtooth from Caribou Mountain

Leaving the idyllic vista behind, you descend short, steep, gravelly switchbacks through sparse, open vegetation. The switchbacks lengthen, but remain just as steep, and the vegetation progressively turns to low shrubs, sparsely distributed conifers, and eventually thicker forest. After 0.75 mile, you reach the intersection of the New Trail coming around the northwest ridge of Caribou Mountain, where a cairn and an old sign mark the junction.

From the Junction of the Old and New Trails to Big Caribou Lake

Proceed southeast from the junction of the Old and New trails, following four long-legged switchbacks in and out of the trees. A few more zigzags at the bottom of the slope lead to a small meadow at the north end of the dike west of Snowslide Lake. Water from a fine spring flows across the trail, halfway down the hill, providing the clearest looking water in the basin, which you should still treat before drinking. Overused campsites cover the top of the dike and carpet the basin around the pond known as Middle Caribou Lake below the south end of the dike. If you decide to camp in this area, be very careful to dispose of human waste and wash water responsibly, well away from the lakes. Less crowded campsites can be found around Big Caribou Lake, but they are more exposed.

Ten-acre Snowslide Lake has no permanent inlet or outlet, resulting in a water level that fluctuates up to 2 feet during the course of the summer. Both eastern brook and rainbow trout live in the cold depths and, if you're lucky, you can still hook the occasional 12-incher during the evening rise.

Use trails branch in virtually all directions through the scrubby mountain hemlocks, firs, and lodgepole pines on the dike above Snowslide Lake, most of them leading to the grass-lined pocket in the rocks holding half-acre Middle Caribou Lake. This tiny lake sits below a scenic waterfall in the stream flowing from Big Caribou Lake. Lower Caribou Lake is a steep-sided, 22-acre lake, very difficult to get around and producing only small eastern brook trout for your trouble. Decent campsites around Lower Caribou Lake are virtually nonexistent.

Big Caribou Lake is the commonly used, and appropriate, name for the 72-acre, deep, subalpine lake at the base of Sawtooth Ridge, although previous maps simply used the name "Caribou Lake." The largest lake in the Trinity Alps, many consider it the most beautiful. The lake is cradled in the bottom of a huge, mostly granite cirque beneath Caribou Mountain, Sawtooth Ridge, and an unnamed spur ridge to the west. Two-thirds of the convoluted shoreline, from the northwest around to almost due south, is granite, with low cliffs overlooking the indigo depths. Moving shadows of small surface waves cross ledges that slope into crystal-clear water, and then rise again as tiny islets offshore. Many "bathtub" lakes and ponds fill hollows and troughs in the glaciated granite around the lake. Erratic boulders perch nearly everywhere, as dwarfed and wind-contorted conifers cling to cracks and crannies.

Where granite gives way to metamorphic rock around the south shore, pocket meadows and other greenery replace bare rock, to some extent, and a few tiny, gravelly beaches offer easier access to the lake. Farther around to the west, fingers of talus from the west ridge slide directly into the water between strips of upright firs and hemlocks. A startlingly white vein of quartz slashes diagonally across the red-stained cliffs toward the top of the west ridge.

Numerous good campsites are in the rocks above the north and east shores, with a few more on the edges of pocket meadows above the south shore. Don't camp directly in the meadows—they are extremely fragile. Firewood is extremely scarce. When the wind isn't blowing too hard, fishing for both rainbow and eastern brook trout is good in Big Caribou, but don't expect to catch any trophy-sized fish.

Side Trip to Sawtooth Ridge

The jagged crest of Sawtooth Ridge fills the southern horizon above Big Caribou Lake. An exceedingly steep trail climbs from the southern shore of the lake up to the crest of the ridge and then drops 2500 feet in 1.5 miles to Portuguese Camp at the bottom of Stuart Fork canyon. Horses are banned from using this trail. Going down from Sawtooth Ridge to Portuguese Flat is certainly preferential to coming up from the canyon below! For a complete description of the route from the flat to the ridge consult Trip 6 (page 77).

No signs mark the trail to Sawtooth Ridge, but you can clearly see the trail heading up and away from Big Caribou Lake. Around the south shore of Big Caribou Lake, however, the trail is crisscrossed by game trails and use trails, but the open topography ensures that you can't get lost. From the meadows near the southeast shore, head southwest through a series of wildflower-filled meadows and over intervening ledges to where the trail should narrow to a single track that climbs southwest, then southeast across a grassy slope. Above a sparse grove of mountain hemlocks, you zigzag directly south up a very steep slope on crumbling rock to a gap in the crest, 0.75 mile from the point where the trail leaves the lake near the southeast shore.

The views from the gap atop Sawtooth Ridge are quite breathtaking but, if you explore a little east and west of the crest, you'll discover even more magnificent views. To the south the incredible bulk of Sawtooth Mountain looms directly above the Stuart Fork canyon below. Down-canyon you can see the wide expanse of Morris Meadow, while up-canyon you have a striking view of Emerald and Sapphire lakes, shimmering like their namesake jewels in a granite basin below rugged, snowcapped Thompson Peak. Behind, Caribou Basin is laid out before you like a raised relief map, on which you can trace your route back to Big Flat.

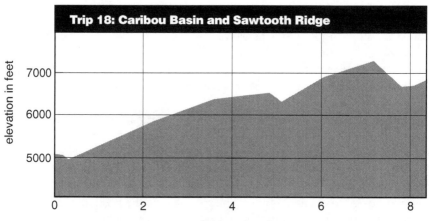

TRIP 19

Sunrise Basin, Horseshoe Lake, and Ward Lake Loop

Historic mines, lofty peaks, high mountain lakes, and flowery meadows remain the chief attractions on this strenuous loop trip.

Trip Type:	Backpack, 3–5 days
Distance:	19.5 miles, loop
Elevation Change:	10,560 feet, average 543 per mile
Difficulty:	Difficult
Season:	Mid-July to late September
Maps:	USGS *Caribou Lake*, *Ycatapom Peak*, and *Siligo Peak*; USFS *A Guide to the Trinity Alps Wilderness*
Nearest Campground:	Big Flat

You may see other recreational enthusiasts on this trip, but certainly not as many as on the Caribou Lakes Trail from Big Flat, or on the alternate route up Swift Creek to Horseshoe Basin and Ward lakes. If you want to escape the crowds and scale some peaks, a whole row of lofty summits is along a crest that this route crosses twice, from Red Rock Mountain on the north end down to Tri-Forest Peak on the south. A side trip to Landers Lake is a relatively straightforward addition as well, via either an off-trail or on-trail route. An extended loop of 29 miles would add Landers Lake, upper Union Creek, Parker Creek, and Parker Meadow to the itinerary (see Trip 11, page 111, for more information). Careful study of a map of the Trinity Alps will reveal even more possibilities for trip extensions.

Fishing in Horseshoe and Ward lakes is apt to be frustrating for anglers—the plentiful eastern brook trout in the lakes sneer at artificial lures. Swimmers will find the water temperature chilly at best.

Which direction to hike the loop is something of a toss-up. With a late start you're perhaps better off walking up the Carter's Lodge road from Big Flat and camping somewhere along Kidd Creek. The major disadvantage to that direction is the steepest and roughest section of trail on the whole loop awaits you at the head of Kidd Creek. The biggest disadvantage of reversing the direction described below is the climb up the ridge past the Yellow Rose and Leroy mines, which can be brutally hot in the afternoon and has almost no water.

Starting Point
From Highway 3, about 40 miles north of Weaverville and immediately past the Coffee Creek bridge, turn west on Coffee Creek Road. The Coffee Creek

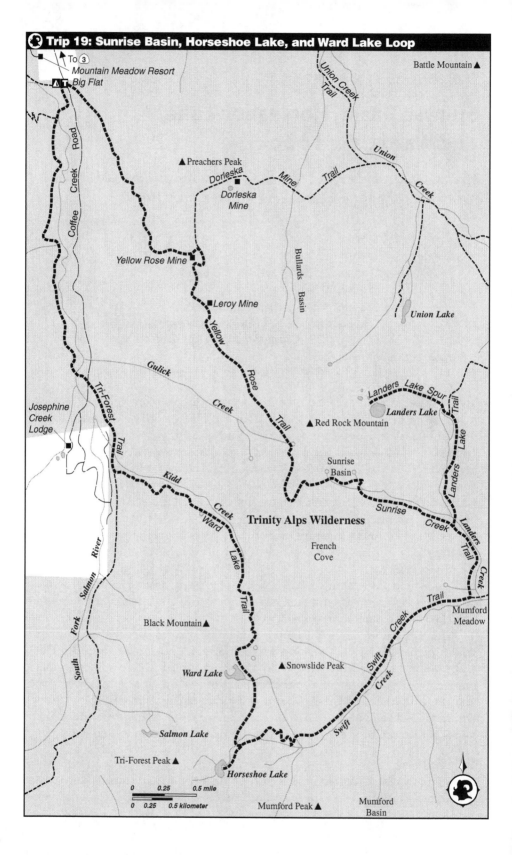

To ③
Mountain Meadow Resort
Big Flat

Battle Mountain ▲

Union Creek Trail

Preachers Peak ▲

Dorleska

Dorleska Mine

Mine Trail

Union

Creek

Coffee Creek Road

Yellow Rose Mine

Bullards Basin

Leroy Mine ■

Union Lake

Yellow

Gulick

Rose

Tri-Forest Trail

Josephine Creek Lodge

Creek

Trail

Landers Lake Spur

Red Rock Mountain ▲

Landers Lake

Landers Lake Trail

Kidd

Sunrise Basin

Creek

Ward

Trinity Alps Wilderness

Salmon River

South Fork

Lake

Sunrise

Creek

Landers Trail

Trail

French Cove

Creek

Mumford Meadow

Black Mountain ▲

Swift Creek Trail

Snowslide Peak ▲

Ward Lake

Swift

Creek

Salmon Lake

Swift

Tri-Forest Peak ▲

Horseshoe Lake

0   0.25   0.5 mile
0   0.25   0.5 kilometer

Mumford Peak ▲

Mumford Basin

ranger station is 300 yards down the first road to the right after you turn off the highway. Continue on well-graded road past Goldfield Campground, and the Boulder Creek, East Fork Coffee Creek/Sugar Pine, North Fork Coffee Creek Union Creek, Hardscrabble, South Fork Coffee Creek, Lady Gulch, Adams Lake, and Packers Peak trailheads to the Big Flat trailhead beside Big Flat Campground, 20.5 miles from Highway 3 and 0.7 mile past the road to Mountain Meadow Ranch. If you reach a gate across the road and signs for a private subdivision, you've gone 0.3 mile past Big Flat. Parking is available for about two dozen vehicles.

While conveniently located near the trailhead, Big Flat Campground is small, primitive, and usually overcrowded—particularly on weekends. Car camping is much more pleasant in developed campgrounds near Trinity Lake.

Description

The trail to Sunrise Basin begins on the east side of Coffee Creek Road above the Big Flat trailhead parking area and proceeds southeast through a couple of groves of Douglas firs alternating with extensive patches of brush and sparse Oregon oaks. A moderate, half-mile climb leads to the crossing of a crystal-clear stream in the bottom of a steep gully. Beyond the crossing the ascent continues through brush and white firs, as you cross several small seeps and streams, all heavily mineralized by the mines above.

After a moderately steep climb, you reach a flat and the Yellow Rose Mine, where, below a large rock dump, an upright boiler and the remnants of a rotary rock crusher provide historic interest. A short walk along the top of the dump bring you to the mouth of a caved-in drift running into the hill. A small stream of water runs from the drift, stinky and mineralized. A leaning, funny-looking, two-story shack to the south up a hill from the drift may not continue to stand through many more winters. Continue 0.2 mile beyond the mine on rough, steep tread to a junction with the Dorleska Mine Trail heading east, 2.5 miles from the trailhead.

Continue south from the junction across a meadow, where a tiny spring is below the trail. Beyond the meadow, you climb a shoulder of the ridge, and then rise more gradually along a bench in open forest of white firs and western white pines. A short, steep, washed-out pitch at the south end of the bench leads up to Leroy Mine, 3 miles from the trailhead, where a clear little stream flows beside the cabins. Several campsites in the vicinity provide the first decent places to camp so far.

A short climb from the Leroy Mine leads to a long contour, turning gradually southeast around the side of the mountain through open forest. The full profile of Caribou Mountain soon comes into view across South Fork Salmon River canyon. Until you see the peak from this perspective, or from an airplane, you have a difficult time realizing the full extent of the massive piece of granite that makes up Caribou Mountain.

An old prospect hole and a spring, badly trampled by cattle lie below a short, steep drop at the entrance to a basin at the head of Gulick Creek, 1 mile from the Leroy Mine, where the tip of Tri-Forest Peak peers over the south wall. The trail contours around the northeast side of the basin to a small meadow just below the headwall. Several springs run across the trail, but if cattle are present you may find the idea of acquiring water here unappealing. The trail snakes east up the headwall without benefit of any real switchbacks. A quarter mile of steep to very steep climbing over broken rock brings you to the crest above Sunrise Basin, 4.6 miles from the trailhead. Western white pines and foxtail pines stand among the rocks on the way up, but only the foxtails seem capable of surviving at the crest.

From the crest above Sunrise Basin, you can see all the way down South Fork Salmon River canyon and up to Packers Peak on the horizon. The fractured red bulk of aptly named Red Rock Mountain rears above the crest to the north. Landers Lake sits in a basin less than a mile away behind the mountain's east shoulder, but only a fairly accomplished mountaineer can scramble down from here. Beyond Sunrise Basin, Parker Meadow on the floor of Swift Creek canyon far below spreads out at your feet.

Heading down into Sunrise Basin, the trail contours south below the crest for about 200 yards, and then turns down to a ravine north of a small ridge composed of shattered rock. Two switchbacks at the bottom of the ravine lead to a dry bench. From the bench, the trail wanders down the north side of the basin, steeply at times, across more benches and both wet and dry meadows.

After skirting the foot of a huge pile of broken red rock that has slid off the side of Red Rock Mountain, descend more steeply across a strip of dry meadow and down a gravelly slope to the foot of a wet meadow, adorned with a mass of California pitcher plants. A substantial stream falls down a lush ravine a mile from the crest. Follow this creek downstream and cross to the far side, cross two more cascading channels above where they disappear into a huge tangle of willows, and then circle the south side of the willows to a large, level meadow on the floor of Sunrise Basin.

Even in late summer, a preponderance of flowers bloom in this meadow— goldenrods, sunflowers, yampa, and several varieties of daisies. The stream course across the meadow is typically dry below the willows by August, but the creek reappears in a ravine in the forest east of the meadow, providing a water source for some excellent campsites. Few people go through Sunrise Basin, making it a fine place to relax and escape the crowds. If you are seeking total solitude, climb over the south wall of the basin and into French Cove. However, neither Sunrise Basin nor French Cove offer any fishing or swimming opportunities. The junction with the trail down to Landers Creek is south of Sunrise Creek.

Side Trip to Landers Lake
From the junction you cross two more small meadows, and then descend moderately steeply through open fir forest to a junction between the Landers Creek Trail and Landers Lake Spur, 6.5 miles from Big Flat.

Landers Lake Spur 9W09A is mucky in spots as it contours around the east side of the wet meadow at the head of Landers Creek. You ascend moderately on a rocky slope north of the meadow and then turn west into a valley with a wall of red rock across the upper end. A short, steep climb leads to a gap at the north end of this dike, from which you continue ascending moderately up a wider valley west to a final, steeper pitch over the rim of the bowl holding Landers Lake, 0.6 mile from the junction.

There is a large, excellent campsite beside the trail where the path first climbs over the rim on the way to the lake. The trail continues a quarter mile to another large campsite northwest of the lake on the edge of the extensive meadows carpeting the upper part of the basin, a site used often by equestrians. There is a small, more secluded site sheltered by trees near the northeast shoreline. In spite of the lake's reduced size by late summer, the water remains cold and clear. Deer congregate in the beautiful meadows most evenings, and a constant chorus of frogs rises from two small ponds on the north- west side of the basin. Small eastern brook trout are plentiful but are difficult to catch. If you have the extra energy, a scramble up the ridge on the north side of the basin affords a fine view directly down toward Union Lake and Bullards Basin 1000 feet below.

The trail becomes a tad rougher below the Landers Creek junction, descend- ing south as the creek falls away southeast, with the last steep, quarter mile washed out and very rocky before you reach the edge of Mumford Meadow. Head south across the expansive meadow to the signed junction with the Swift Creek Trail, 1.6 miles from the Landers Lake Spur junction. The Swift Creek trailhead is 6 miles southeast down the canyon.

After the steep and rough descent down Landers Creek, the trail west up Swift Creek offers very pleasant hiking, with smooth tread rising gradually through alternating forest and meadow not far from the creek. The trail and the canyon turn southwest about a half mile from the junction, and you cross some boggy spots where small streams flow across the trail headed toward Swift Creek. Near the head of Swift Creek canyon, you turn west in a basin and climb moderately through a grove of white firs and across a small meadow toward a granite wall north of a red-colored peak. After a surprising grove of large cot- tonwoods at the edge of the meadow, a little creek runs down a steep pitch of trail, making the ascent a little difficult. You soon leave the creek behind, attack- ing a steep set of zigzags over broken rock and glaciated outcrops and through manzanita brush up to a small flat. A grove of red firs beside a small meadow offers a good spot to rest, but you'll have to travel another quarter mile up the trail to find water in a small creek, lined with shooting stars, lupine, yarrow, and mountain aster. Continue along the creek to a junction with the Ward Lake Trail in a small grove of red firs, 1.9 miles from the Landers Creek junction.

Horseshoe Lake sits in a granite cirque a half mile southwest of the junction. The rough trail snakes up over ledges, through a flat, and over a rock dike to the outlet of the 4-acre lake. The lake bends around a hump of glacier-resistant granite on the floor of the cirque to form a shape roughly resembling a horse- shoe. The outside curve on the west side is very brushy along the shoreline. Sparsely distributed mountain hemlocks, western white pines, and lodgepole

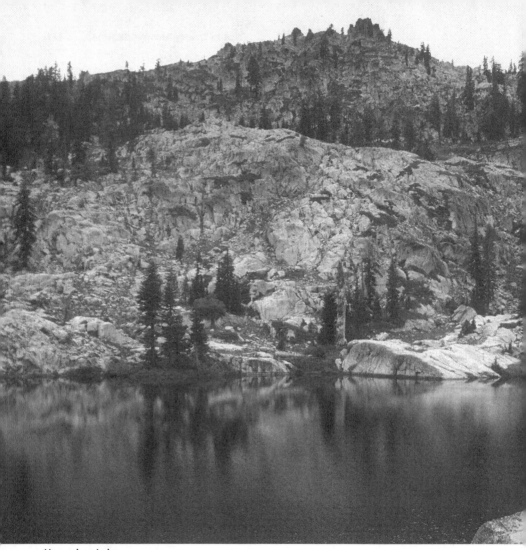

Horseshoe Lake

pines find footing among the rocks above the east shore and on the granite hump extending into the middle of the lake. The inside curve of the horseshoe has a more open shoreline, with rock ledges dropping off into deep water. Fishing is fair for small eastern brook trout. A couple of good campsites will lure overnighters on ledges east of the lake. Please avoid camping on the hump in the middle, as any waste will drain right into the water.

To resume the loop, retrace your steps a half mile to the Ward Lake Trail junction and turn north, ducking to cross a small creek before climbing into a grove of large red firs, snow-bent at the base of their trunks and shading a fair campsite. Small seeps and rivulets muddy the tread across the top of a wet, flower-filled meadow above the grove of firs, where the water streams down into small, deep pothole ponds that reflect the sky.

A steep climb north on rough tread takes you across a brushy hillside and up to some very large, scattered red firs. One or two of these trees must be more than 10 feet in diameter at the base. Beyond strips of meadow and more brush, you ascend very steeply around a granite shoulder and turn west into a red, metamorphic rock basin. Follow a small stream up a narrow, grass-floored gully to the east shore of Ward Lake, 0.7 mile from the Swift Creek Trail junction.

Gorgeous green meadows slope down to the shore of the 5.5-acre lake from the steep south and west sides of the basin. The lake is bent around a hump of rock in the opposite direction from that of Horseshoe Lake, with the outside of the curve to the east, with the outlet draining out of the east part of the curve. The shoreline is rocky, except where the meadows extend all the way to the shore, and the water is quite deep off the rocks on the inside of the curve. Two large, excellent campsites above the south shore and several other fair sites near the outlet and above the north shore offer overnight accommodations. Be prepared for deer wandering through your campsite. Adequate firewood should be available up the sides of the basin. A few spots in the steeply sloping meadow may appear level enough to tempt someone to camp there, but please avoid this temptation, as these subalpine grasslands are extremely fragile—damage to them would take many, many years to repair. Ward Lake seldom warms up enough for comfortable swimming. The large eastern brook trout inhabiting the lake tend to ignore all efforts cast their way. However, the showy sunsets and sunrises, reflected in the still water, are more than worth the price of admission.

After skirting the shore of Ward Lake, the trail dips into the edge of the wet meadow sloping down to the west shore, and then climbs into a grove of firs with a few more campsites. Beyond another strip of meadow north of the trees, you scramble up a very steep, rocky slope. Take the time to catch your breath and look back at the magnificent panorama to the southeast, where a lush, green vale falls away directly into Swift Creek canyon in the middle distance. On the far side of the canyon, hanging valleys decorate the walls leading up to the serrated ranks of the central Alps.

Reach the crest above Kidd Creek at 0.6 mile from Ward Lake. In addition to the panorama back east and south, you can now see all the way down Kidd

Sunset at Ward Lake

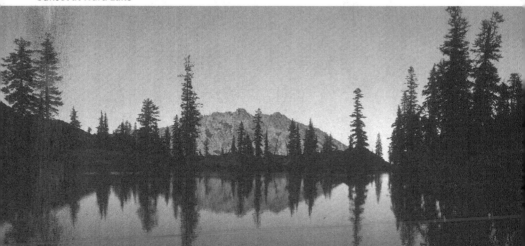

Creek and south across South Fork Salmon River canyon to Mountain Meadow Ranch and Packers Peak. The snowcapped tops of the Marble Mountains spike the horizon to the northwest, and Red Rock Mountain straddles the jagged ridge immediately to the north.

A set of short-legged, very steep switchbacks leads down the north side of the crest and into a cleft filled with huge red and gray talus blocks. Lingering snowbanks here suggest that you should not attempt this descent early in the season, at least not without an ice axe. The trail snakes down the cleft, in and out of talus on tread of broken rock and loose gravel, and then turns out onto a steep hillside on the southwest side of the canyon. The tread is better a half mile from the crest, as you pass a series of little ponds at the head of a meadow sloping north into the main canyon. A good campsite beside Kidd Creek in a grove of red firs and western white pines is another 0.3 mile farther down the trail.

On the southwest side of a large meadow, you continue a moderate descent northwest, and then drop away more steeply into mixed forest. At 2 miles from Ward Lake, you pass a waterfall in Kidd Creek. The next quarter mile of more moderate descent brings you out on a point of rock, with a view directly across South Fork Salmon River canyon of the face of Caribou Mountain. The trail turns south from the point of a ledge, and then descends steeply west down the side of a hill to a set of switchbacks. In predominantly Douglas-fir forest, you reach a junction with the Tri-Forest Trail, 3.8 miles from Ward Lake.

Turn north from the junction and soon cross the rocky bed of Kidd Creek. The creek usually dives underground by midsummer. North of Kidd Creek the trail climbs around the private land of Josephine Creek Lodge and switchbacks down to level tread that leads north through beautiful, open forest to a crossing of the Josephine Creek Lodge road. From the crossing, proceed ahead on good, gently graded tread through pleasant forest for another 2.5 miles to the Big Flat trailhead.

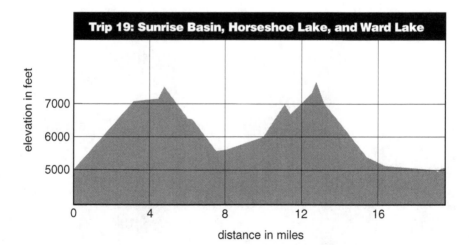

TRIP 20

Stoddard Lake, Doe Lake, and Eagle Creek

Two lovely lakes, eventual solitude, beautiful meadows, abundant wildflowers, climax forest, and good fishing

Trip Type:	Backpack, 3–5 days
Distance:	19.1 miles round-trip, point-to-point
Elevation Change:	13,250 feet, average 693 per mile
Difficulty:	Moderate
Season:	Early July to mid-October
Maps:	USGS *Tangle Blue Lake* and *Billys Peak*; USFS *A Guide to the Trinity Alps Wilderness*
Nearest Campgrounds:	Eagle Creek and Horse Flat

Two lakes, each very different, and a lonely creek canyon with beautiful meadows and climax forest await the adventurous hiker on this trip. Stoddard Lake, although relatively popular, offers plenty of campsites along a forested shoreline, good fishing, and the opportunity to explore off-trail routes to McDonald and Upper Stoddard lakes. Doe Lake, a smaller body of water, promises fewer visitors, dramatic scenery amid rugged surroundings, lush wildflower displays, and good fishing as well.

If solitude is what you're looking for, then upper Eagle Creek is one of the more remote areas in the eastern Trinity Alps. Chances are that you'll see more cows than people there, as cattle graze in a number of the beautiful meadows gracing the floor of the upper canyon and along the Eagle Creek Benches to the south. In spite of the grazing cattle, the meadows put on a marvelous display of wildflowers in midsummer.

Starting Point

Drive north on Highway 3, approximately 45 miles from Weaverville and 4.7 miles from Coffee Creek Road, to a left-hand turn onto County Road 135, signed for Eagle Creek and Horse Flat campgrounds. The narrow, paved road soon crosses the Trinity River on a one-lane bridge and then turns north. At 1.2 miles from the highway, another bridge spans Eagle Creek just before the entrance to Eagle Creek Campground.

Continue along a gravel road a short distance to a left-hand turn onto Forest Road 38N27, signed HORSE FLAT CAMPGROUND 3/4, EAGLE CREEK TRAIL 2, STODDARD LAKE TRAIL 7. Follow this road under dense climax forest cover past the entrance to Horse Flat Campground to another signed junction, 3.2 miles from the highway. Turn left at the junction, cross Eagle Creek again on a single-lane bridge, and then wind steeply up the road toward the Stoddard Lake trailhead. The

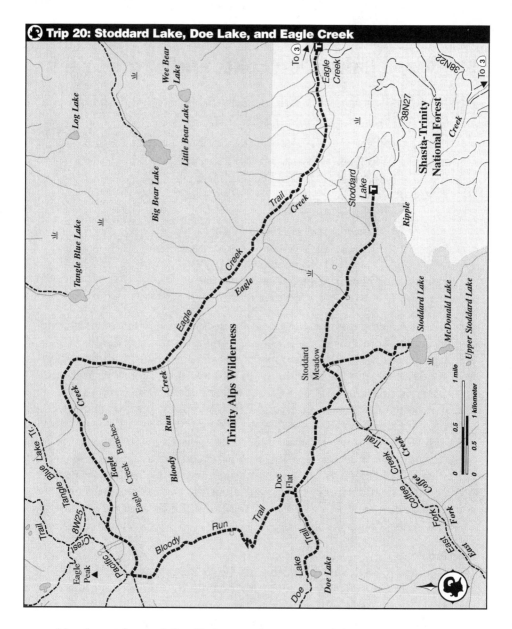

Trip 20: Stoddard Lake, Doe Lake, and Eagle Creek

road levels out for a while, climbs steeply again, and then reaches a fork on a hairpin turn, 5.8 miles from Highway 3.

Without a sign to guide you, follow the obviously more traveled road to the left, reaching a signed, three-way junction at 6.2 miles. Head right, as the road continues a zigzagging climb leading to wide-open views of Eagle Creek canyon and the steep ridge to the north. At 6.6 miles, you reach another junction, where a set of signs for the Stoddard Lake trailhead points your way uphill to the left. Continuing to climb, you pass a couple of spur roads before coming to yet another junction with a gated road straight ahead at 8.4 miles. Follow well-traveled Road 38N27 on steep, rocky switchbacks to the crest of a ridge and the trailhead on the left-hand shoulder, 10.1 miles from Highway 3. Parking is available for a half dozen cars along the side of the road.

Eagle Creek Campground has 17 sites and is equipped with vault toilets and running water ($10 per night fee in 2008). Free Horse Flat Campground has 16 sites with vault toilets but no running water.

Ending Point

At the signed junction 3.2 miles from Highway 3 mentioned above, veer to the right and proceed 0.25 mile to the Eagle Creek trailhead on a hairpin curve. Park your vehicle on the shoulder as space allows.

Description

From the end of the road, dirt and rock tread leads uphill through low brush interspersed with scattered pines and firs past the standard Trinity Alps Wilderness sign. About 0.4 mile into the hike, you reach a wide-open meadow covered with wildflowers and dotted with sporadic incense cedars and white firs. Posted to one of these cedars is a pair of wood signs pointing to the right (northwest) marked STODDARD LAKE, DOE LAKE. Without the aid of these signs, you might miss this junction; the faint, unmarked path on the left is the shorter, steeper, older route to Stoddard Lake. The signed, well-traveled path on the left is the newer, longer, and preferred trail, built by the U.S. Forest Service to replace the previous trail.

Continuing on the newer trail, follow good tread through the meadow before passing between two large cedars into deeper forest cover, where the meadow gives way to azaleas and ferns and the trail climbs again. The vegetation shifts to drier shrubs, primarily manzanita, after a quarter mile, where the grade eases to an ascending traverse across the shoulder of a ridge. Along this traverse, you have good views across the valley of the steep ridge on the north side of Eagle Creek and all the way to snowcapped Mt. Shasta on the horizon. The gentle ascent continues, as the terrain alternates between small meadows filled with wildflowers and grasses, and groves of evergreens floored with manzanita and ceanothus.

At 1.2 miles from the trailhead, you enter a large, lush, green meadow, carpeted in midsummer by colorful wildflowers. An icy-cold, spring-fed stream flows across the track, with California pitcher plants adorning the banks as the stream follows a meandering course through the meadow. Leaving the serenity of the meadow behind, the trail resumes a mild ascent beneath forest cover before beginning an equally mild descent toward Stoddard Meadow. Where the trail levels out, you reach the broad expanse of Stoddard Meadow, covered with tall wildflowers and meadow grasses and rimmed by tall, mature firs. Campsites beside the trail near the west end of the meadow will lure overnighters, with water nearby from the upper tributary of East Fork Coffee Creek. After crossing the tributary, you continue 0.1 mile to a flat, formerly the site of Stoddard Cabin, and reach a junction with the East Fork Coffee Creek Trail. Pay close attention on the approach to this junction, as the tread of the Stoddard Lake Trail turning sharply left vanishes in the tall grass for 50 feet or so (if you reach the next tributary of East Fork Coffee Creek, you should turn around and go back about 500 feet).

At the junction, 2.2 miles from the trailhead, turn left (south) and soon pick up more defined tread again near a trail sign. Immediately cross and then follow alongside the lushly vegetated banks of the creek beneath cool forest before crossing back over the creek. Leaving these pleasant surroundings behind, the tread becomes steep and rocky on the climb up to Stoddard Lake, as the vegetation shifts to manzanita, ceanothus, and pine forest. After climbing for 0.3 mile you reach a flat, with a glimpse of the rugged cliffs above the lake. The level reprieve is short-lived, as the climbing quickly resumes, eventually leading you to the north shore of the 25-acre, tree-rimmed lake.

A use trail encircles the entire shoreline, although a short rock scramble is required to successfully negotiate a cliff along the northwest shore. The path leads to many fine, widely spaced campsites, as well as access for anglers to fair to good fishing for small to medium eastern brook trout. Swimmers will find the water temperature acceptable by early summer. The drawbacks to the Stoddard Lake basin are few but noteworthy, including the area's popularity with both backpackers and equestrians, clouds of mosquitoes in early summer, and the possibility of having to share the area with grazing cows. With some planning and a little luck, you should find these minor hindrances.

Around the lake on the southeast shore lies a fair-sized meadow with a vigorous stream. Use trails alongside the stream lead on a nearly level, short stroll to much smaller McDonald Lake. If campsites are crowded at Stoddard Lake, the short hike to McDonald Lake may provide campers with more solitude. The more adventurous could opt for a short and easy climb up cliffs to a shelf on a shoulder of Billys Peak to tiny Upper Stoddard Lake, an almost surefire location for a little privacy.

Stoddard Lake

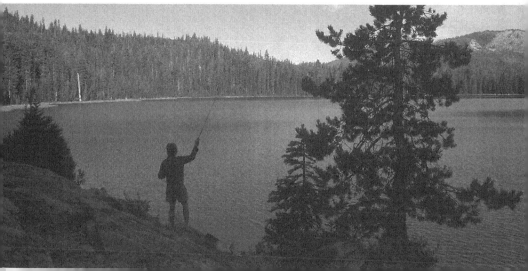

To continue your journey, retrace your steps 1 mile to the junction at Stoddard Meadow, turn left (west) onto the East Fork Coffee Creek Trail, cross the creek, and descend under forest cover 0.4 mile to a signed junction of the Doe Lake Trail.

From the junction, turn right and head northwest toward Doe Lake on a steep climb that attacks the hillside under the cover of white fir forest. Continue the climb, coming alongside another tributary of East Fork Coffee Creek, until you cross the tributary and head away from the creek's roaring cascades. The trail crosses a minor ridge, descends slightly, and then traverses a hillside covered with grass to the crossing of another stream. Climb away from the stream on the way to a ridge with a fine view. Traverse the far side of the ridge in and out of forest cover, gradually ascending into the meadows of Doe Flat.

Entering the meadows, you cross a small stream and pass a small flat on your left with campsites and a set of trail signs attached to a couple of pines, 6 miles from the trailhead; the signs denote a junction with the Bloody Run Trail heading north over a divide toward Eagle Creek. Plenty of evidence of animals can be found at Doe Flat: Cow pies are spread about, and many of the trees have scratch marks from bear claws. Although you stand a fair chance of hearing cowbells ringing, the odds of seeing a black bear are fairly remote.

Turn left (west) at the junction and head toward Doe Lake, which nestles into a basin scooped out of the cliffs above. Hop across a small creek near some campsites and come to a large field covered with corn lilies. More than likely, you'll encounter some muddy patches of trail as you cross this field; the condition of the tread depends on snowmelt and the amount of bovine traffic. Past the corn lily field, the trail heads back under forest cover and begins a moderate descent toward the lake. Alder thickets and stream channels greet you on the lower section until just before a stream crossing, where the terrain shifts to a dry, open hillside littered with granite glacial erratics. Reaching the top of a cliff, the grade moderates on a traverse to the right, and then the trail turns up a canyon to soon reach the north shore of 4.5-acre Doe Lake, 7.2 miles from the trailhead.

Doe Lake is an attractive little subalpine lake cradled into a granite cirque with a rugged, serrated peak to the southwest as a backdrop. The east side of the lake is forested, sheltering many excellent campsites, with the rest of the shoreline carpeted with lush vegetation. A rockslide above the southwest shore provides a particularly pleasing garden of wildflowers that include such species as aster, leopard lily, angelica, and heather. The lake offers the opportunity for solitude. Firewood is scarce, but fishing should be good for medium-sized eastern brook trout. Swimming in the 7000-foot lake is chilly until mid-August.

To resume the circuit, retrace your steps back to the trail junction at Doe Flat. From there, head north on the Bloody Run Trail and climb on dry, dusty tread straight uphill. Cross a creek coursing through an alder grove and then traverse the open hillside above. Along the ascent, fine views open up into the Doe Lake basin and the Coffee Creek drainage. Reach the crest of a ridge dividing the

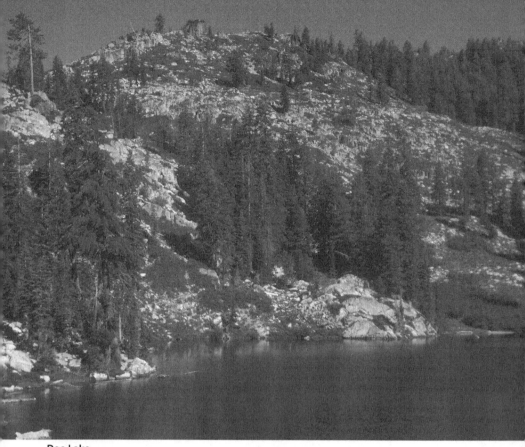

Doe Lake

drainages of Granite and Eagle creeks, where a rock knob offers good views of distant Mt. Shasta and the neighboring terrain.

Descend from the crest on good, sandy tread 0.3 mile to a patch of alders and wildflowers, where a piped spring offers clear, cold water and a lone campsite is nearby. Beyond the spring, you traverse the head of Bloody Run Creek canyon through open terrain composed of scattered firs and manzanita. The descent resumes, in and out of cool forest, until you reach the crossing of a seasonal stream. The trail climbs once more and, after two, short-legged switch-backs, reaches the top of a pass (located southwest of Peak 7272). Unfortunately, views from the pass are mostly obstructed by the forest.

The trail drops steeply from the pass through dense, primarily white-fir forest. After a mile or so, you begin a gradual ascent, which increases to moderate on the way toward a notch in the ridge above. At the top of a shady saddle, 2.6 miles from Doe Flat and 11 miles from the trailhead, you reach the rather undistinguished four-way junction with the Eagle Creek Trail. Signs at the junction provide directions to a variety of destinations, including the well-trod Pacific Crest Trail, 0.1 mile straight ahead to the north.

Turning right (south-southeast) you drop from the forested saddle into more open vegetation, which allows many magnificent views of lofty Mt. Shasta. A short distance farther, you pass through a series of small meadows sprinkled with colorful wildflowers. Upon reaching a larger meadow, the tread disappears, for the first but not last time in the lush meadows of Eagle Creek canyon; the trail becomes distinct again near a white fir tree with a blaze cut into the bark. Stay alert to blazes and cairns while traveling through the meadows, which may help guide you through several stretches of disappearing tread.

After negotiating another couple meadows by such means, a more defined section of trail skirts a patch of alders and then winds past a large downed tree into another large, open meadow, where the trail once again disappears. By staying headed in the same direction, you'll pick up defined tread again, paralleling Eagle Creek for a distance before crossing over to the north bank through a break in the alders, next to a very large, lone red fir. Fortunately, a large cairn also marks this crossing.

After crossing Eagle Creek, you locate the trail again by gazing straight up the meadow to the far hillside in front of you, where you can spy a very well-defined track leading steeply up the hill. Your first inclination may be to assume that this track is the route to Tangle Blue Lake and that the Eagle Creek Trail must be somewhere lower downstream. (You may even find a trail in that location—a use trail leading back across the creek and up onto Eagle Creek Benches, a fine area for off-trail exploration of wildflower-filled meadows, deep green forests, and tiny ponds). Your tired legs may push you toward the downstream route, but let wisdom prevail and head for the steep climb up the hillside away from the creek. Fortunately, the steep climb ends after 0.2 mile, as you reach a small flat and a signed junction with the Tangle Blue Lake Trail.

Turn to the right (east) at the junction and head downhill, paralleling Eagle Creek below on a moderate descent aided by a couple of switchbacks. Cross over a seasonal stream and enter a small meadow, where the track once again disappears—watch for cairns. After the meadow, the trail becomes distinct again until you reach another, much larger meadow covered with abundant wildflowers. This beautiful meadow is quite moist, which accounts for the preponderance of flowers, and travel can be a very soggy experience through here, especially in early summer. In general, this trail does not receive a lot of maintenance (a recent trail report listed 100 downed trees across the trail). Fortunately, the trail builders were kind enough to construct a raised section of trail in the upper part of the meadow, which helps keep your feet from becoming completely mud-soaked. Watch for ducks in the lower, drier portion of the meadow.

Your trail down the canyon continues to wander through more meadows and open forest north of Eagle Creek, past many excellent campsites between the trail and the creek. Few people visit this part of the canyon but, for a couple months each summer, numerous cows graze here. As you enter dense white-fir forest, 2 miles from the junction, the canyon closes in and bends south. Another half mile of hiking brings you onto a steep slope far above the creek. Work your way down 0.7 mile of boulders and ruts on the way back toward the creek. As you descend, the trail makes a short detour around some trees knocked over by an avalanche. A number of good campsites appear on the benches beside Eagle

Creek, where the floor of the canyon levels a little. Stealthy fishing may reward you with a pan full of native trout up to 8 to 9 inches long.

As the canyon veers southeast and you descend moderately, Douglas firs dominate the mature forest and head-high ferns crowd the trail in moist spots. You continue the descent, well away from the creek again. Plenty of water is available from numerous creek crossings on your way down the canyon. The approach of civilization becomes a reality at the wilderness boundary, where you may notice several property-line and survey markers nailed to trees just beyond a stand of black oaks on a steep hillside about 100 yards above the creek. Even without the posted signs, you sense almost immediately that you're leaving the wilderness behind, as you step out of virgin forest onto a logged flat and, directed by a trail sign and steel posts, step onto a graded and graveled haul road. The only good thing to say about this road, other than providing some easy walking, is that it doesn't appear to be open to public vehicles.

At a junction a mile or so down the road, keep right for another quarter mile to a log-loading flat, where a signed trail turns up the hill on the left, 50 yards before the end of the road. Climb steeply through tall grass, and then turn to contour southeast again through beautiful mixed forest, which now includes ponderosa pines and sugar pines. This welcome section of trail provides a pleasant change from the hot, dusty road. After detouring into two deep ravines with little creeks shaded by dogwoods and bigleaf maples, you descend moderately steeply across a dry hillside, where canyon oaks appear for the first time on the way down the canyon.

About 8 miles from the PCT junction, you come close to the creek, pouring through a wide bed of boulders, and then climb up the side of the canyon again to where a creek falls over a concrete wall just above the trail—part of the former water system for Horse Flat Campground. The exit trailhead is another 0.2 mile ahead, 7.4 miles from the Tangle Blue Lake Trail junction at the upper end of Eagle Creek canyon.

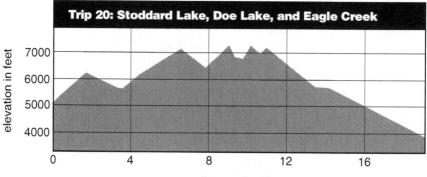

TRIP 21

Big, Little, and Wee Bear Lakes

Gorgeous Trinity Alps Lakes near the wilderness's eastern boundary

Trip Type:	Dayhike or 2- to 3-day backpack
Distance:	9.4 miles round-trip, out-and-back
	(plus 1.5 mile round-trip cross-country to Little Bear Lake)
Elevation Change:	3200 feet, average 561 per mile
Difficulty:	Moderate
Season:	Late June to early October
Maps:	USGS *Tangle Blue Lake*
	and USFS *A Guide to the Trinity Alps Wilderness*
Nearest Campground:	Eagle Creek

Big Bear Lake, along with off-trail companions Little Bear, Wee Bear, and Log lakes, are the easternmost of all the Trinity Alps lakes. Thanks to a 4-mile jog of the wilderness area boundary, these four lakes enjoy wilderness protection. Had the powers that be not approved this boundary deviation, the Trinity Alps Wilderness would have been greatly diminished.

Outstanding examples of Trinity Alps lakes, Big Bear and Little Bear are both set in granite cirques on the north sides of rugged peaks visible from Highway 3 north of Eagle Creek. Wee Bear is a diminutive, forest-rimmed pond, which shares Little Bear's cirque but not its stature. Although not particularly high in elevation (5800 and 6240 feet, respectively) the steep-sided cirques face north, oftentimes retaining patches of snow well into midsummer. The deep waters are correspondingly cold. Seclusion appears to be the main attraction of diminutive Log Lake.

Despite the nearly 50-mile distance from Weaverville, the trip to Bear Lakes is fairly popular. Campsites at Big Bear Lake (by far the easiest of the four lakes to reach) are limited and competition may be fierce on weekends—check with the Weaverville ranger station to see how many wilderness permits have been issued for the time you'd like to visit). The slightly less than 10-mile round-trip distance makes dayhiking to Big Bear a distinct possibility, although the area might be overcrowded. Fishing is good for eastern brook trout up to 12 inches, and an abundance of granite offers excellent climbing and scrambling opportunities.

Starting Point

The Bear Lakes Road veers left from Highway 3 at Sunflower Flat, near a sign reading BEAR LAKES TRAIL 1 1/2. This junction is just below a bridge to the east bank of the Trinity River, 8 miles north of the Coffee Creek junction and

⟳ Trip 21: Big, Little, and Wee Bear Lakes

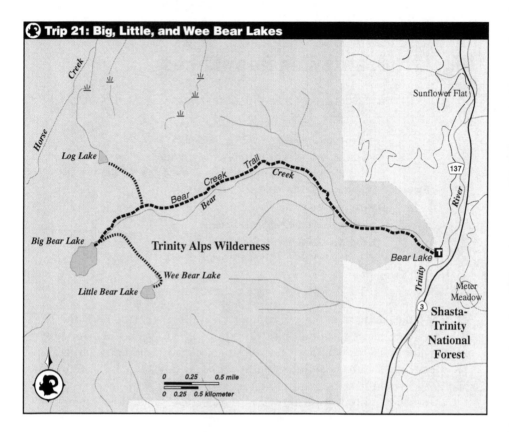

approximately 48 miles north of Weaverville. Pass Sunflower Flat Cabins and continue to where the road is blocked by boulders, 1.2 miles from the highway and just before a bridge over Bear Creek. Limited parking is available near the trailhead signboard.

Description

Walk across the bridge and continue up the dirt road about 200 yards to the start of single-track trail on the right, where a sign marked simply TRAIL points you uphill. The path climbs steeply away from the road via a pair of short-legged switchbacks and then continues northwest along the side of Bear Creek canyon to a flat, where the ascent moderates through an open forest of Douglas firs, incense cedars, and canyon oaks. Farther up, the narrowing canyon pushes the trail closer toward the stream on the way to a stout bridge across Bear Creek.

Beyond the crossing the trail climbs more steeply to a switchback and then up to a ridge separating the main branch of Bear Creek from the much smaller northern branch. Follow the crest of this razorback ridge to four long-legged switchbacks, followed by an upward traverse northwest across the side of the canyon through scattered western white pines, huckleberry oaks, and manzanitas.

Now you turn north away from the creek on steep, worn, and washed-out tread through mixed forest until the trail turns west among granite boulders and then levels out headed southwest in a pleasant valley adorned with patches of fern-covered meadow. Beyond, a short climb through dense forest is interrupted briefly by a narrow avalanche swath, followed by more dense forest, and then another, wider avalanche swath. Through momentary openings in the vegetation, you catch fleeting glimpses of the vertical granite headwall at the head of Bear Creek canyon. Before midseason, you'll see ribbons of water streaming down rocks to the southwest (the outflow from Wee Bear and Little Bear lakes).

Steep to very steep trail traverses the side of the canyon southwest through alder thickets, where rills periodically spill across and sometimes down the trail. Wildflowers and water-loving plants are present in abundance here, and parts of the trail are nearly overgrown with the thick, tall brush. Proceed up the canyon through dense foliage to a small flat shaded by mountain hemlocks and western white pines and then emerge onto open, tilted slabs of bare granite. Bear Creek raucously spills down the canyon about 200 yards to the south, as you follow ducks along the right-hand edge of the slabs toward the lake. Past the field of granite, you continue through low brush, boulder hop the outlet, and make a short climb from there to the lake.

Big Bear Lake, at 28 acres, is one of the larger Trinity Alps lakes. The nearly vertical granite walls of the lake's cirque rise directly from the water in semicircular fashion. Crevices in the north-facing wall may hold onto snowbanks

Big Bear Lake

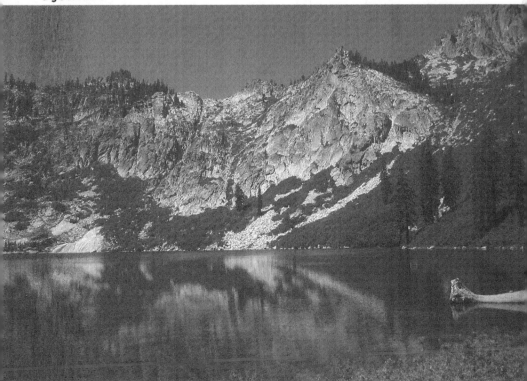

well into August in some years. The northeast shoreline is covered with thick brush that grows right up to the water's edge, accented by scattered white firs, Jeffrey pines, mountain hemlocks, and western white pines. A few campsites are jammed between the brush along the north shore close to the outlet and above on a granite shoulder. Due to the open nature of the surroundings, privacy may be hard to come by unless you happen to be alone at the lake. Fishing for eastern brook trout to 12 inches is best from the log jam at the outlet and off the steep, rocky shoreline on the east side.

At the conclusion of your stay at Bear Lakes, the rewards haven't completely ended, as you'll have fine views of Mt. Shasta from the upper part of the canyon on the return leg.

Cross-Country Route to Wee Bear and Little Bear Lakes

When contemplating the easiest route to Wee Bear and Little Bear lakes, the first temptation may be to travel around the east shore and ascend a broad gap up to the ridge. While reaching the lakes is possible this way, an easier route ascends the northeast ridge a short distance back down the canyon from Big Bear Lake. Ascend granite benches east above the lakeshore camping area to game trails crisscrossing through brush that lead to granite shelves above. The goal is to bisect the top of the ridge at approximately the midpoint near some dead trees. From the ridgecrest you can see a notch about 0.5 mile away through which the outlet of Wee Bear Lake flows.

Make a straightforward traverse toward this notch, which may necessitate some minor ups and downs along the way, aided by ducks and cairns. Views down Bear Creek canyon along the traverse are quite impressive. At the notch you arrive at Wee Bear Lake, which in contrast to Big Bear and Little Bear lakes is not particularly dramatic. If you choose to camp here rather than around the more impressive lake above, there are certainly places to do so.

The route between Wee Bear and Little Bear lakes requires little time or effort. Simply follow the lakeshore to the southeast end of Wee Bear Lake and cross the marshy patch to where an obvious use trail ascends the west side of a creek flowing from the upper lake. In no time at all, you will reach the north shore of Little Bear Lake.

Little Bear Lake appears to be a smaller version of Big Bear Lake. The clear, cold waters are ringed on three sides by impressive granite cliffs, where snowbanks may linger late into the season as well, and the conifers seem to be of the same type and arrangement. However, there are two important differences between the two lakes: Little Bear Lake's east shore has fine campsites without the shrubby vegetation that nearly covers Big Bear Lake's shore, and you'll likely see far fewer campers than at the more popular lower lake. The cross-country route will require an expenditure of time and effort, but the route is not difficult and you'll be well rewarded. Fishing is much better at Little Bear, more than likely due to less pressure.

Cross-Country Route to Log Lake

The off-trail route to Log Lake is easy to see but hard to accomplish for one reason: the unrelenting battle of the brush, but while I was camped at Big Bear Lake, a group of junior high students from Camp Unalayee descended this route without incident. From

Big Bear Lake, descend the trail about a quarter to half mile and then make an angling ascent toward the obvious (although not always visible from below) saddle directly southeast of Log Lake. At the saddle, pick your way down to the lake, which is nestled in a delightful cirque. Camping is limited.

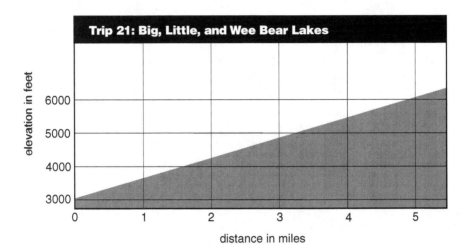

TRIP 22

Tangle Blue Lake

The lake is even more charming than the name.

Trip Type:	Dayhike or 2-day backpack
Distance:	6.6 miles round-trip, out-and-back
Elevation Change:	940 feet, average 930 per mile
Difficulty:	Moderate
Season:	Mid-June to mid-October
Maps:	USGS *Tangle Blue Lake* and USFS *A Guide to the Trinity Alps Wilderness*
Nearest Campgrounds:	Eagle Creek and Scott Mountain

What self-respecting hiker can resist a moderate 3.3-mile stroll to a lake with such a charming name? Legend suggests that Tangle Blue Lake and Creek were named by an early resident of the area who started his trip into the wilderness after awaking from a long night of partying to find his feet tangled and the air blue. No matter what it's named, this lake is a worthy destination for both dayhikers and backpackers. The final approach travels through a large, lush meadow, where nearly ideal campsites nestle under large firs.

A picturesque inlet creek tumbles down the rocks above the south shore to meander through a riot of colorful wildflowers in a wet meadow before flowing into the lake. Additional smaller meadows alternate with rock ledges and brush around the rest of the shoreline. Anglers can walk around the entire lake with relative ease to fish for fair-sized eastern brook trout and rainbows.

Rugged pinnacles top the crests on the west, south, and east sides of Tangle Blue Lake's basin, where rock climbers and scramblers will find the views from the ridgetops quite rewarding. The lake itself offers excellent swimming opportunities. Tangle Blue Lake might not be the best place for solitude, but the distance from Weaverville ensures that it's not overrun. Groups of youths from Camp Unalayee, located at Mosquito Lake, hike to the lake with some regularity, but otherwise the lake receives less visitation than hikers might expect.

Starting Point

Unfortunately, vandals seem to covet the Tangle Blue Lake sign marking the junction between the road to the trailhead and Highway 3, which creates some difficulty for first-timers attempting to find the right turnoff. Highway 3 turns northwest away from the upper Trinity River at a junction with Forest Road 17, approximately 51 miles north of Weaverville, and begins a climb toward Scott Mountain Summit, located at the northeast corner of the Trinity Alps. After a mile of climbing, you cross Scott Mountain Creek on a steel-culvert and

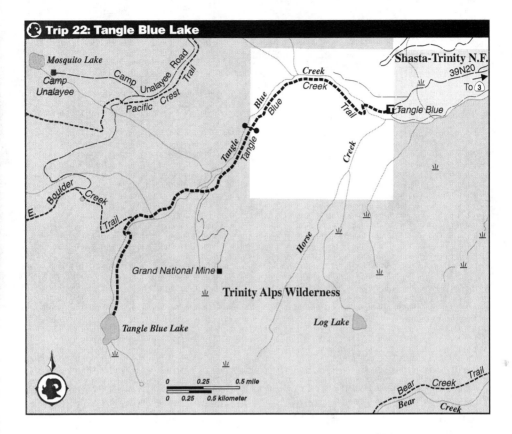

Trip 22: Tangle Blue Lake

Mosquito Lake

Camp Unalayee

Camp Unalayee Road

Pacific Crest Trail

Creek

Creek

Shasta-Trinity N.F.

39N20

To 3

Tangle Blue

Tangle Blue

Tangle Blue

Creek

Boulder Creek

Trail

Horse

Grand National Mine

Trinity Alps Wilderness

Tangle Blue Lake

Log Lake

0   0.25   0.5 mile

0   0.25   0.5 kilometer

Bear Creek Trail

Bear Creek

concrete bridge in the middle of a hairpin turn. The wide, dirt haul road that leads to the trailhead forks left from the very next curve above the bridge. If you reach a second bridge across Scott Mountain Creek, you've gone 0.25 mile too far up the hill.

The initial stretch of Forest Road 39N20 crosses private land, as you climb very steeply for about 200 yards and then turn west across the side of Tangle Blue Creek canyon. The road draws near the creek around the 1.2-mile mark, where you cross a seasonal creek and then turn north uphill again. At 2.0 miles, Road 39N20A takes off to the right as your road continues left and traverses the side of the canyon far above the creek. Near the high point of this traverse, about 2.8 miles from Highway 3, Road 39N59 forks right (north) up the hillside. Stay left at this intersection, and travel another 0.75 mile to the trailhead at a broad, sweeping intersection, 3.6 miles from the highway. The trail begins beyond the ample parking area, past a locked gate across the roadway.

Description

From the trailhead, descend along the road about 200 yards to a steel and wood bridge across Tangle Blue Creek. Once across the creek, you climb steeply up a dry and dusty roadbed with the aid of a couple of switchbacks, where seeps

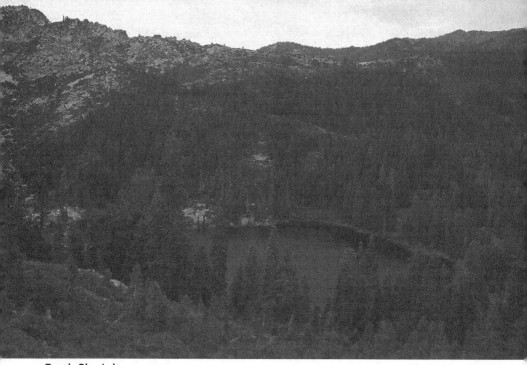

Tangle Blue Lake

refresh a narrow strip of lush plants and wildflowers along the edge. The climb continues through scattered forest beside the tumbling waters of the creek, never more than a stone's throw away, reaching the signed wilderness boundary at a steel gate, 1.5 miles from the trailhead. In former days, driving all the way to this point was possible, but fortunately the Forest Service wisely relocated the trailhead some time ago.

Away from the wilderness boundary the climb continues up the old roadbed, passing some primitive campsites and a lushly vegetated hillside covered with green grasses and colorful wildflowers. A short climb up the hillside leads to an informal junction, 1.9 miles from the trailhead, with an overgrown road that formerly took miners a steep mile up to the Grand National Mine. A brief descent away from this old road leads through drier vegetation and across a tributary stream. A short distance farther, you cross the main branch of Tangle Blue Creek and then turn upstream on single-track trail.

Passing through a mixed forest composed of Douglas firs, incense cedars, and sugar pines, the trail switchbacks and rejoins the old road for another 0.25 mile. Back on single-track trail, you proceed to a crossing of the creek draining Little Marshy Lake—in early season a footlog crossing may be necessary to avoid wet boots. On the far side of the creek, pick up the road again and make a moderately steep climb on rocky tread to a signed junction with the East Boulder Lake Trail, 2.5 miles from the trailhead.

Turn left (southwest) and leave the road behind for good, proceeding on the Tangle Blue Lake Trail to a beautiful sloping meadow filled with tall grasses and dotted with seasonal wildflowers. Through the trees you have your first glimpse of the rock cliffs of Tangle Blue Lake's cirque, now less than a mile away. Toward the far end of the meadow the trail dives to a crossing of Tangle Blue Creek. On the opposite bank is a tangled pile of old boards and rusty stove parts, all that remains of the Messner Cabin.

Away from the creek the trail begins a moderately steep climb through a light, mixed forest on the way to a lush area filled with willow thickets, alders, ferns, grasses, and wildflowers. A number of rivulets trickle across the path, giving life-sustaining moisture to leopard lilies, columbines, and other assorted wildflowers. At 0.5 mile from the site of Messner Cabin, the grade eases at the large meadow just north of the lake. A pleasant stroll across the meadow leads to the north shore of lovely Tangle Blue Lake.

Nearly surrounded by steep, gray cliffs, Tangle Blue Lake sits in the bottom of a deep basin, the placid surface reflecting the walls and pinnacles towering above. Just above the north shore, a lake view, mortared rock fireplaces, and level spots beneath grand white firs near a stream add up to a highly coveted camping area. Additional campsites, perhaps offering a little more solitude, may be available west of the outlet stream near a small meadow, or above the far end of the lake. A use trail encircles the lake but may be muddy or overgrown with brush in parts. Anglers will appreciate the relatively easy access to the shoreline, but the fair-sized trout may test their skill and patience. Swimmers will find that the cool lake water provides a refreshing break from the normally warm afternoon temperatures. Rock climbers and scramblers will find plenty of challenges scattered around the cirque. Marshy and Boulder lakes are close enough for day trip extensions.

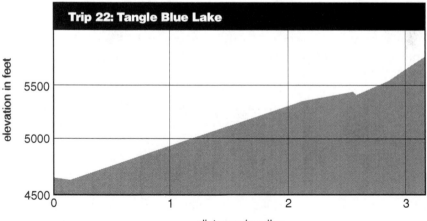

TRIP 23

Pacific Crest Trail: Scott Mountain Summit to Carter Meadows Summit

This section of the famed PCT is a marvelous way to see the eastern Trinity Alps on some of its best trails.

Trip Type:	Backpack, 3–5 days
Distance:	18.4 miles, point-to-point (plus 1.6-mile side trip to Telephone Lake and 1.3-mile side trip to Upper South Fork Lake)
Elevation Change:	6785 feet, average 369 per mile
Difficulty:	Moderate
Season:	Early July to early October
Maps:	USGS *Scott Mountain, Tangle Blue Lake, Billys Peak*, and *Deadman Peak*; USFS *A Guide to the Trinity Alps Wilderness*
Nearest Campgrounds:	Scott Mountain and Hidden Horse

The 18 miles of Pacific Crest Trail within the Trinity Alps Wilderness is without question the best-built 18 miles of trail in the area. Paradoxically, this stretch of trail receives much less use than many of the area's other trails, despite being very scenic, easy to hike, and close to a string of lakes. One reason for this lack of traffic is the location near the 2,600-mile trail's midpoint and far from any population center. Consequently, only very serious PCT thru-hikers, starting from either Mexico or Canada, get this far. The lack of attention is certainly a boon for those who opt to hike this section.

The PCT comes within a mile of each of a beautiful series of lakes north of the Scott River crest. From east to west, they include East Boulder, Middle Boulder, Telephone, West Boulder, Mavis, Fox Creek, Section Line, Virginia, and upper and lower South Fork lakes. Although many of these scenic lakes are not described in this particular trip, they all can be easily reached from the PCT, along with Marshy and Mosquito lakes, south of the Scott River crest.

Along with the strong potential for solitude, the PCT offers ridgecrest hiking abounding in spectacular vistas of such notable mountains as Mt. Shasta, Lassen Peak, and the central Trinity Alps. Much of the trail has been constructed to be a relatively mild grade, which, in combination with the excellent tread, makes for pleasant hiking. Also, this section of the PCT passes through a variety of vegetative zones, including meadows, chaparral, and evergreen forests. You will have to descend into various drainages to locate decent campsites, but because of the attractions of the aforementioned lakes, doing so can hardly be considered a drawback. Solitude, panoramic vistas, and diversity make hiking this 18-mile stretch of the PCT well worth the effort.

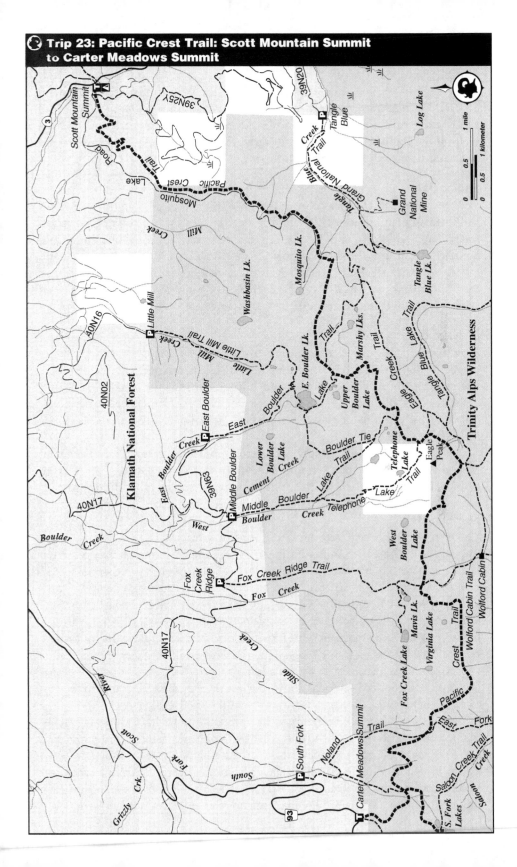

Starting Point

The Pacific Crest Trail crosses Highway 3 at the very top of Scott Mountain Summit, 56 miles north of Weaverville, and then continues west to the north of Scott Mountain Campground. Following signs for the PCT, park your vehicle well off the highway but not in the campground. The free 5-site campground has vault toilets but no running water or trash pickup.

Ending Point

Continue north on Highway 3 from Scott Mountain Summit and drop 8.5 miles to the small community of Callahan. Immediately north of town, turn left at the junction of Forest Road 93, heading toward Cecilville, Forks of Salmon, and Somes Bar. Climb 11.7 miles on Forest Road 93 to Carter Meadows Summit and the signed Pacific Crest Trail parking area on the left, which is also the trailhead for Hidden Lake (Trip 25, see page 207). The paved parking area is equipped with a vault toilet and is located just below a heliport.

Description

From the Scott Mountain trailhead, follow good tread across a flat to two long-legged switchbacks and a shorter one leading to the top of a hump (6380 feet). Away from the hump, continue west through manzanita and open woods along the crest of the ridge. An unusual combination of sugar pines and lodgepole pines appears before you enter a sparse forest of red firs on the way to a saddle.

Mountain mahogany, usually considered more of an eastern Sierra or Great Basin tree, grows on a rocky hump after more switchbacks. Cross to the north side of the divide in fir forest, 2.7 miles from the trailhead, and emerge onto more open slopes before returning to red-fir forest just before the signed wilderness boundary.

From the boundary you circle the side of a mountain to turn southwest into a saddle, 4 miles from the trailhead, where the PCT crosses the crest right beside, but not on, the Mosquito and Marshy lakes road. From there, the PCT drops away from the road and traverses an open and brushy slope, with excellent views across Tangle Blue Creek canyon to the jumble of peaks beyond the Grand National Mine hanging on the side of a ridge. Lassen Peak juts into the horizon far in the distance, and the backside of Castle Crags is nearer and a little farther down. Cross a pair of small streams and another, slightly larger rill a short distance farther, which waters a large garden of California pitcher plants on the hillside above. After rounding the shoulder of a ridge, you turn west to cross the Marshy Lakes Road, 6.1 miles from the trailhead.

Away from the road, you cross a tiny stream lined with California pitcher plants running across a flat to the west and continue another 250 yards to a ravine. The ravine holds a much larger stream that drains from Mosquito Lake above, which is home to Camp Unalayee, a summer camp with two-week sessions for kids between ages 10 and 17. Since hundreds of campers swim each day in Mosquito Lake, you may want to consider acquiring water elsewhere.

Beyond Mosquito Lake creek, the PCT contours to the shoulder of a ridge overlooking the upper end of Tangle Blue Creek canyon and the lower end of Marshy Lakes basin, although the Marshy Lakes remain out of sight. The road to Marshy Lakes is directly below, and you should be able to see Tangle Blue Lake shimmering in a cirque farther south. Regal Mt. Shasta crowns the horizon back to the northeast.

The PCT rises gradually from the shoulder, heading generally west along the north side of the Marshy Lakes basin. Cross over a path connecting Camp Unalayee and Marshy Lakes, marked only by cairns above and below the tread, 1 mile from the road crossing. After another 0.5 mile along the side of the basin, both Marshy Lakes spring into view below. You may notice that Upper Marshy Lake is aptly named, as the lake is indeed surrounded by marshes.

Great effort was expended in making this section of the PCT across this steep hillside a first-class trail. Brush was cut back three feet on both sides of the tread, large rocks were removed to avoid steep detours and, where the trail crosses talus slides, the tread was blasted, dug out, and leveled, and dirt was hauled in to fill the cracks. Time will tell if the trail will be maintained as well as it was built. The metasedimentary rock is rosy red to rust-colored on the surface, but when broken appears grayish dark blue to indigo, mixed with flecks of light blue and white.

As you turn southwest around the head of a basin, a trail from Marshy Lakes, marked by signs nailed to a large tree, crosses the PCT on the way toward East Boulder Lake. The crest is merely 200 yards up this little-used trail, with East Boulder Lake 0.6 mile down the north side. Even if you don't want to make the side trip to the lake, you should at least climb up to the ridge for the view of East Boulder's wide-open basin: Three little ponds, surrounded by meadows as green as billiard-table felt, sit on a wide shelf a quarter mile below the crest, and a long strip of grass runs up through red rock strata almost to the crest farther west. Bordered by more meadows, 32-acre East Boulder Lake fills the lower end of the basin below a drop-off. East Boulder Lake receives a fair amount of traffic from the north side because a road comes within 2 miles of the lake. Anglers can test their skill on some fairly large eastern brook, rainbow, and brown trout. The only drawback to this otherwise delightful haven is the possibility of cattle grazing nearby.

Mt. Shasta from Marshy Lakes Road

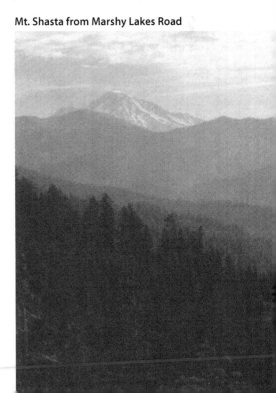

The PCT continues contouring around the head of Marshy Lakes basin through rough terrain behind some knobs and across the face of cliffs, where the tread has been blasted out of the rock. A beautiful little spring trickles down the rocks beside the trail, 0.3 mile from the East Boulder Lake Trail. After contouring around the basin, you're headed almost due east, and then you climb moderately south to a spur ridge between Marshy Lakes and Eagle Creek canyon, 7 miles from the trailhead. From there, the trail turns west to ascend another spur ridge and along the side of the main ridge through brush, open forest, and talus slides. Several small ponds occupy a wide bench a quarter mile below the trail, offering a good place to camp if you're ready to stop for the day. After rounding the shoulder of another spur ridge, you reach a junction with the Middle Boulder Lake Trail right on top of the Scott River Divide, 2.4 miles from the East Boulder Lake Trail junction. The Middle Boulder Lake Trail heads north down the divide slope past two small ponds to Middle Boulder Lake, a repeat of East Boulder Lake on a smaller scale. The Middle Boulder basin is not as big, or as verdant, as the East Boulder basin.

From the Middle Boulder Lake junction, the PCT drops away from the divide through a forest of foxtail pines that changes to red firs as you go farther down the side of the ridge. The trail skirts the edges of two meadows, and then rises slightly to run across a third meadow, from where you have a fine view of 7790-foot Eagle Peak. Continue to the upper, southwest edge of the meadows, enter back into forest cover, and soon reach a junction with the Telephone Lake Trail, 0.4 mile from the Middle Boulder junction.

Side Trip to Telephone Lake

Once you locate the rather indistinct beginning of the Telephone Lake Trail, the path is not hard to follow. A cairn in the edge of the meadow and blazed trees mark where the trail turns west to zigzag up a hill away from the meadow. Look for blazes on large foxtail pines at the upper end of a smaller meadow higher up the slope, which lead to the crest of the divide, 0.25 mile from the junction. West of the crest, the trail drops very steeply to a heavily grazed meadow, and then turns northwest to descend steeply again, not far from a small stream that drains the meadow. As you emerge on a low ridge that trends north-south, 0.4 mile from the crest, look east for the lake.

Telephone Lake is an irregularly shaped, 3.5-acre pothole lake with no outlet or permanent inlet. Consequently, the water level fluctuates 3 to 4 feet during the course of the summer. A little bay at the north end, separated from the rest of the lake, gets warm enough for good swimming by late summer. Anglers can test their skill on large rainbow trout that occasionally rise.

Just beyond the Telephone Lake junction, the PCT passes a junction with a trail descending toward Eagle Creek, and then descends around the southeast flank of Eagle Peak, mostly through thick fir forest. A fair-sized creek flows across the trail through a tangle of alders 0.5 mile farther. Beyond the creek, a fine spring flows from an iron pipe above the trail. There's a fair campsite below the trail past the spring, on a site that once held a miner's cabin. A second spring, a quarter mile farther along the trail, is piped through a piece of old, riveted sheet-iron mining pipe. Climb away from this spring to an obvious junction with the Bloody Run Trail heading south. About 100 yards down this trail, the Eagle Creek Trail heads east down Eagle Creek canyon and the Granite Lake Trail heads west toward Wolford Cabin.

The PCT continues on an ascending traverse along the south ridge of Eagle Peak to an open saddle on top of the divide. A small rock knob (7511 feet) east of the saddle presents a grand opportunity for some magnificent views, north down the West Boulder Creek drainage, south across to the central Trinity Alps peaks, and east toward Lassen Peak. For more adventurous peakbaggers, a 475-foot climb to the summit of Eagle Peak is possible through low, open brush up the west ridge, where you'll have even grander views.

A short descent bottoms out at another saddle, above West Boulder Creek canyon. Campsites with nearby water are available down in this pastoral canyon, but, without a trail, you'll have to travel cross-country to reach them. Another mountainside traverse, beginning in open vegetation and then through fir forest, crosses a lushly lined creek before coming to the junction of the Wolford Cabin Trail in yet another saddle on top of the ridge, 1.2 miles from the previous saddle. By turning north on this trail, you can access Mavis and Fox Creek lakes.

The PCT contours around another unnamed peak, breaks out of the trees briefly onto a manzanita-covered slope around a spur ridge, and then makes a long, descending traverse to a three-channeled tributary of Granite Creek, 1.7 miles from the previous junction. Another 1.2-mile traverse leads around another ridge and over to an open saddle, where you meet the junction of the East Fork Saloon Creek Trail.

From the junction, the PCT crosses the crest to the north side of the Scott River Divide and then heads downhill to follow the course of an old roadbed, as you enjoy this trip's last views of the central Trinity Alps peaks. In another 0.2 mile, you reach a junction with the little-used Noland Trail, which descends on the continuation of the old road to the site of the abandoned Loftus Mine.

Back on newer, single-track trail, the PCT trends slightly uphill across the head of a meadow basin strewn with wildflowers and rimmed by rock cliffs. Cresting a ridge, the trail rounds the head of the next basin and descends to the crossing of the east branch of South Fork Scott River, 1.1 miles from the Noland Trail junction. A spring a short distance upstream gives birth to this lovely watercourse. The trail drops away from the stream crossing and continues 0.8 mile to a junction with the South Fork Lakes and South Fork Ridge trails in a lush green meadow covered with wildflowers.

Side Trip to South Fork Lakes
The route to the lakes is short but quite steep. Begin the ascent amid lush underbrush beneath tall firs, reaching a small basin with a steep rock headwall rising straight up from the basin floor after 0.2 mile. A lone campsite is at the near edge of this basin, quite suitable if you're not interested in continuing the arduous ascent up to the lakes.

If you decide to go on, the trail proceeds through some tall grass, winds up along the stream, and then immediately crosses over to the far bank. From there, the trail bends sharply uphill and then abruptly traverses to the right (northwest) through tall, dense vegetation, passing many seeps and rivulets flowing down from springs above. A series of switchbacks leads to the top of a rise, where the grade mercifully eases. From there, the first lake is just a short jaunt away.

Lower South Fork Lake is a pleasant, but rather uninspiring, little lake. Plenty of the necessities for camping are present here in abundance, but the little extra effort required to reach the upper lake is well worth the expenditure. To reach the upper lake, walk around the lower lake to the inlet, follow the trail along the west bank, and reach the north shore of the upper lake in 0.1 mile.

Upper South Fork Lake is certainly more picturesque than its lower neighbor, with a steep slope rising up out of the opposite shore and leading to rugged, rock cliffs above. The abundant vegetation along the shore may slightly hinder your ability to enjoy the views or fish the waters, but doing either is certainly possible with a little effort. Rainbow trout up to 15 inches and smaller eastern brook trout will keep any anglers in your group quite busy. Camping is limited to excellent sites along the northeast shore near the outlet. The fir- and hemlock-forest surrounding the lake provides adequate firewood.

From the junction, your descent on the PCT continues west until the crossing of South Fork Scott River. As the trail climbs away from the crossing, you cross another smaller, wildflower-lined stream before an extended, almost mile-long climb leads to the Carter Meadows Summit trailhead. Immediately prior to the trailhead, you meet the Hidden Lake Trail junction and then continue a very short distance up to the parking area.

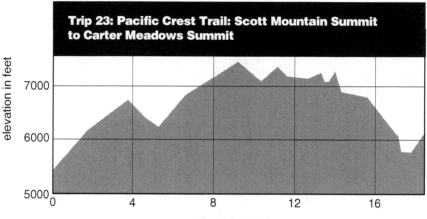

TRIP 24

Mavis, Fox Creek, and Virginia Lakes

An uncrowded, gorgeous trio of lakes with excellent fishing

Trip Type:	Dayhike or 2- to 3-day backpack
Distance:	9.4 miles round-trip, out-and-back
Elevation Change:	1460 feet, average 311 per mile
Difficulty:	Moderate
Season:	Early July to mid-October
Maps:	USGS *Billys Peak* and USFS *A Guide to the Trinity Alps Wilderness*
Nearest Campground:	Hidden Horse

You'll likely spend more time driving than hiking on this trip; the upside is that you'll likely have this area mostly to yourself. Even Mavis Lake, the easiest of the lakes to reach from both the north and south sides, is generally not overcrowded—if you don't count the cows. Fortunately, the cows don't get all the way to Virginia Lake, and neither do many bipeds either. All three lakes are bordered by picturesque meadows with wider and more open basins than around many other Trinity Alps lakes. All three have excellent campsites and good fishing. The catch will probably be pan-sized eastern brook trout, but an occasional lunker brown, left over from a long-ago planting, may thrill anglers in Mavis or Fox Creek lakes. Mavis Lake warms up first, but even Virginia Lake is usually warm enough for swimming by mid-August.

Starting Point

Once at Callahan (along Highway 3, about 65 miles north of Weaverville), watch for a road turning south just west of the bridge across East Fork Scott River and before the general store on the north side of the main drag. This road becomes Forest Road 40N16 on the way through the upper part of town to a junction. Following signed directions toward McKeen Divide, turn right and proceed 2 miles to another junction on top of McKeen Divide. Keep left here, following Forest Road 40N17, the obvious main road where several lesser roads branch away to the left and right.

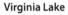

Virginia Lake

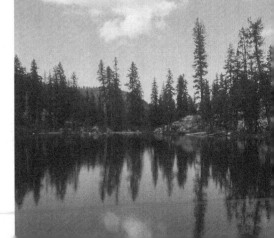

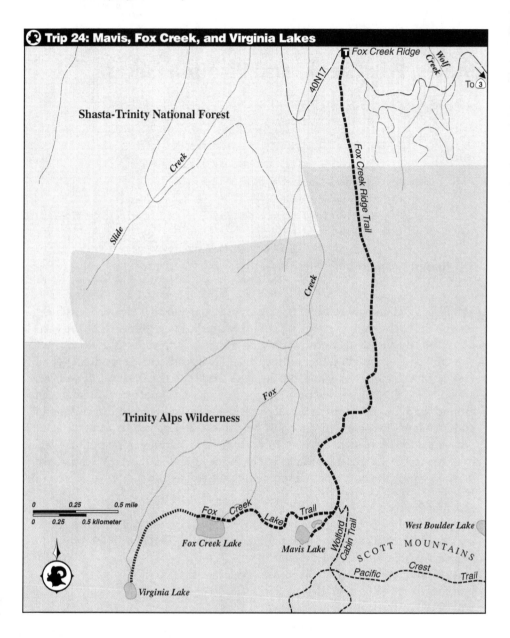

Trip 24: Mavis, Fox Creek, and Virginia Lakes

Fox Creek Ridge

Wolf Creek

40N17

To ③

Shasta-Trinity National Forest

Creek

Fox Creek Ridge Trail

Slide

Creek

Creek

Trinity Alps Wilderness

Fox

0   0.25   0.5 mile
0   0.25   0.5 kilometer

Fox   Creek   Lake   Trail

Fox Creek Lake

Mavis Lake

Wolford Cabin Trail

West Boulder Lake

SCOTT   MOUNTAINS

Pacific   Crest   Trail

Virginia Lake

At 3 miles above McKeen Divide, you reach a junction with Forest Road 39N10, signed for East Boulder Lake, and turn right, remaining on Road 40N17 toward Mavis Lake. A corral beside Boulder Creek, 0.2 mile farther, marks the Middle Boulder trailhead for trips to Middle Boulder Lake, Telephone Lake, and Eagle Creek. Continuing on, you cross Wolf Creek, 7 miles from Callahan, and climb steeply for a half mile to the signed Fox Creek Ridge trailhead on the point of a spur ridge. Parking should be available off the road to the right, where the road turns left around the point toward Fox Creek.

Description

A steep, 50-yard pitch leads from the south side of the road to the top of the ridge, from where the trail ascends south moderate to moderately steep along the ridgecrest. At 0.6 mile from the trailhead, you cross the signed wilderness boundary and continue through selectively logged forest of Douglas firs, white firs, sugar pines, and Jeffrey pines up to the former boundary of the old Primitive Area, 1.2 miles from the trailhead. A small stream trickles down a gully east of the trail. Along the way you may notice some orange metal markers with a black diagonal between two dots nailed 12 feet up the trunk of the trees, markers for a snow-gauging course.

Around 1.5 miles, the spur ridge on which you've been climbing merges with a large mountain. The trail jogs west, and then continues climbing south across a west-facing slope. At about 2 miles from the trailhead, you emerge from the forest cover into a sloping meadow full of angelica and other wildflowers, where an alder patch shelters two small springs, which may dry up by late summer.

Away from the meadow, the grade eases through open white-fir forest for a half mile on the way to a little alder-lined seasonal creek. Delphiniums bloom beside this crossing and a good campsite may be available in a grove of firs on the north side. Now you climb again up to a junction with the Wolford Cabin Trail, 2.8 miles from the trailhead. A short distance farther, about 300 yards, is a second junction with a trail on the left to Mavis Lake and a trail on the right to Fox Creek Lake.

Veering onto the left-hand trail, you climb a short pitch and then level out past the east shore of a lily pond. Beyond a tiny stream, you climb southwest over a moraine and then drop down to the northeast shore of 3.5-acre Mavis Lake, 0.4 mile from the last junction.

Mavis Lake is surrounded by a thick forest of firs, mountain hemlocks, and lodgepole pines behind a narrow border of boulders and grass, except where meadows run down to the south shore. Good campsites beside the trail on the approach to the northeast shore offer legal camping, while a campsite with a built-up fireplace and sawed blocks for sitting upon near a tiny inlet stream is too close to the southeast shore. Additional, excellent campsites occupy a ledge above the west shore. Plenty of firewood should be available. Trees crowding the shore make fly-fishing difficult, but the lake seems to have plenty of fish. When your time at Mavis Lake is over, retrace your steps 0.4 mile to the junction

From the junction of Mavis and Fox Creek lakes trails, follow the right-hand trail toward Fox Creek Lake on a contour to the west. Stay above an alder thicket and a wet meadow, and then cross two alder-choked stream channels. On good tread, you turn northwest around a large hump of granite and then descend the side of a wide valley before turning southwest. After a quarter mile of moderate ascent along the side of the valley the trail leads to the southeast shore of Fox Creek Lake, 0.8 mile from the junction.

More than twice the size of Mavis Lake, 9.5-acre Fox Creek Lake is bordered by wet meadows that, unfortunately, have been subject in the past to heavy cattle grazing. Thick forest covers the sides of the wide basin above the meadows, except on the west shore, where a rock face rises up to a ridge. A ring of lily pads 25 to 50 feet offshore makes fishing difficult around the east and south shores. Better fishing can be found off some rocks at the west end. There are good to excellent campsites above the north shore just west of the outlet. A number of other sites near the end of the trail and around the south shore are way too close to the water.

Although there is not a maintained trail from Fox Creek Lake to Virginia Lake, a use trail, of sorts, has evolved over the years. The 0.9-mile route begins above a patch of alders near the northwest corner of the lake, and then runs up a gully to a saddle in the ridge west of Fox Creek Lake. From there, follow another gully down the other side to a granite shelf, where ducks mark the way to the floor of a wide, heavily forested valley. Continue to climb moderately southwest, then south, between dense forest and a steep slope littered with large granite boulders. Keep to the east of an alder thicket, a wet meadow, and another alder thicket farther up the valley, and then follow ducks up the final, steep, quarter-mile climb generally southeast through big boulders to the shore of the lake just east of the outlet.

Although Virginia Lake is in a deep cirque close to the top of the divide, grass and meadows ring the shoreline, backed by a dense forest of red firs, mountain hemlocks, lodgepole pines, and western white pines. Labrador tea grows at the edge of the forest. All in all, Virginia Lake is a beautiful little 3-acre lake, more pristine than the previous two lakes due to the lack of cattle. There are only a few poor to fair campsites up in the rocks east of the lake, but you should be able to find plenty of better sites in the valley below. Fishing should be excellent for pan-sized eastern brook trout.

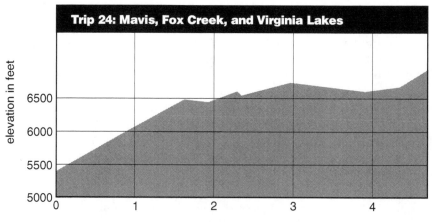

TRIP 25

Hidden Lake

An excellent, easy hike for those new to hiking or others short on time

Trip Type:	Dayhike or overnight backpack
Distance:	1.8 miles round-trip, out-and-back
Elevation Change:	450 feet, average 500 per mile
Difficulty:	Moderate
Season:	Late June to mid-October
Maps:	USGS *Deadman Peak* and USFS *A Guide to the Trinity Alps Wilderness*
Nearest Campground:	Hidden Horse

The almost mile-long trip to Hidden Lake is an excellent choice for young children or beginner backpackers, and the lake is far enough away from population centers to protect it from the use a lake of this caliber would normally receive. You should be able to find a decent campsite, take a dip, drop a line, and generally have a good time without having to battle the masses. Although not as dramatic as many of the Trinity Alps lakes, Hidden Lake is a nice spot to enjoy a couple hours, or even days. The trail dead ends at the lake, but the truly adventurous will find the peaks above the lake to be sufficiently challenging.

Starting Point

Highway 3 crosses the Scott River Divide at the very top of Scott Mountain Summit, 56 miles north of Weaverville, and then continues north on Highway 3, dropping 8.5 miles to the small community of Callahan. Immediately north of town, turn left at the junction of Forest Road 93,

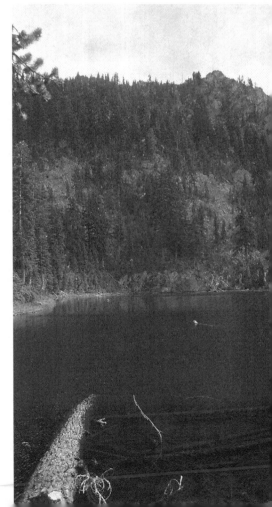

Hidden Lake

Trip 25: Hidden Lake

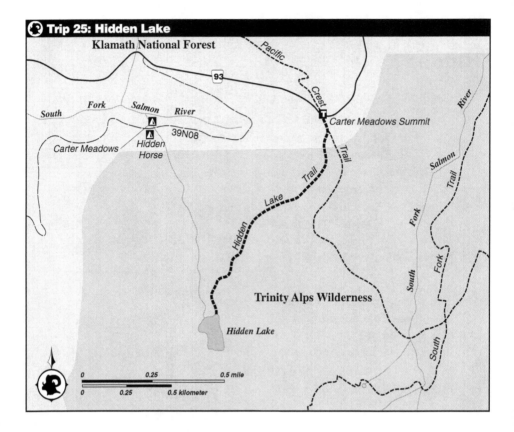

heading toward Cecilville, Forks of Salmon, and Somes Bar. Climb 11.7 miles on Road 93 to Carter Meadows Summit and the signed Pacific Crest Trail parking area on the left, which is also the trailhead for Hidden Lake. The paved parking area is equipped with a vault toilet and is located just below a heliport.

Description

Immediately down the hill from the parking area is a junction with the Pacific Crest and Hidden Lake trails. Cross the PCT and head southwest toward the lake on well-graded tread. Initially, fir forest shades your path, but, as you gain a ridge, the trees diminish, allowing for fine views across the canyon. As you round the ridge, the foliage thins even more to patches of manzanita with an occasional pine poking out of the brush. Also, the trail becomes much steeper here, resulting in a hot and dry ascent on the clear and sunny days typical during summer and early fall in the Trinity Alps. Mercifully, fir forest cover resumes after a while, providing some much-appreciated shade, although the ascent remains brutally steep. After topping out on the lip of Hidden Lake's basin, a very brief descent leads to the north shore.

Hidden Lake is a pleasant body of water surrounded by firs, with steep hillsides along the south and east shores. There are plenty of campsites on the west shore, enough for a number of parties. Firewood should be in adequate supply. Swimming in the 6658-foot lake is usually comfortable by midsummer.

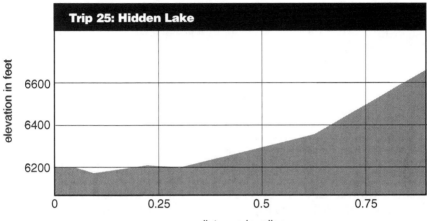

TRIP 26

Trail Gulch and Long Gulch Lakes

Dramatic scenery and plenty of excellent campsites

Trip Type:	Dayhike or overnight backpack
Distance:	8.4 miles, loop
Elevation Change:	5330 feet, average 635 per mile
Difficulty:	Moderate
Season:	Early June to early October
Maps:	USGS *Deadman Peak* and USFS *A Guide to the Trinity Alps Wilderness*
Nearest Campground:	Hidden Horse

There are two excellent reasons to take this trip: Long Gulch Lake and Trail Gulch Lake at the head of their respective "gulches," or very pleasant valleys filled with meadows and forests and threaded by delightful creeks. The lakes are virtual twins, cradled in spectacular cirques beneath crenellated peaks rising more than 1200 feet above the surface of the water. Bare rock and talus cover the south shores of both lakes, while stands of red firs and mountain hemlocks, interrupted by meadows and patches of willows, cover the rest of the shorelines. Despite their stunning beauty, both lakes were excluded from the original Salmon-Trinity Primitive Area, a glaring mistake corrected by their inclusion in the current Trinity Alps Wilderness.

The extensive meadows around the lakes provide plenty of potential forage, which makes Long Gulch and Trail Gulch lakes relatively popular with equestrians. However, this area still sees far fewer visitors than other areas of the Alps, like Caribou Basin, for example. Many campsites, spread over a large area north of each lake, can accommodate a fairly large number of visitors without undue crowding.

The names of the two gulches were reversed at some point in the past. Subsequent maps and guidebooks perpetuated the errors until they were corrected on the Forest Service's *A Guide to the Trinity Alps Wilderness* map, which now correctly shows Long Gulch Lake to the southwest of Trail Gulch Lake.

Starting Point

Highway 3 crosses the Scott River Divide at the top of Scott Mountain Summit, 56 miles north of Weaverville, and then continues north on Highway 3, dropping 8.5 miles to the small community of Callahan. Immediately north of town, turn left at the junction of Forest Road 93, heading toward Cecilville, Forks of Salmon, and Somes Bar. Climb 11.7 miles on Road 93 to Carter Meadows Summit and continue on Road 93 for another 0.7 mile to a left-hand turn onto

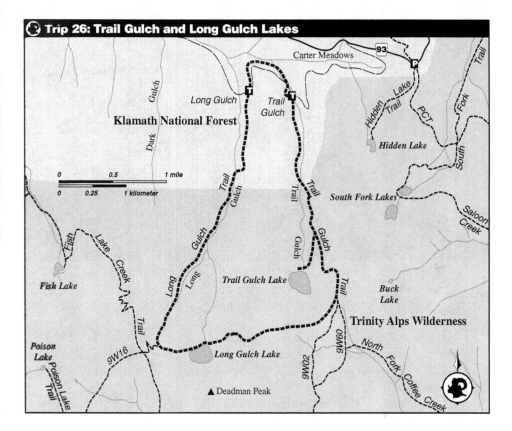

Trip 26: Trail Gulch and Long Gulch Lakes

Forest Road 39N08, signed CARTER MEADOWS TRAILHEADS. Pass turnoffs to Carter Meadows Horse Camp and Hidden Horse Campground, circle the upper end of Carter Meadows, cross Long Gulch Creek, and then immediately reach the Trail Gulch trailhead, 1.8 miles from Road 93. Parking is available for about a half dozen vehicles. An informal car camp is in a grove of trees beside the creek.

If you want to access the Long Gulch trailhead, continue west on Road 39N08 around the shoulder of a ridge for 0.75 mile. Road 39N08 continues west past a turnoff to the Fish Lake trailhead, and Trail Creek Campground before intersecting Forest Road 93, 14 miles east of Cecilville and 3.2 miles west of the Trail Gulch trailhead.

Description

Good tread leads south away from the Trail Gulch trailhead up the west side of a wide valley and into a grove of mature Douglas firs. Continue ascending southeast across a meadow and through some alders alongside Trail Gulch Creek before crossing to the east bank, 0.8 mile from the trailhead. Beyond the crossing, you pass more alders and through another wildflower-covered meadow. Steeper trail leads through red-fir forest cover and across a seasonal stream flowing down from the east side of the canyon. A series of switchbacks

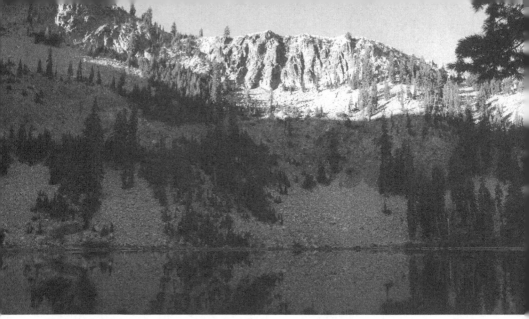

Trail Gulch Lake

takes you up to a junction with a lateral to Trail Gulch Lake, 1.8 miles from the trailhead.

Turning right (southwest), you ascend more gradually past a large alder thicket to a meadow beside the outlet of Trail Gulch Lake. Just before the lake, you cross this stream and rise slightly to a large camping area on a flat above the north shore.

Dramatic Trail Gulch Lake is set in a dark cirque of granite and metamorphic rock. So close to a trailhead, the lake is a popular destination for both hikers and equestrians, which makes for scarce firewood and keeps the resident rainbow trout small. Swimming should be comfortable by mid-August. Once your stay at Trail Gulch Lake is over, retrace your steps 0.4 mile to the junction.

Continuing the loop, you climb generally south up the canyon through a large, open meadow on good tread and a series of eight steep switchbacks to the top of the divide and a junction with trails south to North Fork Coffee Creek and southwest to Steavale Creek.

Turn right at the junction and head west toward Long Gulch Lake on a slightly ascending traverse along the south side of the divide through cover of forest. Past a pair of switchbacks, the trees part enough to allow a fine view to the south of the central Trinity Alps peaks. Eventually the grade becomes steeper and then the ascent abruptly ends at a saddle in the ridge above unseen Long Gulch Lake. From the saddle, you have excellent views of the Marble Mountains to the north.

Eight long-legged switchbacks lead down the forested hillside from the saddle to an extensive meadow near Long Gulch Lake and then into an alder grove. Proceed across the lake's outlet to the north shore of 10-acre Long Gulch Lake, 0.8 mile from the saddle.

Long Gulch Lake is set in another dramatic cirque, rimmed by granite cliffs, talus slopes, and the 7617-foot summit of Deadman Peak. Nearly twice the distance from a trailhead, Long Gulch Lake receives far fewer visitors than its neighbor to the east. With less pressure, fishing should be much better for rainbow trout up to 10 inches. Plenty of campsites provide tempting overnight havens along the north shore, and firewood is not as scarce as at Trail Gulch Lake—at least for now. Swimming in the 6436-foot lake is good by August, and a small island off the south shore makes a fine destination for good swimmers.

From the outlet of Long Gulch Lake, continue west for 0.5 mile through forest and broken rock to a junction with the South Fork Coffee Creek Trail heading south, the Fish Lake Creek Trail heading northwest, and Trail 9W16 heading southwest. (For the curious adventurer enticed by the route to Fish Lake, the trail is infrequently maintained, difficult to find, and hard to follow—sections could be considered an off-trail route).

From the junction, head north down Long Gulch on good tread through dense forest. Continue descending past a large alder patch, across meadows, and through open forest to the crossing of Long Gulch Creek at 1.7 miles from the junction. Continue the descent through ferns and young firs, passing through a gate in a split-rail fence at the wilderness boundary, and then proceeding a short distance to the Long Gulch trailhead, 7.6 miles from the Trail Gulch trailhead and 3.1 miles from Long Gulch Lake.

To return to the Trail Gulch trailhead, follow the relatively new connecting trail across Forest Road 39N08 and then climb away from the road through dense forest, eventually reaching Long Gulch Creek. Ascending along the west bank, the pleasant, forested climb continues until you come alongside the road again. After a short climb, cross the road to the north side and follow a trail sign pointing toward the Trail Gulch trailhead. The terrain opens up as you follow a more gradual ascent 0.1 mile to the trailhead, 0.9 mile from the Long Gulch trailhead. Thankfully, the Forest Service built this much more enjoyable option that replaced hiking the road between the two trailheads.

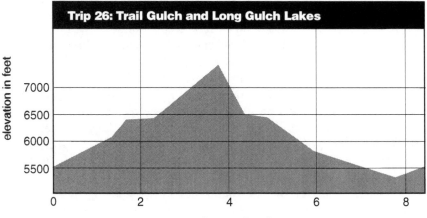

TRIP 27

China Gulch to Grizzly Lake

The short but torturous way to the dramatic scenery of Grizzly Falls and Grizzly Lake

Trip Type:	Backpack, 2–5 days
Distance:	14 miles, out-and-back
Elevation Change:	5540 feet, average 791 per mile
Difficulty:	Moderate to difficult
Season:	Mid-July to late September
Maps:	USGS *Thompson Peak* and USFS *A Guide to the Trinity Alps Wilderness*
Nearest Campground:	East Fork

This trip follows a shortcut to Grizzly Lake. The only positive aspect to the grueling, hot, and dry climb over the Salmon River divide is that at least there's some shade on the north side. Get an early start to avoid climbing the open, brushy slope under the blistering afternoon sun. The popularity of this route has grown exponentially during the last couple decades. Apparently, many backpackers don't mind the combination of a long drive and a tough climb. Don't expect to be alone during peak season.

Grizzly Lake, Grizzly Falls, and Grizzly Meadow, and the high country around the highest peak in the Trinity Alps, 9002-foot Thompson Peak, are more than satisfactory reasons for a little torture in order to get there sooner, but, if you have the time, the longer approach along North Fork Trinity River is much more pleasant (see Trip 33, page 247). Also, unless you're driving in from Oregon, the driving time to the Hobo Gulch trailhead will be much less than the time involved in getting to the remote China Gulch trailhead.

Grizzly is the Trinity Alps' quintessential high mountain lake, with deep blue waters reflecting perpetual snowfields and remnant glaciers draping the north side of Thompson Peak. Small pockets of red firs, whitebark pines, and mountain hemlocks shelter a few campsites, as well as soften the harsh outlines of the granite bowl cradling the lake. As magnificent as both the peak and the lake are, the most spectacular feature is found at Grizzly Lake's outlet, where Grizzly Creek leaps clear of the top of an overhanging granite cliff and plunges nearly 100 vertical feet, crashing upon the rocks below and cascading another 100 feet through a rocky cleft to a picturesque meadow.

Hauling a backpack up the steep and rough last mile to Grizzly Lake on the designated scramble route is tedious. In addition, the ecosystem surrounding the lake is quite fragile, so you may want to consider camping near the meadow below the falls and dayhiking up to the lake instead. If you have your heart set

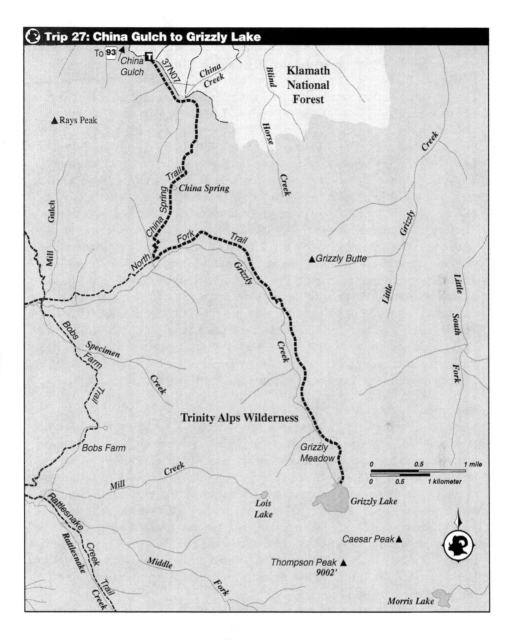

Trip 27: China Gulch to Grizzly Lake

To 93
China Gulch
37N07
China Creek
Klamath National Forest
Rays Peak
Horse Creek
Blind
Creek
China Spring Trail
China Spring
North Fork Trail
Grizzly
Grizzly Butte
Little
Little South Fork
Gulch
Mill
Bobs
Specimen Farm
Creek
Trail
Grizzly Creek
Trinity Alps Wilderness
Bobs Farm
Creek
Mill
Grizzly Meadow
Grizzly Lake
Lois Lake
Caesar Peak ▲
Rattlesnake
Creek
Rattlesnake Creek Trail
Middle
Fork
Thompson Peak ▲ 9002'
Morris Lake

0   0.5   1 mile
0   0.5   1 kilometer

on camping near the lake, please limit your stay and take extra precautions to minimize your impact. Cross-country enthusiasts will find the off-trail route to Lois Lake a short and pleasant diversion; peakbaggers will find the route along the southwest ridge of Thompson Peak to be a straightforward ascent route to the summit.

Starting Point

Follow Forest Road 93 west from Callahan to Cecilville and continue another 1.4 miles northeast of the small town to a left-hand turn onto South Fork Road leading to East Fork Campground (the junction is 4.5 miles east of Shadow Creek Campground). East Fork Campground is beside the road just before you cross a bridge over East Fork Salmon River. The free six-site campground near the river has vault toilets but no running water.

The paved South Fork Road wanders south through old dredge piles and brush for 3.7 miles before turning to cross to the west bank of the river. Another 100 yards leads to a four-way intersection, where the left fork accesses ranches and trailheads along the river, the right fork heads back to Cecilville, and the middle road, Forest Road 37N07 proceeds toward your trailhead. Follow Road 37N07 past a side road leading to a log deck, around a ridge, and then generally southwest up a canyon to a junction, 2.3 miles from the four-way intersection.

Turn right at the junction on the continuation of Road 37N07 and head across the ridge through a road cut, passing by a side road as you wind up the hill to another junction. Following signs, turn left at the junction and come around the east side of a ridge to spectacular views ahead of South Fork canyon, Packers Peak, and Caribou Mountain. Cross China Creek at 5.6 miles from South Fork Road (if your water containers are empty, you better get water here for the steep and dry ascent waiting for you ahead) and continue another 0.3 mile to the trailhead. Park along the shoulder of the road as space allows.

Description

The China Spring Trail starts with a bang, climbing straight up the bank on the uphill side of the road and then zigzagging up steep and very steep tread through madrones and ponderosa pines on the way to a stand of Douglas firs farther west. The climb moderates a tad where you double back over the nose of a ridge, but steep and very steep tread returns as the trail turns south. The forest becomes predominantly composed of white firs over the next mile, as you switch sides of the ridge three more times. A couple of long-legged switchbacks, west and then southeast, lead to the top of a knob, approximately 1 mile from the trailhead, where the ascent temporarily eases again. More switchbacks take you to the flat summit of the divide, 1.2 miles from the trailhead. A few dry campsites are nearby.

Old, deeply worn tread heads southwest off the summit and continues southwest. Hunters Camp and China Spring are 100 yards or so down the hill from the crest and about 50 yards west of the trail. A stand of ponderosa pines beside the trail a quarter mile below the summit makes a notable landmark on the otherwise open slope, which offers good views of Thompson Peak and the snowfield on the north side. Rougher trail turns more to the south and zigzags steeply and very steeply down through thick brush and sparse forest to a junction with the North Fork Trail along Grizzly Creek, 2.5 miles from the China Gulch trailhead. A most welcome, clear and cold little creek rushes down the side of the canyon a short distance west down the North Fork Trail.

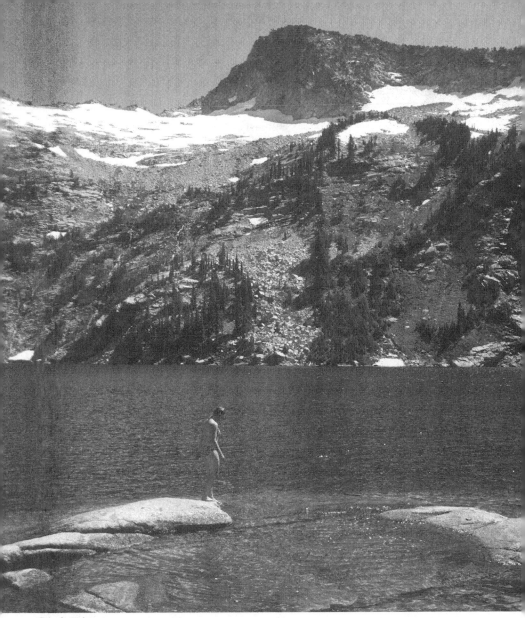

Grizzly Lake

Turning left (northeast) up Grizzly Creek canyon, you follow the course of the canyon, which eventually turns south in thick timber well away from the course of the creek. At 1.3 miles from the China Spring junction, you climb out of the woods and over the top of a glaciated metamorphic rock outcrop, which provides a vantage point for some long views of the valley above, revealing the typical U-shape of a glacier-carved canyon.

You follow the trail on traverses across the east side of the more open upper canyon alternating with switchbacks in order to gain altitude across patches of broken rock and brush. From openings 3 miles above the China Spring junction you have your first glimpses of Thompson Peak and the perpetual snowfields clinging to the north face since the open slopes below the divide. Small meadows, willow flats, and groves of red firs soon replace brush on the more level floor of the upper valley, with good campsites appearing above and below a spring flowing across the trail. Beyond the spring, you climb moderately steeply for a half mile over exposed rock and through belts of firs to the north edge of Upper Grizzly Meadow, one of the most serene locales in the Trinity Alps.

Directly ahead, beyond the lush grasses and wildflowers of Upper Grizzly Meadow, the outlet of Grizzly Lake is forcefully propelled over a precipice of granite to dissolve in a flurry of cascades of white foam and mist in the jumbled granite blocks below. The south and west fringe of the meadow offers good to excellent, sheltered campsites in groves of firs. Additional sites may be available between the trail and the creek below the meadow. Make sure to fully protect your food and equipment while camped near the meadow; deer and rodents seem to be more of a problem here than the bears, but food should definitely be hung away from the reach of all critters, provided you're not using bear canisters.

The trail continues past Upper Grizzly Meadows through the trees and into the pile of talus on the east side. The Forest Service has improved the condition of the trail from this point over the years, but the path is still a long way from what you would generally expect from a trail. The route from the meadow up to Grizzly Lake has been designated a "scramble" trail, the purpose of which is to define a single route up the very steep slope (rather than a multiplicity of boot-beaten paths), but not to encourage visitors to carry backpacks up to camps around the lake (to prevent environmental degradation). The route is steep, strenuous, and for experienced hikers only.

Above the lower section of talus, a virtual granite staircase has been constructed and marked by cairns. Approximately halfway up the slope, a spring-fed little stream flows down a rocky channel, a welcome spot to slake your thirst and catch your breath. Pass over the stream, pick up dirt tread, slick and muddy in spots, and proceed to a rock outcrop. Beyond the outcrop follow a steep path through a cleft, marked by ducks, leading alongside the upper channel of the stream before crossing over the watercourse to a field of vibrant wildflowers. Higher up, cross another branch of the stream. Now on more gently graded tread, indistinct at times, pass over boulders, stroll through lush vegetation, and hop over another tiny watercourse before following an angling traverse across the slope. The trail becomes more distinct again on the way to the north shore of dramatic-looking Grizzly Lake, where the full breadth of deep, blue Grizzly Lake and the magnificent basin finally lies before you.

Nearly level slabs of granite ease into the water just west of the outlet, offering splendid opportunities for sunbathing, quick dips into the chilly water, or simply admiring the stunning scenery. Mountain hemlocks, red firs, and whitebark pines eke out an existence in cracks and on ledges around the nearly solid granite basin. Lush gardens of wildflowers bloom in tiny meadows long after the blooms of their counterparts have faded in Grizzly Meadow below. Above the first set of cliffs to the southeast, a large, higher cirque and shelf on the north face of jagged, 9002-foot Thompson Peak holds a glacier and permanent snowfields.

There are a handful of useable campsites sprinkled on the rock slabs along the north shore, and among small groves of conifers on a ridge and peninsula above the northwest shore. If you decide to camp near the lake, don't burn firewood if you even find any. Old-timers in the Trinity Alps may tell tales of taking limits of rainbow trout, all exceeding 12 inches, but heavier visitation has taken a harsh toll on the fish population in Grizzly Lake. Today you'll be fortunate to catch enough pan-sized trout for breakfast.

Rock climbers and scramblers will find an abundance of good vertical and overhanging granite both above and below the lake. For the more prosaic who desire to stand atop the summit of the highest peak in the Trinity Alps, the route up the arcing northwest ridge is a straightforward ascent—you may want an ice ax in early season. From the north shore of the lake, work above the granite cliffs to the southwest. You angle across granite slabs above, which may be covered with snow in early season, to the low point on the ridge leading up to the summit. From there, follow the backside of the ridge to the top, where the far-ranging views are utterly superb.

Cross-Country Route to Lois Lake

For cross-country enthusiasts, the route to diminutive Lois Lake, directly west of the much larger Grizzly Lake, is a short and straightforward endeavor. To reach Lois Lake, climb clefts in the ridge southwest of the north shore of Grizzly Lake until gaining the top of the ridge. Turn left (west) along the ridge and climb to a saddle at the intersection of another ridge from the northwest. Carefully drop down southwest from the ridge to where you can see Lois Lake below, sitting serenely in a rock basin, and then descend about 350 feet to the shore. The ridge above Lois Lake includes a panorama across a 2700-foot-deep cleft of Mt. Shasta in the distant east and excellent views of Thompson Peak.

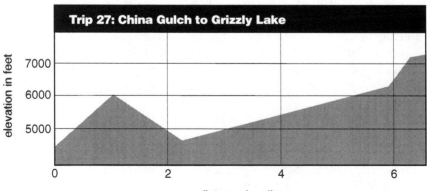

TRIP 28

High Point to Rock and Red Cap Lakes

This remote, beautiful corner of the Trinity Alps is especially appealing to plant lovers.

Trip Type:	Dayhike or 2- to 3-day backpack
Distance:	7.6 miles, out-and-back to both lakes;
	4.2 miles, out-and-back to Rock Lake;
	4.4 miles, out-and-back to Red Cap Lake
Elevation Change:	5560 feet, average 732 per mile;
	2320 feet, average 552 per mile to Rock Lake;
	3940 feet, average 895 per mile to Red Cap Lake
Difficulty:	Moderate
Season:	Late June to early October
Maps:	USGS *Salmon Mountain* and *Youngs Peak*;
	USFS *A Guide to the Trinity Alps Wilderness*
Nearest Campground:	Hotelling

About 1300 feet of this trip's elevation change occur in the 0.6 mile from the top of the ridge above Red Cap Lake to the shore and back. Of course, you could skip Red Cap Lake and climb Salmon Summit instead, or head out along the ridge to Eightmile Camp, one of the most remote places you'll ever find. However, if you skip Red Cap Lake, you'll miss out on the chance to fish for some large eastern brook trout. The abundant meadows and open hillsides along this isolated section of the Salmon River Divide and the ridge south of Salmon Mountain are normally covered with a solid carpet of wildflowers, including many unusual and interesting species, around the end of June. Virgin, climax forest, predominantly composed of red firs, covers the remainder of the crest.

You most likely won't see many other people in this area, with the possible exception of during hunting season. What you will find are black bears and black-tailed deer, or, more accurately, numerous tracks and copious piles of their scat. Be sure to keep a clean camp and adequately hang your food, or use a bear canister.

Difficult and somewhat complicated access combined with a lack of publicity account for the paucity of visitors to this remote, beautiful corner of the Trinity Alps. From the south side a long and strenuous trip on poorly maintained trail up New River and Virgin Creek to the Salmon River Divide awaits you (see Trip 38, page 285); from the north side a whole day's drive from just about anywhere is required to reach the High Point trailhead. Simply reaching the tiny burg of Forks of Salmon from any direction is tedious.

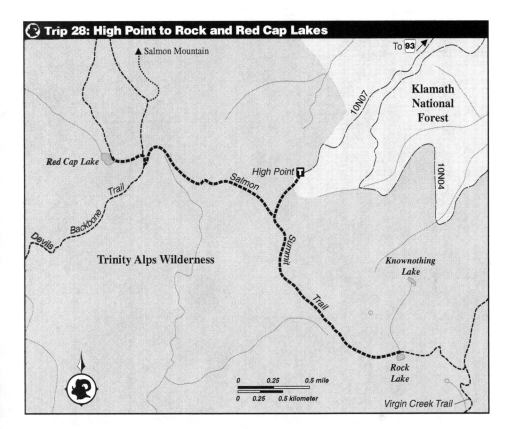

Trip 28: High Point to Rock and Red Cap Lakes

▲ Salmon Mountain

To 93

Klamath
National
Forest

10N07

Red Cap Lake

High Point

10N04

Salmon

Trail

Backbone

Devils

Trinity Alps Wilderness

Summit

Knownothing
Lake

Trail

Rock
Lake

Virgin Creek Trail

0   0.25   0.5 mile
0   0.25   0.5 kilometer

Starting Point

Forest Highway 93 from Cecilville down alongside South Fork Salmon River canyon to Forks of Salmon is about the most thrilling, and slowest, 18.5 miles of pavement you'll ever see. One-lane, blind, hairpin curves, hung on the sides of steep cliffs, are common, as many as a half-dozen per mile. The same "highway" coming up the main stem of the Salmon River from the west to Forks of Salmon from Somes Bar (at the confluence of the Salmon and Klamath rivers) is just as crooked, if not more so. If you're tempted to circumvent Highway 93 by traveling southwest from Etna and Sawyers Bar, think again—that road is the worst of all. Unfortunately, an easy route to Forks of Salmon by automobile simply does not exist.

From Forks of Salmon head south upriver and cross over the South Fork bridge to reach a three-way junction. Turn onto the farthest left road, signed 10N04 and head south up a canyon. Cross a creek and then switchback up the nose of a ridge before turning south again far up the side of the canyon. Several little-used roads branch off along the way but the main road is obvious at all forks.

Climb another set of switchbacks into a large burned area and proceed to a junction, 6.4 miles from Highway 93. Proceed straight ahead from the

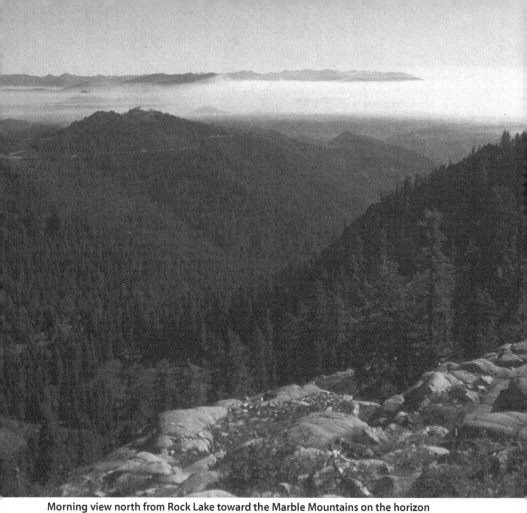

Morning view north from Rock Lake toward the Marble Mountains on the horizon

junction, remaining on Road 10N04, and follow a curve past Road 10N05 on your right on the way to a three-way junction at 8.7 miles. Veer left onto Road 10N04, entering live forest after nearly 4 more miles, which is quite beautiful in contrast to the previous burned area. After traversing the southwest side of a long ridge overlooking the upper basin of East Fork Knownothing Creek, you reach the knob known as High Point and your next road junction at 14.7 miles. From High Point, the highest hump you see on the summit directly south is just above Rock Lake.

Leaving Road 10N04, which turns left down into the valley, you turn up Road 10N07 and follow along the side of the ridge for another 0.8 mile to an old log landing. Some vehicles may have to stop here, as the road beyond diminishes to a narrow, one-lane track, lined with creeping brush. Your road follows a rough, steep pitch climbing straight up the side of the ridge to the west of the landing, and then turns up the crest to the trailhead on an almost level area overgrown with tall grasses, 14.9 miles from the three-way junction back at Forks of Salmon. Right at the wilderness boundary, the trailhead has more than enough parking for the few vehicles that come this far.

Description

From the trailhead, follow the course of an old four-wheel-drive track climbing moderately on the east side of the ridge for 0.5 mile to a saddle in the crest of Salmon River Divide and a junction with the Salmon Summit Trail. Just above the junction, nailed to a dead fir is a trail sign with an arrow to the right pointing toward Eightmile Camp and an arrow to the left pointing the way to Rock Lake.

Turning left, you head south along Salmon River Divide on well-defined tread that climbs away from the saddle through open fir forest with an understory of grasses and low brush. The ascent, steep at first, eases where the trail turns southeast across the face of the ridge. Beyond another steep pitch, you head south again on a moderate descent along the crest before dropping down more steeply across the southwest side. A mile from the junction, break out into the open above a steeply sloping meadow and begin a climb back toward the crest through brush and thickets of young incense cedars. Farther on, a moderately steep climb through red firs leads to a gorgeous little meadow in a saddle, where a profusion of sulfur flowers and naked eriogonums bloom through midsummer. Before you leave the meadow, take the time to look up at the ledge below Rock Lake and the steep-sided mountains behind.

Considering the little trail maintenance done in this area, the Salmon Summit Trail is in reasonably good shape. Head away from the meadow on a moderately steep ascent southeast up the ridge. A profusion of wildflowers, including paintbrush, lupine, valerian mint, and wallflower, bloom beside rough tread, as you turn more east across a north-facing slope. As you climb higher, little Knownothing Lake, bordered by brush, springs into view at the lower end of the valley below. Although there's no trail, heading cross-country from the vicinity of the saddle to the lake is possible, provided you're amenable to doing some bushwhacking. A half mile of moderate to moderately steep climbing around the head of a valley leads to the metamorphosed rock ledge that forms the north lip of the cup holding 2-acre Rock Lake. Step across the tiny, willow-lined outlet, where the lake pops into full view, and then climb a short distance to the north shore.

Almost perfectly round Rock Lake sits right under the precipitous north face of a granite mountain on the divide. Granite talus falls into the water on the south side, but metamorphic rock slopes up from the rest of the shoreline. How the lake's cup was formed is hard to imagine, appearing as a glacial cirque, but there's no evidence of past glaciation along this part of the Salmon River Divide. One good campsite and a few more fair ones under scattered red firs and western white pines may lure overnighters along the east shore. Late in the season the water drops below the level of the outlet and the lake loses some of its aesthetic appeal. Fishing is good for eastern brook trout up to 10 inches. Red newts may surprise you by rising to the surface to breathe. The top of a spur ridge east of the lake offers breathtaking views of sunrises and sunsets over Salmon River canyon. Coastal fog often creeps up the canyon at sunrise to set a series of ridges adrift on a pink sea.

Other Options for Trips in the Area

This trip doubles back from Rock Lake past the High Point Trail junction in order to reach Red Cap Lake at the other end, then doubles back again to the trailhead. With careful study of the related topographic maps, a variety of other routes and destinations could be incorporated into your trip, but be aware that some of the trails shown on some of the maps in this area can't be found on the ground. For example, the unmaintained trail to Knownothing Lake shown on the Forest Service's wilderness map absolutely does not exist.

To further complicate matters, pertinent information about the actual condition of these trails is awfully hard to come by, since a particular path may pass through two national forests and three different ranger districts, not to mention the fact that the Forest Service's budgets for trail maintenance are woefully underfunded. All in all, you definitely need a pioneering spirit to venture into this remote and isolated section of the Trinity Alps Wilderness. Fortunately, in spite of lack of use and little to no trail maintenance, trails along the top of the Salmon River Divide are, for the most part, in surprisingly good condition.

To reach Red Cap Lake, retrace your steps 1.6 miles to the High Point junction in the saddle. From there, follow an old road northwest down the other side of the ridge, along the upper edge of a wide meadow dotted with clumps of ceanothus and willow. Carpets of wildflowers cover the meadow and the sides of the old road trace. Skullcap, appearing somewhat like a tiny white penstemon, is one of the more unusual varieties found here. The road becomes a washed-out gully farther down the slope, until the tread improves where the old track levels out. A fair campsite is beside a little stream that has cut through the road, 0.5 mile from the junction.

Raw red dirt that appears to be a mine dump from farther up the hill turns out to be a massive slide at the head of Eightmile Creek, as you rise slightly and reach the edge of the slide. You have to climb very steeply up the east side to negotiate the crossing, and then drop down to pick up the road again on the west side. Continue a moderate rise northwest across the head of the basin above a mass of willows, and then climb more steeply through red-fir forest to the ridgecrest and a junction with the Devils Backbone Trail, 1.3 miles from the High Point junction. (The old road on the ridgecrest runs north 0.5 mile from here to High Spring at the foot of Salmon Mountain, and then south 1.25 miles to Eightmile Camp and a series of beautiful, ridgecrest meadows.)

From the Devils Backbone junction, head north down the road approximately 200 yards to a signed junction with a spur heading down to Red Cap Lake. Turn left here and head downhill, with the lake coming into view as soon as you start zigzagging down the very steep hillside. The lake is a gorgeous and colorful sight from this vantage, with lush green meadows bordering most of the shoreline, red cliffs and talus providing some contrasting color on the south side, and the deep blue northern California sky reflecting in the placid water. The 13 switchbacks leading down to the lake are interrupted by a long traverse across meadows and gullies. Through scattered firs, the remaining switchbacks lead down to the bottom of the basin, where a traverse across meadows takes you to the north shore near a campsite sheltered beneath a grove of firs, 0.3 mile from the junction.

On close inspection, the gorgeous lake seen above turns out to be shallow and weedy, with a very soft mud bottom crisscrossed by large, waterlogged trees that jut out of the surface, which makes the 2- to 3-acre lake undesirable as a swimming hole. However, anglers will be delighted by the good fishing for large eastern brook trout, although they may become frustrated by all the weeds and logs.

Plenty of opportunities exist for further exploration, including a nontechnical ascent of 6956-foot Salmon Summit. The route out to wild and lonely Eightmile Camp and the remote country beyond is described in Trip 38 (page 285).

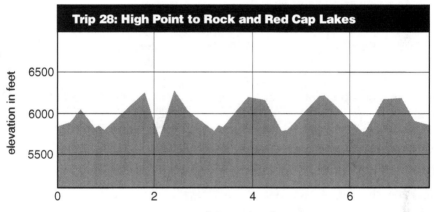

Salmon Summit Trail to Red Cap Lake

A gentle, forested path to a seclusion-drenched lake

Trip Type:	Dayhike or 2- to 3-day backpack
Distance:	8.2 miles, out-and-back
Elevation Change:	3920 feet, average 361 per mile
Difficulty:	Easy
Season:	Late June to mid-October
Maps:	USGS *Salmon Mountain* and USFS *A Guide to the Trinity Alps Wilderness*
Nearest Campground:	Hotelling

The Salmon Summit National Scenic Trail provides the wilderness traveler with solitude, relatively gentle hiking through cool forest, and occasional ridgetop views of the wild and remote western Trinity Alps. Red Cap Lake is a long way from any population center, but this route to the Salmon Summit trailhead avoids the tedious, serpentine drive to Forks of Salmon and the High Point trailhead described in the previous trip, which provides the other access to the lake. For the relative few who reside west of the Alps, this hike may be one of the closer trips for them.

Red Cap Lake is a serene body of water set below a forested ridge, bordered by meadows that are ablaze with colorful wildflowers in early summer. Backpackers have a good chance of having the lake all to themselves, even on weekends. A base camp at the lake offers the opportunity to dayhike to other remote destinations in the area, including Rock Lake, Salmon Summit, or Eightmile Camp. However, be forewarned that some of the area's trails are seldom used and infrequently maintained. The more daring might be inclined to follow the full length of the Salmon Summit Trail to the Cecil Lake trailhead, but this route requires some tremendous logistics for driving between the two trailheads.

This section of the Salmon Summit Trail to Red Cap Lake is mostly through forest, providing some escape from the typically hot summer sun, but the trees part enough on occasion to reveal some panoramic views of the surrounding ridges and valleys, as well as some more distant mountains. Despite the lack of use, the tread is generally in good condition, well graded, and easy to follow.

Make sure your water containers are full before you reach the trailhead, since none will be available along the drive, at the trailhead, or anywhere near the trail until you reach the lake.

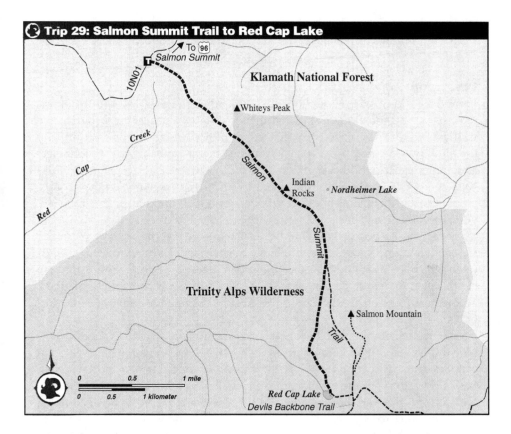

Trip 29: Salmon Summit Trail to Red Cap Lake

To 96
Salmon Summit

10N01

Klamath National Forest

▲Whiteys Peak

Cap Creek

Red

Salmon

Indian
▲ Rocks
Nordheimer Lake

Summit

Trinity Alps Wilderness

▲ Salmon Mountain

Trail

0   0.5   1 mile
0   0.5   1 kilometer

Red Cap Lake
Devils Backbone Trail

Starting Point

Follow Highway 299, either west from Weaverville or east from the Eureka-Arcata area, to the town of Willow Creek and the junction of U.S. 96. Head north on U.S. 96 for 40 miles to the town of Orleans. (If you are coming from Oregon, Orleans is 102 miles southwest on U.S. 96 from the Interstate 5 junction north of Yreka.) Continuing north on U.S. 96, cross the Klamath River on a suspension bridge immediately north of town and then turn right (east) onto Red Cap Road.

Follow paved Red Cap Road, with conveniently placed road markers every mile and sometimes every half mile, along the east bank of the Klamath River, passing several homes and ranch homes spread about the river valley. The road narrows after 1.5 miles and begins a long, winding ascent that continues all the way to the trailhead. Cross a one-lane bridge over Boise Creek at 4 miles from U.S. 96, leaving the last of the private homes behind. After another mile, you reach a junction where County Road 532 heads west toward the Klamath River down Red Cap Creek. Continue straight ahead from the junction on Forest Road 10N01 in the direction of LePerron Peak, Sheldon Butte, and Hoopa. Remain on this road for several more miles, which turns to gravel near the 15-mile mark. At 18.4 miles, you reach the trailhead at the top of a ridge north-northwest of

Whiteys Peak. With a definite sense of overkill, plenty of parking is available for a high number of vehicles. Up the hill from the trailhead there's a horse corral.

Description
From the parking area the trail quickly descends into forest cover of white firs, incense cedars, and Douglas firs and then maintains a nearly level course on a well-graded dirt path covered with needles. Minor ups and downs accompany the slightly ascending tread beneath a cool forest canopy, with wildflowers and underbrush periodically lining the trail. This trailside vegetation varies considerably along the way, from sparse to dense, representative of the variable amount of light reaching the forest floor. About 0.75 mile from the trailhead, you cross the Trinity Alps Wilderness boundary, just prior to Baylor's Camp, a dry camp used primarily by hunters in the fall. Tucked beneath dense forest, the camp has places to tie stock and hang meat, as well as numerous log rounds upon which to sit around the campfire. Immediately beyond the camp, the trail bends left and 5 yards farther comes to a signed junction with an old roadbed. To the north, the old road follows the crest of the Salmon Mountains toward Orleans Mountain.

Veer right (southeast) at the junction and climb more steeply, eventually topping out on the divide, 1.3 miles from the trailhead. On the ridge the vegetation changes from dense forest to primarily manzanita, dotted with an occasional fir. Your first view from the trail includes the realization that the area behind was once logged over and the area ahead fell victim to a more recent fire. Following the ridge, you proceed ahead with views to the east and west until you encounter an old downed log with an almost equally aged sign attached reading RED CAP LAKE. From here, the trail drops away from the top of the ridge across a previously burned hillside, where young white firs are attempting to succeed the extensive brush. Soon you find yourself back in dense forest, where the grade eases again. Continue as the trail drops down the south side of the ridge once more to bypass the weathered diorite outcrop of exposed rock straddling the ridge known as Indian Rocks. You reach a junction, 2.75 miles from the trailhead, where the Salmon Summit Trail continues south toward High Spring below the southwest flank of Salmon Mountain, but your trail drops away to the right toward Red Cap Lake.

A trail makes a steady, moderate descent away from the junction through alternating pockets of open and dense forest. After a mile, the trail levels off and then makes an almost imperceptible climb through forest and meadows on the way across the lake's basin. Red Cap Lake soon appears, resting peacefully at the head of the basin. The trail continues to a junction with the High Point Trail above the east shore, near a large campsite.

Red Cap Lake is a shallow pond with a mud bottom that is crisscrossed by several dead snags, making it unsuitable for swimming. Reportedly, large eastern brook trout inhabit these waters, but the weeds and snags might make it difficult for anglers to land any fish they snag. However, for those who want nice scenery, the lake won't disappoint. Meadows, carpeted with colorful wild-flowers in season, ring a good part of the shoreline around Red Cap Lake, the lush vegetation attracting some of the wary wildlife of the area. The rest of the terrain around the lake is lightly forested and shelters a number of good campsites. Perhaps the best site is in a grove of conifers near the southeast edge of the lake just beyond the meadows. Almost any time you visit the lake you should have your pick of campsites. A spring on the southwest side of the lake is a fine source of water.

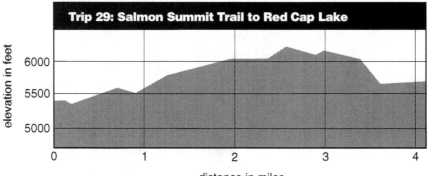

TRIP 30

East Weaver and Rush Creek Lakes

Even the drive to the trailhead is awe-inspiring.

Trip Type:	Dayhike or 2- to 3-day backpack
Distance:	8 miles round-trip, out-and-back
Elevation Change:	3720 feet, average 930 per mile
Difficulty:	Moderate to East Weaver Lake; difficult to Rush Creek Lakes
Season:	Early July to mid-October
Maps:	USGS *Rush Creek Lakes* and USFS *A Guide to the Trinity Alps Wilderness*
Nearest Campground:	East Weaver

In 9 miles from Weaverville to the trailhead you climb 5000 vertical feet. The last 1.7 miles are on one-lane road, hanging rather precariously on steep-sided Weaver Bally Mountain. Another 0.9 mile past the trailhead is the Weaver Bally Lookout from where you can gaze straight down Weaverville's chimneys and enjoy a lofty view of several hundred square miles of forests, mountains, and canyons. A trip to Monument Peak and East Weaver and Rush Creek lakes won't be complete without a stop at the lookout.

The hiking part of this trip offers a bonus opportunity to scale Monument Peak and enjoy a 360-degree panorama that includes *all* of the Trinity Alps. East Weaver Lake is a pleasant place to enjoy lunch along the way and, under other circumstances, would be a fine destination. However, the lake is completely outclassed by the neighboring Rush Creek Lakes, pristine and diminutive jewels strung down a rugged canyon of the magnificent, pinnacled cirque below aptly named Monument Peak.

Gazing from the narrow crest above the Rush Creek cirque near the trip's midpoint across at several miles of brutally steep, dry Rush Creek Lakes Trail snaking up the ridge from Kinney Camp to Rush Creek Lakes, you may feel justifiably proud of yourself for having arrived at this spot so easily. Of course, you'll still have to descend the almost vertical wall of the cirque (and get back up again), but the extra effort is fully rewarded when you bask in the sheer beauty of these magnificent lakes.

Starting Point

From the historic district of Weaverville, proceed westbound on Highway 299 toward Eureka, passing the ranger station on your left and a large complex of sheriff's facilities on your right. Immediately past the sheriff's complex, turn right onto Weaver Bally Road and continue for a block or so to a stop sign, where the paved road turns right but you should go straight ahead onto Forest

Trip 30: East Weaver and Rush Creek Lakes

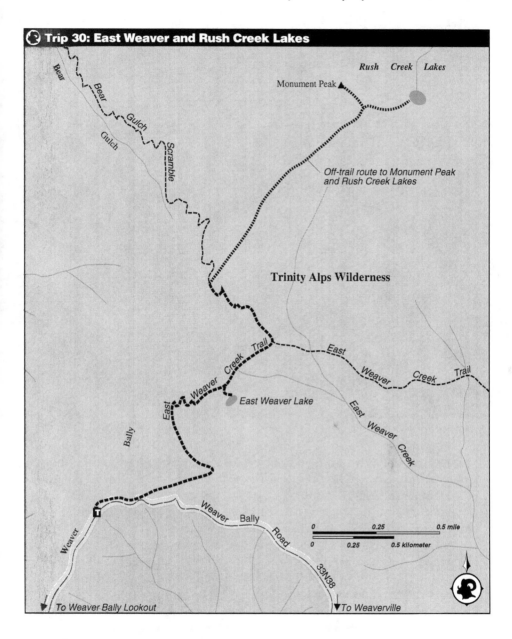

Rush   Creek   Lakes

Monument Peak ▲

Off-trail route to Monument Peak
and Rush Creek Lakes

Trinity Alps Wilderness

East Weaver Creek Trail

East Weaver Creek Trail

East Weaver Lake

East Weaver Creek

East Bally

Bear

Bear Gulch

Gulch

Scramble

Weaver Bally Road

Weaver

0   0.25   0.5 mile
0   0.25   0.5 kilometer

33N38

▼ To Weaver Bally Lookout   ▼To Weaverville

Road 33N38, signed WEAVER BALLY LOOKOUT, EAST WEAVER LAKE TRAILHEAD. The dirt
road is potholed in places but should be passable for any vehicle, unless recent
rains have muddied up the surface. The condition of the road improves beyond
the first mile or so, where you start to climb seriously in Munger Gulch.

The ascending road offers a good opportunity to observe changes in the
flora as you climb from 2000 feet near Weaverville to more than 7000 feet at
the top of Weaver Bally. The vegetation at the start includes ceanothus brush
beneath a forest of ponderosa pines, incense cedars, and Douglas firs. Bigleaf

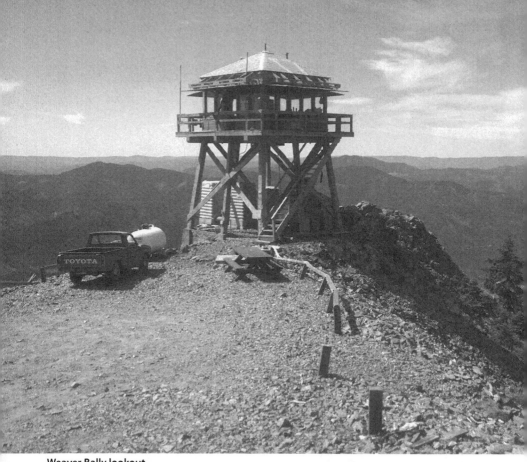

Weaver Bally lookout

maples, madrones, live oaks, and canyon oaks grow in Munger Gulch. Above the gulch, you first see black oaks, followed by white firs and sugar pines as you continue climbing. Near the top of the ridge, ceanothus, huckleberry oak, and manzanita carpet the open hillside, as Jeffrey pines, lodgepole pines, western white pines, and Shasta red firs make up the forest.

The road switchbacks to the top of a spur ridge and, at 7.5 miles from Highway 299, dips down briefly to reach Low Gap in a grove of white firs. A number of side roads branch off from 33N38 on the way up the mountain but the main road should be obvious. After you keep left at a fork in Low Gap, the road narrows to one lane and climbs steeply across a brush-covered ridge with very few turnouts along the way. At 8.8 miles from 299, a pipe trickles icy water from a boxed spring on the uphill (north) side of the road. Continue another half mile to where the road meets the ridgecrest. In 2008, a broken trailhead sign was propped up on the ground on the right, barely visible from the road. Despite the lack of a clearly visible sign, you'll know you've reached the trailhead where you see the only place on the ridge possibly wide enough to provide parking for a few vehicles.

Having traveled this far, you might as well drive to the end of the ridge and enjoy the view from the lookout.

Description

Stroll briefly along the ridgecrest, passing a picnic table and fire ring on the way to a weathered sign about the 1987 fire. The trail leaves the top of the ridge here and embarks on a descending traverse through thick brush across the right-hand hillside above the road to the trailhead. The dense vegetation threatens to overgrow the trail in places and you may want to consider wearing long pants for the first quarter mile or so. Eventually the grade switches to a gently ascending traverse before a short section of steeper trail leads to a switchback near the top of the ridge.

Tree-filtered views of two of the trip's destinations, sparkling East Weaver Lake below and rugged Monument Peak across the gorge, can easily be had by leaving the trail and strolling a short distance along the ridge. Continuing on the trail, you drop off the ridge and traverse the head of East Weaver Lake's basin, initially through a grove of firs and hemlocks and then across open shrub- and rock-covered slopes. Soon the path zigzags more steeply down to a ledge overlooking the west shore of the mossy 1-acre lake. A couple of poor to fair campsites ring the brushy shoreline, but this destination is perhaps better suited for a dayhike than an overnight backpack. The lake supports a healthy population of eastern brook trout, but the profuse vegetation may inhibit shore-line access.

On the way down to the lake, you may be tempted by a shortcut across the side of the basin to the saddle north of East Weaver Lake, where the Bear Gulch Trail crosses the ridge. However, don't try this route, as very thick, tall brush makes the steep hillside virtually impassable. The better course is to follow faint tread down the side of the canyon below the lake about 0.3 mile to inter-sect the Bear Gulch Trail. From there, a moderately steep climb leads through meadows, patches of brush, and open forest to the top of the ridge, 2.0 miles from the trailhead. From the ridge, views up to the head of Canyon Creek are quite spectacular.

Off-Trail to Monument Peak
and Rush Creek Lakes

Where your route intersects with the Bear Gulch Trail, you head cross-coun-try toward a gap just east of the highest point of Monument Peak, the rocky sum-mit a mile northeast that dominates the horizon. The route follows the firebreak created to halt a 1987 fire and becomes steeper the closer you get to the peak. A final quarter mile of very steep climbing leads you to a narrow crest overlooking the beautiful cirque at the head of Rush Creek.

One of the Rush Creek Lakes

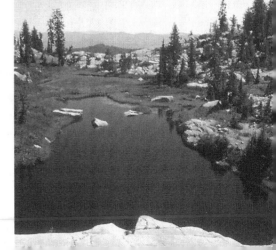

To reach the summit of Monument Peak, climb west over broken blocks of metamorphosed rock. As you climb higher, Upper Rush Creek Lake springs into view on the floor of the cirque below. Although the elevation is a mere 7771 feet, the top of Monument Peak offers unrestricted views of all the higher Trinity Alps peaks to the north and overlooks the vast canyons of Canyon Creek and North Fork Trinity River farther west. The Cascade volcanoes of Mt. Shasta and Lassen Peak can be seen to the east over Trinity Lake and the Trinity Divide.

Rush Creek runs out the open north side of the deep cirque below through grassy meadows and over rock ledges to connect a string of little lakes and tiny ponds known as the Rush Creek Lakes—eight of them in all. A row of slanted pines tops the east wall above the largest lake, out of sight from the ridge behind tall firs and rock outcrops. The west wall leads up to crags below the pyramidal summit of Monument Peak.

Reaching the floor of the cirque and the shore of Upper Rush Creek Lake requires scrambling down some very steep slopes of loose dirt, rock, and talus, and of course, you'll have to climb back up again to return to the trailhead. However, with shuttle arrangements, traveling downstream on the poorly maintained Rush Creek Lakes Trail is possible, although not preferred. From the gap just east of the highest point on Monument Peak, head west, then north, and finally east along a ledge to the bottom of the cirque. Occasional ducks and traces of a use trail mark the way.

The deep, nearly round, 2-acre upper lake lies beneath the nearly vertical east wall of the cirque. Direct sun warms the water for only a short time even in midsummer, and slivers of snow may linger in the cracks until August of some years, both of which discourage swimming. The shoreline is rough and brushy, but anglers who find a suitable perch from which to cast should expect a good catch of eastern brook trout.

Farther down the canyon, the smaller and shallower lakes should be warm enough for a refreshing swim by late summer. However, no obvious trail connects the string of lakes, requiring you to find your own way over rough terrain to see them all.

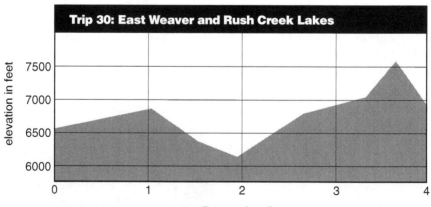

TRIP 31

Canyon Creek and El Lakes

If you can take only one trip in the Trinity Alps, Canyon Creek is your best bet.

Trip Type:	Backpack, 2–5 days
Distance:	16.6 miles round-trip, out-and-back to El Lake
Elevation Change:	3810 feet, average 459 per mile
Difficulty:	Moderate
Season:	Early July to mid-October
Maps:	USGS *Mt. Hilton* and USFS *A Guide to the Trinity Alps Wilderness*
Nearest Campground:	Ripstein

This trip samples the sights and activities that make the Trinity Alps unique and marvelous. Thompson Peak, highest of the Alps, soars in snowcapped splendor above the deep, blue waters of Canyon Creek lakes nestled in the upper basin. Above Canyon Creek lakes in a side pocket of granite, contorted, diminutive "El" Lake reflects the permanent snowfields and rugged minarets on the north side of Sawtooth Mountain. A relatively cold microclimate contributes an almost alpinelike character to this basin and the three lakes despite the relatively low elevations, ranging from 5606 feet at Lower Canyon Creek Lake to 6529 feet at El Lake.

Big brown, rainbow, and eastern brook trout reside in the two lower lakes and occasionally yield to the hooks of experienced anglers, while smaller eastern brook trout succumb to almost anyone with a pole at El Lake. The lower reaches of Canyon Creek support an excellent population of native rainbow trout. The cliffs, peaks, and steep granite faces surrounding the lakes offer opportunities for all classes of rock climbing.

Hikers pass three notable sets of waterfalls and dozens of lesser cascades on the Canyon Creek Trail. Oaks, madrones, dogwoods, and bigleaf maples of the lower forests give way to white and red firs, Jeffrey pines, and sugar pines farther up the canyon. Deer are most prevalent in the lush meadows and forests near the midpoint of the Canyon Creek drainage. Hikers are sure to be greeted by a wide variety of birds any time, along with a host of wildflowers during midsummer, and might even spy a black bear.

If all these fantastic attributes seem too good to be true, you're right! The Canyon Creek area is to the Alps as Yosemite Valley is to Yosemite National Park, with many of the same problems, albeit on a different scale. In the past, people have loved this area nearly to death. Don't expect to be alone and don't camp at the lakes, as sanitation is a major concern in the granite basin; find a

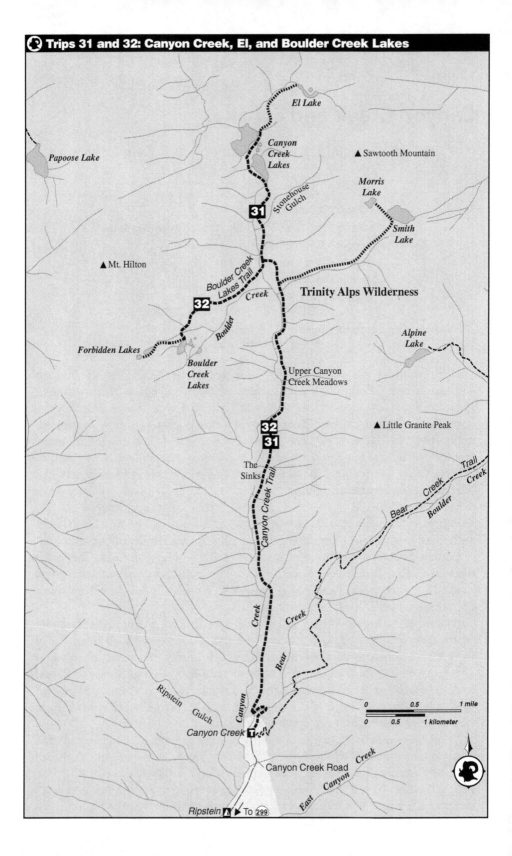

El Lake

Papoose Lake

Canyon Creek Lakes

▲ Sawtooth Mountain

Morris Lake

31

Stonehouse Gulch

Smith Lake

▲ Mt. Hilton

Boulder Creek Lakes Trail

Creek

Trinity Alps Wilderness

32

Boulder

Alpine Lake

Forbidden Lakes

Boulder Creek Lakes

Upper Canyon Creek Meadows

▲ Little Granite Peak

32

31

The Sinks

Bear   *Creek*   *Trail*

Canyon Creek Trail

Boulder   *Creek*

Creek

Creek

Bear

Ripstein   *Gulch*

Canyon

0   0.5   1 mile

0   0.5   1 kilometer

Canyon Creek 🆃

Creek

Canyon Creek Road

East   *Canyon*

Ripstein 🏕 ▶ To (299)

campsite along Canyon Creek below the lakes and dayhike to them instead. Observe the campfire ban, which begins 500 feet above the junction with the Boulder Lakes Trail. If possible, plan your trip for the middle of the week, or after Labor Day to help minimize the crowds. Despite the high level of use, Canyon Creek and the lakes are still breathtakingly beautiful and shouldn't be missed. Just don't wear out your welcome.

Starting Point

Canyon Creek Road turns north from Highway 299 in the tiny burg of Junction City, just shy of 8 miles from Weaverville and 0.1 mile east of the highway bridge over Canyon Creek. The narrow road is paved but unsigned on the way past an old hotel, post office, and residences of Junction City. If you are traveling east on Highway 299 from Eureka and Arcata, a shortcut forks left 3 miles west of Junction City, just before the Junction City Bureau of Land Management campground. This paved road, also unsigned, snakes over a ridge to meet the Canyon Creek Road on the east side of the canyon, 2.5 miles above Junction City.

From this intersection, narrow and sometimes steep pavement continues up the east side of the rugged canyon, overlooking a variety of rustic miner's shacks clinging precariously to the rocks below. Cross a bridge to the west side of the creek at Fisher Gulch, 8.6 miles from Junction City and veer right at a fork with Grasshopper Flat Road 1.3 miles farther. A one-lane bridge soon leads back to the east bank and passes a right-hand turnoff to the East Fork trailhead on Forest Road 35N47Y. Continue up the canyon to an open flat where the old town of Dedrick once stood.

At 12.1 miles from Junction City, small, undeveloped, and very pleasant Ripstein Campground sits between the road and Canyon Creek. Continue to a loop at the end of the road, 13 miles from Junction City, where numerous parking spaces are provided for the most popular trailhead in the Alps. There are vault toilets near the south end of the loop. The trail begins up the hill at the opposite end of the loop, where a sign points north to the wide, well-trod Canyon Creek Trail and the seldom-used Bear Creek Trail.

Description

A short distance from the trailhead sign, another sign provides destinations and mileages: CANYON CREEK TRAIL, THE SINKS 3, LOWER CANYON CREEK LAKE 8, BOULDER CREEK LAKES 9. The first quarter mile rises slightly, beyond which the tread levels off well up the side of the canyon before turning east into the shady side canyon of Bear Creek. Lush stands of dogwood and bigleaf maple line the descent to the crossing of Bear Creek. Beyond the boulder hop, you climb a short, steep pitch to a shoulder far above Canyon Creek, where you will see the first signs of a fire that closed the trail for a number of weeks midsummer in 2008. Continue north across an open, dry hillside forest of canyon oaks, black oaks, ponderosa pines, Douglas firs, and a few incense cedars. Approximately 1.5 miles from the trailhead, a few fair campsites can be seen on a bench in more lush forest, with the obvious drawback of a long and steep descent to the creek for water.

At 2.5 miles you skirt the top of a cliff above boulder-strewn Canyon Creek. A half mile farther you reach a junction, unsigned except for a tiny sign marked TRAIL pointing the way up the main trail, with a path heading down to an area along the creek bottom known as The Sinks, a large flat—actually more of an island between two channels of the creek. Both channels are typically dry by midsummer and the creek disappears upstream in The Sinks, buried by an enormous rockslide, only to reappear again at the downstream end of the island. A number of excellent campsites on the island and one on a flat west of the creek will lure overnighters.

Back on the wide, smooth tread of the Canyon Creek Trail, you climb moderately, far up the east side of the canyon. A half mile from the junction, a fresh-looking rivulet spills across the trail, a tempting little stream. You may want to wait to gather water, as the trail soon switchbacks to cross the stream two more times. Not far above the switchbacks, you will first hear, then glimpse the high cascade known as Canyon Creek Falls. In the old days, the main trail was located on the floor of the canyon and passed right beside the falls, but the modern route of the trail bypasses this scenic feature; you'll have to crawl back down the creek to see the falls nowadays. The present Canyon Creek Trail draws closer to the creek at 3.8 miles, just below another, less spectacular fall, now referred to as Lower Canyon Creek Falls. A lovely swimming hole at the base of this fall will certainly tempt you with the prospect of a refreshing swim, particularly if it's hot, as it oftentimes is in midsummer.

Canyon Creek Falls

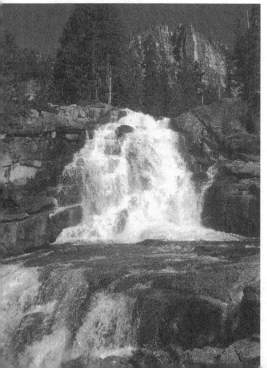

Pass some campsites before the nearly level trail passes along the east side of Upper Canyon Creek Meadow through shoulder-high ferns carpeting the forest floor. Masses of flowers typically bloom in the marshy meadows during mid-July. Above the meadow a moderate climb leads away from the creek. About 5 miles from the trailhead, you ascend some granite ledges directly above the creek, then turn up a side canyon on rough tread through rocks and brush. A large, heavily forested flat, littered with boulders and crossed by a number of watercourses (generally dry in midsummer), begins at 5.2 miles, with several fair to good campsites amid boulders not far from Canyon Creek. An extremely difficult, steep, strenuous cross-country

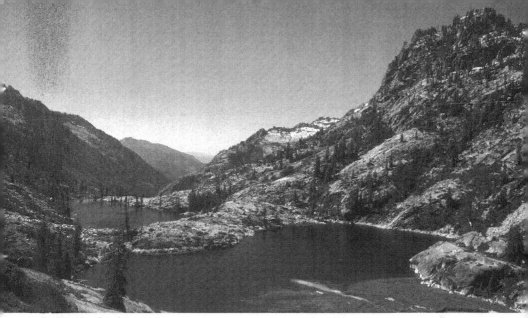

Canyon Creek Lakes

route to Morris and Smith lakes runs up the south side of a gulch east of this flat and over the top of the ridge south of Sawtooth Mountain. On the approach to a cliff at the north end of the flat, a faint use trail branches west toward the foot of Middle Falls, a spectacular cascade spilling down rock ledges into a deep granite bowl.

The trail turns east at the base of a cliff at the flat's north end and soon begins a series of moderately steep switchbacks north beside a small, thin stream. At the top of the switchbacks you enter a forested, azalea-floored dell and a junction with the Boulder Creek Lakes Trail forking west at 5.75 miles. This junction is poorly marked by a small, old sign attached to a snag and is easily missed if you're not paying attention.

Continuing ahead on the Canyon Creek Lakes Trail, you draw near the creek again above the azalea dell, pass more good campsites, and then turn east to ascend another set of switchbacks around the next set of falls. A grove of firs near the top of the falls shelters a small, fair campsite, as you once again approach the creek. After climbing above the falls, the grade eases on the way to a ford of Canyon Creek.

Beyond the ford, you proceed up the canyon on a winding, mostly level course through dense forest to a large camping area big enough for four or five parties. Continue through a patch of azaleas and ferns to another picturesque fall cascading down a narrow side canyon. Nearby, there are more campsites alongside the creek. From the falls, follow a ducked route straight up some granite slabs to a band of dark gray cliffs and then make a long ascending traverse below the cliffs and up some switchbacks to Lower Canyon Creek Lake, 2 miles from the Boulder Creek Lakes junction and 6.8 miles from the trailhead.

The very deep, blue, 15-acre lake sits in a bowl of solid granite. The bowl is very steep on the west side, rising to the massive hulk of Sawtooth Mountain, but is lower and shelving on the other three sides. Only a few clumps of brush and a smattering of scattered weeping spruces, Jeffrey pines, and red firs break the wide expanse of smooth, glaciated granite sloping up the west shore to a row of cliffs. Beyond more cliffs and rugged ridges, snowcapped Mt. Hilton towers into the western sky. To the north, the jagged tip of Mt. Thompson fits neatly into a notch at the head of the canyon.

Near the outlet of Lower Canyon Creek Lake, the route to the upper lake heads directly west over granite slabs, climbing up into the cliffs above the west shore. Beyond the lower lake, the route leads to a gully, through which you climb northwest to the first awe-inspiring view of Upper Canyon Creek Lake. From this viewpoint at the west end of a granite dike between the two Canyon Creek lakes, you gaze north to vertically tiered strata resembling irregular slices of toasted bread rising directly from a deep bay. Jagged Wedding Cake and Mt. Thompson top the granite skyline beyond. Canyon Creek flows in several meandering channels across a lush green delta before entering the upper lake from the northeast. A frozen cascade of glacier-rounded granite falls to the east shore from the cirque holding El Lake.

A strip of grass and gravelly beach, backed by willows and alders, runs from the outlet at the east end of the granite dike between the lower and upper lakes around to the bare granite south of the meadow that's bisected by the inlet. The outlet of the upper lake courses through a steep-sided gash. A wood-timbered dam once raised the lake level by six to eight feet and, although no evidence of flumes or ditches related to mining activity downstream remains, an obvious bathtub ring mars the shoreline to this day.

You must either be a very accomplished long jumper or ford the creek at this point to get across the outlet from the upper lake. This crossing is not recommended in early season when the water is swift and the level is high. Beyond the crossing, a use trail continues briefly around the east shore to a pocket of sandy

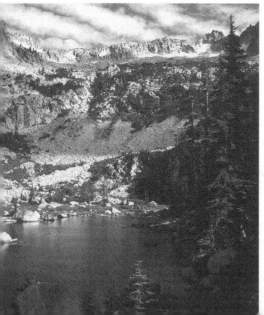

El Lake

beach and a campsite that's too close to the water. Please consider camping in the canyon below the lakes—the walk to the lakes from there is not long, campsites are much better, and you'll help preserve the fragile beauty of the basin. Brown and rainbow trout will provide anglers with plenty of challenges at the upper lake.

Off-Trail to El Lake

There is not a maintained trail up the steep granite slopes between Upper Canyon Creek Lake and the secluded cirque of little El Lake, but a ducked route with stretches of a discernible path has evolved over years of repeated use. To find the beginning of this route, walk north along the strip of grass and beach on the east side of Upper Canyon Creek Lake to where vertical granite seemingly blocks your way. Climb up a gully and turn northeast across the top of the first granite knob, where you should soon pick up ducks marking the route south of some cliffs. Continue generally northeast, very steeply at times, up and over ledges, through gullies, and past a pair of small ponds. Along the way are spectacular views across Canyon Creek lakes up to Mt. Hilton. About a half mile from the start of the route, you top out on a ledge overlooking a very green valley, through which the outlet from El meanders. Turn upstream above the chasm of the outlet stream and head northeast toward the lake, which is beyond a shoulder of rock to the east, located in a cirque surrounded by an amazing tableau of cliffs and peaks.

Permanent snowfields clinging to the towering north face of Sawtooth Mountain form the south wall of the cirque and reflect in the serene, rock-studded surface of El Lake. The 2-acre lake was obviously named for its shape, a contorted L wrapped around shoreline rocks and plush meadows. Weeping spruce, mountain hemlock, and red fir fill pockets of soil along the steep west shore and up the cirque walls to the base of some cliffs. Abundant wildflowers fill the meadows around the lake through midsummer. Talus slopes at the base of the upper cliffs are so white that they appear to be snowfields at first glance.

A small, poor campsite in the rocks where you first reach the shoreline should not be used. Look for better sites along the edge of the meadows below the lake, or for exposed sites (with good views) on top of the rocky hill south of the outlet. Small eastern brook trout rise to almost anything that touches the surface, but travel around the shoreline is hampered by brush along the far shore.

The timbered ridge across the valley to the north of the lake is the divide separating the Canyon Creek and Stuart Fork drainages. A strenuous cross-country route runs through a saddle in this ridge and down to Mirror and Sapphire lakes in the large cirque beyond. The part of this route running around the head of the Stuart Fork cirque to Mirror Lake is potentially dangerous due to unstable rock and should be attempted only by experienced parties.

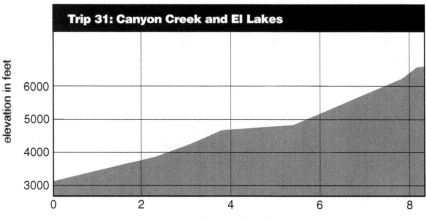

TRIP 32

Canyon Creek to Boulder Creek Lakes

Three beautiful lakes await the determined explorer.

Trip Type:	Dayhike or 2- to 4-day backpack
Distance:	14.8 miles round-trip, out-and-back
Elevation Change:	2987 feet, average 409 per mile
Difficulty:	Moderate to difficult
Season:	Early July to mid-October
Maps:	USGS *Mt. Hilton*
	and USFS *A Guide to the Trinity Alps Wilderness*
Nearest Campground:	Ripstein

see map on p. 236

Boulder Creek basin and the lovely lakes that mirror the serrated peaks above are a mere 2 miles off the heavily traveled Canyon Creek Lakes Trail, but receive far fewer visitors than the much more popular Canyon Creek lakes. Forbidden Lakes, tucked into a granite cleft 500 vertical feet above Boulder Creek Lakes see hardly anyone at all, thanks to the absence of a maintained trail and a nasty patch of nearly impenetrable brush, but the beautiful, diminutive lake and even smaller tarn are bordered by a permanent snowfield and worth the effort.

Boulder Creek Lakes consist of three lakes and a half dozen murky ponds hosting a sizable population of tadpoles and frogs. All of the lakes and ponds fill depressions scooped out by glaciers halfway up a granite ridge directly west of the Middle Falls of Canyon Creek. Very widely scattered conifers dot the polished granite shoreline, and the only viable (and scarce) shelter is under overhanging ledges—don't forget your tent and don't stay here during a thunderstorm. The wide-open basin allows you to see virtually forever, with the spectacular scenery towered over by the summits of jagged Sawtooth Mountain and rugged Mt. Hilton. The wide-open skies should reward stargazers handsomely.

Fishing is fair for small eastern brook and rainbow trout in the Boulder Creek Lakes. Nearby Mt. Hilton will certainly appeal to climbers, who can ascend to the summit from the northwest edge of the basin without needing more than Class 2 climbing skills. More challenging climbing is available on an abundance of vertical granite pitches surrounding the basin. Unlike Canyon Creek lakes, Boulder Creek lakes provide water warm enough for swimming by midsummer, and granite slabs offer fine spots for sunbathing. Fair, exposed campsites appear on ledges and in pockets of granite soil between rocks around Boulder Creek Lakes, but there are absolutely no adequate campsites anywhere around Forbidden Lakes. Campfires are banned a short distance above the

Canyon Creek lakes junction, but even if they were allowed you'd be hard-pressed to find any wood to burn anywhere in the basin.

Starting Point

Canyon Creek Road turns north from Highway 299 in the tiny burg of Junction City, just shy of 8 miles from Weaverville and 0.1 mile east of the highway bridge over Canyon Creek. The narrow road is paved but unsigned on the way past an old hotel, post office, and residences of Junction City. If you are traveling east on Highway 299 from Eureka and Arcata, a shortcut forks left 3 miles west of Junction City, just before the Junction City Bureau of Land Management campground. This paved road, also unsigned, snakes over a ridge to meet the Canyon Creek Road on the east side of the canyon, 2.5 miles above Junction City.

From this intersection, narrow and sometimes steep pavement continues up the east side of the rugged canyon, overlooking a variety of rustic miner's shacks clinging precariously to the rocks below. Cross a bridge to the west side of the creek at Fisher Gulch, 8.6 miles from Junction City and veer right at a fork with Grasshopper Flat Road 1.3 miles farther. A one-lane bridge soon leads back to the east bank and passes a right-hand turnoff to the East Fork trailhead on Forest Road 35N47Y. Continue up the canyon to an open flat where the old town of Dedrick once stood.

At 12.1 miles from Junction City, small, undeveloped, and very pleasant Ripstein Campground sits between the road and Canyon Creek. Continue to a loop at the end of the road, 13 miles from Junction City, where numerous parking spaces are provided for the most popular trailhead in the Alps. There are vault toilets near the south end of the loop. The trail begins up the hill at the opposite end of the loop, where a sign points north to the wide, well-trod Canyon Creek Trail and the seldom-used Bear Creek Trail.

Description

A short distance from the trailhead sign, another sign provides destinations and mileages: CANYON CREEK TRAIL, THE SINKS 3, LOWER CANYON CREEK LAKE 8, BOULDER CREEK LAKES 9. The first quarter mile rises slightly, beyond which the tread levels off well up the side of the canyon before turning east into the shady side canyon of Bear Creek. Lush stands of dogwood and bigleaf maple line the descent to the crossing of Bear Creek. Beyond the boulder hop, you climb a short, steep pitch to a shoulder far above Canyon Creek, where you will see the first signs of a fire that closed the trail for a number of weeks midsummer in 2008. Continue north across an open, dry hillside forest of canyon oaks, black oaks, ponderosa pines, Douglas firs, and a few incense cedars. Approximately 1.5 miles from the trailhead, a few fair campsites can be seen on a bench in more lush forest, with the obvious drawback of a long and steep descent to the creek for water.

At 2.5 miles you skirt the top of a cliff above boulder-strewn Canyon Creek. A half mile farther you reach a junction, unsigned except for a tiny sign marked TRAIL pointing the way up the main trail, with a path heading down to an area along the creek bottom known as The Sinks, a large flat—actually more of an island between two channels of the creek. Both channels are typically dry by midsummer and the creek disappears upstream in The Sinks, buried by an enormous rockslide, only to reappear again at the downstream end of the island. A number of excellent campsites on the island and one on a flat west of the creek will lure overnighters.

Back on the wide, smooth tread of the Canyon Creek Trail, you climb moderately, far up the east side of the canyon. A half mile from the junction, a fresh-looking rivulet spills across the trail, a tempting little stream. You may want to wait to gather water, as the trail soon switchbacks to cross the stream two more times. Not far above the switchbacks, you will first hear, then glimpse the high cascade known as Canyon Creek Falls. In the old days, the main trail was located on the floor of the canyon and passed right beside the falls, but the modern route of the trail bypasses this scenic feature; you'll have to crawl back down the creek to see the falls nowadays. The present Canyon Creek Trail draws closer to the creek at 3.8 miles, just below another, less spectacular fall, now referred to as Lower Canyon Creek Falls. A lovely swimming hole at the base of this fall will certainly tempt you with the prospect of a refreshing swim, particularly if it's hot, as it oftentimes is in midsummer.

Pass some campsites before the nearly level trail passes along the east side of Upper Canyon Creek Meadow through shoulder-high ferns carpeting the forest floor. Masses of flowers typically bloom in the marshy meadows during mid-July. Above the meadow a moderate climb leads away from the creek. About 5 miles from the trailhead, you ascend some granite ledges directly above the creek, then turn up a side canyon on rough tread through rocks and brush. A large, heavily forested flat, littered with boulders and crossed by a number of watercourses (generally dry in midsummer), begins at 5.2 miles, with several fair to good campsites amid boulders not far from Canyon Creek.

Sawtooth Mountain from Boulder Lakes Basin

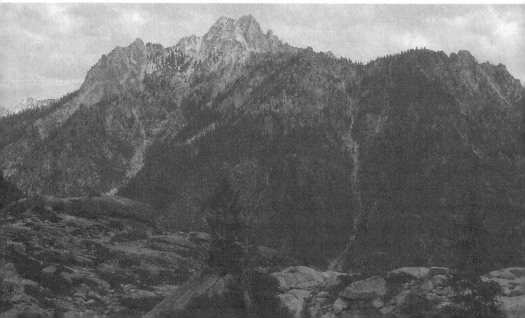

Off-Trail to Morris and Smith Lakes

An extremely difficult, steep, strenuous cross-country route to Morris and Smith lakes runs up the south side of a gulch east of the flat you reach at about 5.2 miles from the Canyon Creek trailhead. You can follow it over the top of the ridge south of Sawtooth Mountain.

On the approach to a cliff at the north end of the flat, a faint use trail branches west toward the foot of Middle Falls, a spectacular cascade spilling down rock ledges into a deep granite bowl.

The trail turns east at the base of a cliff at the flat's north end and soon begins a series of moderately steep switchbacks north beside a small, thin stream. At the top of the switchbacks you enter a forested, azalea-floored dell and a junction with the Boulder Creek Lakes Trail forking west at 5.75 miles. This junction is poorly marked by a small, old sign attached to a snag and is easily missed if you're not paying attention.

Now heading west on the Boulder Creek Lakes Trail, you gently ascend for a short distance through the azalea dell, cross a shelf of bare granite, and then descend through low brush to a ford of Canyon Creek. Be aware that this crossing may be very dangerous during the high waters of early season. Except in late season, you will have to ford the stream or find a footlog to negotiate this ford. There are many excellent campsites upstream on either side of the ford.

Good tread turns south from the ford and climbs moderately through open forest and some brush around a buttress of the west ridge and up into the lower valley of Boulder Creek, passing into the signed no fires zone along the way. Where the trail turns southwest at the lower edge of the wide, flat-floored valley a half mile from the junction, you can see the ribbon of Boulder Creek spilling over an escarpment to the south. Beyond the flat section of valley, the tread deteriorates as you ascend more steeply over slabs and around boulders and through thick brush that threatens to overgrow the trail in places. As you crest a hump of granite, the lower lakes spring into view directly south, separated from you by a wide crack in the floor of this broad amphitheater. Little Boulder Creek froths through the bottom of this vertical-walled slot after cascading down from Forbidden Lakes. Follow ducks and cairns southwest across bare rock to a point where the chasm is only a few feet deep and relatively easy to cross.

From the crossing, pick your way around a large hump of granite and down to the largest lake, 1.5 mile from the Canyon Creek lakes junction. The 5-acre, shallow lake reposes in a depression scoured out of solid granite by the last glacier to flow from the ridge into Canyon Creek. Geologists theorize that a later glacier carved out the valley below and left the pronounced escarpment below the lakes. A 1-acre lake to the east is joined to the largest lake in early season when the water level is high. Patches of brush grow in pockets of soil around the lakes, but only a few solitary Jeffrey pines, red firs, and weeping spruces interrupt the broad expanse of rock.

Slabs of granite that slope down into the lake offer excellent sunbathing opportunities and easy access for a refreshing swim. However, an easily stirred layer of silt on the bottom will likely cloud the otherwise clear water. Bashful skinny dippers will have a problem in this wide-open basin—there's absolutely no place out of view. Small rainbow and eastern brook trout rise morning and evening to well-placed dry flies. Many fair to good campsites are scattered among the rocks, but make sure your tent is free standing, as there is very little soil for anchoring tent stakes. Avoid spots too close to the water and be very careful about disposing of your waste.

Off-Trail to Forbidden Lakes

From Boulder Creek Lakes you can easily spot the location of Forbidden Lakes, tucked into the notch above the basin on the west wall from which pours Boulder Creek. However, locating the lakes and getting there are two very different propositions. To reach the lakes, travel around the largest Boulder Creek Lake to the north shore. Cross between the biggest lake and the next lake in the chain and head up the first rock rib emerging from the headwall around the largest lake. Continue heading straight up toward the lakes along this rock rib, attempting to avoid as much brush as possible. Keep climbing until you reach the level floor of the notch holding the outlet stream. The stream valley is narrow and choked with brush, making travel through here difficult. The lesser of two evils seems to be heading along the south side of the stream and clambering over large talus blocks until you reach the northeastern shore of the main lake.

Small trout feed on the surface all day in the deep shade of the larger lake, but access to the shoreline is difficult, as heavy brush chokes the north shore and large talus blocks line the opposite side. The determined adventurer can travel to the small upper lake, bordered by a permanent snowfield that drops down from the steep-walled slopes of the upper canyon. Since there are no reasonable campsites at either lake, the old adage applies: Forbidden Lakes is a beautiful place to visit, but you wouldn't want to stay there.

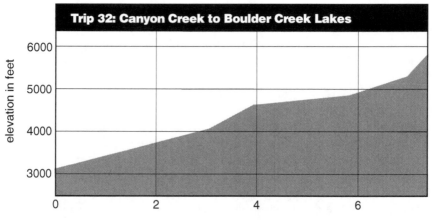

TRIP 33

North Fork Trinity River to Grizzly Lake

This is the "relaxed" route to Grizzly Lake, for those who have enough time to enjoy the pleasant journey.

Trip Type:	Backpack, 4–7 days
Distance:	35 miles round-trip, out-and-back
Elevation Change:	4650 feet, average 266 per mile
Difficulty:	Moderate
Season:	Mid-July to early October
Maps:	USGS *Thurston Peaks*, *Cecil Lake*, and *Thompson Peak*; USFS *A Guide to the Trinity Alps Wilderness*
Nearest Campground:	Hobo Gulch

The trail starts out easy, climbing only 1000 feet within the first 10 miles of excellent tread in lush, deep canyons that follows the course of North Fork Trinity River and Grizzly Creek. You will see an amazing variety of trees, ferns, and flowers along the way and maybe even a school or two of big steelhead or salmon. Picturesque old cabins on benches along the river and a plethora of relics along the way hearken back to the heyday of the old mining period. You may even see some present-day miners in wet suits working Venturi dredges on a few active claims. Don't expect to be alone at Grizzly Lake or Grizzly Meadows—the drama of Grizzly Falls and the stunning beauty of Grizzly Lake and Thompson Peak lure many admirers. However, one of the advantages of the longer route described here is that you'll more than likely have the first 13.5 miles of trail substantially to yourself. If you're limited by time, the strenuous 13-mile round-trip from the China Creek trailhead on the north side of the Salmon River divide will be your best alternative (see Trip 27, page 214).

Grizzly is the Trinity Alps' quintessential high mountain lake, with deep blue waters reflecting perpetual snowfields and remnant glaciers draping the north side of the area's highest summit, 9002-foot Thompson Peak. Small pockets of red firs, whitebark pines, and mountain hemlocks shelter a few campsites. As magnificent as both the peak and the lake are, the most spectacular feature is at Grizzly Lake's outlet, where Grizzly Creek leaps clear of the top of an overhanging granite cliff and plunges nearly 100 vertical feet to crash upon the rocks below and cascade another 100 feet through a rocky cleft to the meadow below.

Hauling a backpack up the steep, rough last mile to Grizzly Lake is difficult, and the ecosystem surrounding the lake is quite fragile, so you may want to consider camping near the meadow below the falls and dayhiking up to the lake instead. If you have your heart set on camping near the lake, please limit

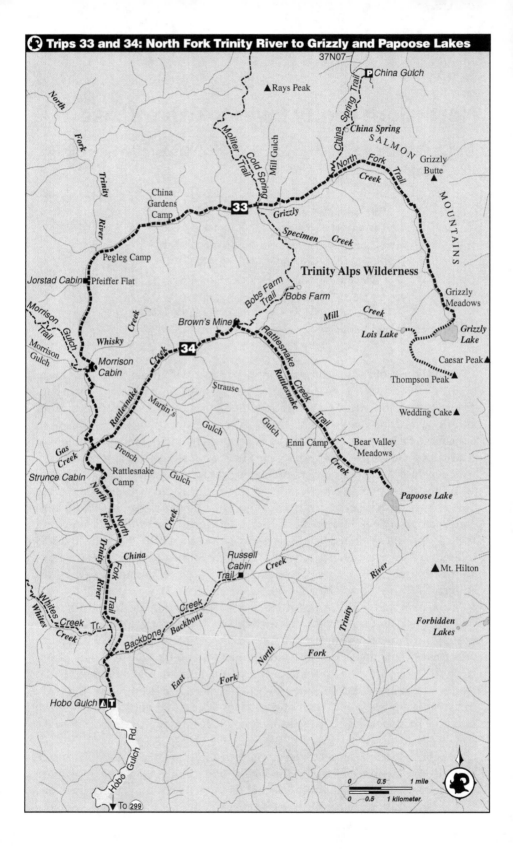

the duration of your stay and take precautions to minimize your impact as much as possible. Cross-country enthusiasts will find the off-trail route to Lois Lake a pleasant diversion; peakbaggers will find the route along the southwest ridge of Thompson Peak a straightforward ascent.

Starting Point

The Hobo Gulch trailhead is 17 miles north of the turnoff to the ghost town of Old Helena from Highway 299. Driving west from Weaverville on Highway 299, you top Oregon Mountain Summit at 4 miles and, 0.4 mile farther, pass a historical monument on the left featuring a hydraulic miners "Long Tom." Although nature has done a great deal of healing over the last century, keen eyes can still see where the entire side of the mountain south of the highway was washed down Oregon Gulch by hydraulic mining activity. At 8 miles from Weaverville, you pass through tiny Junction City, dating from the early mining days, beside the Trinity River at the bottom of the Oregon Mountain hill. In 7 more miles you reach a bridge over North Fork Trinity River and, immediately beyond, your turnoff, which is signed OLD HELENA.

Leaving Highway 299, head north of the town site, following a narrow, paved road, which crosses the North Fork and then continues along the East Fork of the North Fork for 2.7 miles to a junction with the Hobo Gulch Road. Turn left at the junction and follow a narrow, very crooked, and sometimes steep gravel road that climbs more than 8 miles to the top of a ridge between the North Fork and East Fork of the North Fork. A steeper downgrade of 5 more miles leads to the trailhead, 0.3 mile above Hobo Gulch Campground.

Large ponderosa pines and Douglas firs shade the primitive Hobo Gulch Campground, placed on a quarter-mile-long flat beside the river, which is the only water source. The free year-round campground has vault toilets but no trash pickup and is often crowded during the height of the season.

Description

The trail starts out almost level through dense mixed forest on the way to a junction with a spur trail from the campground. Beyond the junction, you climb moderately steeply for a short stretch before descending the east slope to cross Backbone Creek, 0.6 mile from the trailhead, where you reach a somewhat confusing three-way junction on the north bank.

Farthest to the right, Backbone Creek Trail 11W07, signed RUSSELL CABIN, heads northeast up Backbone Creek. The trail to the left, leading almost straight beside the river and signed PAPOOSE LAKE—LOW WATER TRAIL, BEAR WALLOW MEADOWS, is the North Fork Low Water Trail, which travels upstream a short distance, fords the North Fork, and then comes to a trail junction, 0.5 mile from this junction. From there, the Whites Creek Trail heads northwest toward Bear Wallow Meadows, and the North Fork Low Water Trail continues north another 0.3 mile, fording the North Fork again and reconnecting with the main trail. The middle trail, your route, signed PAPOOSE LAKE, is the main North Fork Trail, veering slightly to the right and climbing steeply uphill.

The steep climb along the main trail moderates eventually, as you head along a spur ridge between Backbone Creek and the North Fork, and then travel north along the east side of the canyon. Climbing above the canyon, you encounter a very pleasant open forest, which includes madrones, canyon oaks, and an occasional sugar pine, as well as the more common Douglas firs and ponderosa pines. A descent leads to a beautiful flat shaded by incense cedars and Douglas firs. Beyond the flat, you soon drop down to meet the trace of the Low Water Trail, 0.6 mile from Backbone Creek. Seemingly, an entire army could set up camp between here and China Creek and still have an adequate supply of firewood. Another flat with excellent campsites is higher above the river just north of China Creek, 2.3 miles from the trailhead.

At the upper end of the flat, the northern section of the North Fork Low Water Trail veers down toward the river and more campsites. The main trail on the right climbs up and down several times, passing the remnants of Strunce Cabin on the way. Approximately 0.25 mile past the cabin remnants, you reach the junction of the Rattlesnake Creek Trail to Papoose Lake in a broad flat with plenty of campsites nearby, 4.5 miles from the trailhead.

Your trail on the left, signed GRIZZLY LAKE, fords Rattlesnake Creek, which is a good-sized creek that may be difficult to ford in early season. Pass an excellent campsite on the north bank of Rattlesnake Creek, and then climb the ridge north of the creek in five, moderately steep switchbacks before turning around the nose of the ridge and continuing north well up the east side of the North Fork canyon. After a contour, follow a steeply descending traverse across a nearly vertical rock face, contour again, and then drop to a flat below Morrison Gulch and Morrison Cabin. Reach a junction with the Morrison Gulch Trail on the left, signed RATTLESNAKE LAKE.

Veer right at the junction, following a sign marked GRIZZLY LAKE, and climb above the east bank of the river, which makes a horseshoe-shaped bend around the spur ridge upon which sits Morrison Cabin. The cabin, which nestles beneath ponderosa pines and Douglas firs, was built in conjunction with a mining claim and was abandoned in 1989. Almost level trail runs through deep woods until emerging into the open again at Pfeiffer Flat, 8.2 miles from the trailhead.

At the flat, the trail almost delivers you to the doorstep of Jorstad Cabin, built by George Jorstad in 1937. Mr. Jorstad lived in the cabin and placer-mined his claim by hand until his death in 1989. The cabin, now under the care of the U.S. Forest Service, has escaped the calamities of fire and vandalism—at least so far. This idyllic site deserves your utmost consideration and respect. Away from the cabin, an easy amble beneath ponderosa pines, incense cedars, and Douglas firs leads to Pegleg Camp at the confluence of the North Fork and Grizzly Creek, where there is room for three or four tents with plenty of firewood nearby.

Leaving the North Fork behind, you turn east from Pegleg Camp and head up the narrower canyon of Grizzly Creek on good tread, built up on the south slope to avoid the steep canyon bottom choked with alders. A ford without a footlog, 0.9 mile from Pegleg Camp, takes you to the north side of the canyon, where you climb moderately steeply above more alders and willows, before leveling off in a jumble of rock piles that marks the old mining site of China Gardens.

Beyond the diggings, you climb steeply for 200 yards to an old ditch and walk alongside this relic for a quarter mile to a tributary stream. After another steep pitch, you ascend more gradually to Mill Gulch and a pair of trail junctions, 3 miles from Pegleg Camp.

At the creek, the seldom-used and never maintained Moliter Cold Springs Trail climbs north toward the Salmon Mountains divide and Cecil Lake. Just beyond the creek, the Bobs Farm Trail fords Grizzly Creek, climbs steeply southeast up Specimen Creek over a divide, and then down to a junction with the Rattlesnake Creek Trail. Your trail, which continues east up Grizzly Creek, is clearly marked at both junctions.

Shortcut to Papoose Lake?

On the way out from Grizzly Lake, if you plan to visit Papoose Lake, you should probably avoid the temptation to shorten the distance by using Bobs Farm Trail, since this rough path is one of the steepest trails in the entire wilderness. Just about anyone who's attempted this route will tell you that traveling the full distance back down the North Fork and then up Rattlesnake Creek is a much better alternative. Cursory study of the map reveals a site just over the south side of the ridge named Bobs Farm. An old-timer named Bob really did grow vegetables for the early miners here, carting his produce down to the mines by burro and returning with a tiny bit of gold for all his trouble.

The North Fork Trinity Trail gets steeper along Grizzly Creek between the Bobs Farm Trail junction and the China Spring Trail junction, 1.7 miles farther up the canyon, just beyond a clear, cold little creek cascading down a gully from the north. From the China Spring junction, the China Spring trailhead is 2.5 miles north over the Salmon Divide, 1350 vertical feet up to the crest and 1600 feet down the other side.

Continuing up Grizzly Creek canyon, you begin to turn south in thick timber well away from the course of the creek. At 1.3 miles from the China Spring junction, you climb out of the woods and over the top of a glaciated metamorphic rock outcrop, which provides a vantage point for the first long views since leaving the trailhead, nearly 14.5 miles ago. The higher valley above reveals the typical U-shape left by glaciers, in contrast to the V-shaped canyon below.

You follow the trail on traverses across the east side of the more open upper canyon, alternating with switchbacks in order to gain altitude across patches of broken rock and brush. From openings 3 miles above the China Spring junction you have your first glimpses of Thompson Peak and the perpetual snowfields clinging to the north face. Small meadows, willow flats, and groves of red firs soon replace brush on the more level floor of the upper valley, with good campsites appearing above and below a spring flowing across the trail. Beyond the spring, you climb moderately steeply for a half mile over exposed rock and through belts of firs to the north edge of Upper Grizzly Meadow, one of the most serene locales in the Trinity Alps.

Directly ahead, beyond the lush grasses and wildflowers of Upper Grizzly Meadow, the outlet of Grizzly Lake is forcefully propelled over a precipice of granite to dissolve in a flurry of cascades of white foam and mist in the jumbled granite blocks below. The south and west fringe of the meadow offers good to excellent campsites sheltered in groves of firs. Additional sites should be available between the trail and the creek below the meadow. Make sure to fully protect your food and equipment while camped near the meadow; deer and rodents are more of a problem here than the bears, but you should definitely hang your food away from the reach of all critters or use a bear canister.

The trail continues past Upper Grizzly Meadows through the trees and into the pile of talus on the east side. The Forest Service has improved the condition of the trail from this point over the years, but the path is still a long way from what you would generally expect from a trail. The route from the meadow up to Grizzly Lake has been designated as a "scramble" trail, the purpose of which is to define a single route up the very steep slope (rather than a multiplicity of boot-beaten paths), but to discourage visitors from carrying backpacks up to camps around the lake (to prevent environmental degradation). The route is steep, strenuous, and for experienced hikers only.

Above the lower section of talus, a virtual granite staircase has been constructed and marked by cairns. Approximately halfway up the slope, a spring-fed little stream flows down a rocky channel, a welcome spot to slake your thirst and catch your breath. Pass over the stream, pick up dirt tread, slick and muddy in spots, and proceed to a rock outcrop. Beyond the outcrop follow a steep path through a cleft, marked by ducks, leading alongside the upper channel of the stream before crossing over the watercourse to a field of vibrant wildflowers. Higher up, cross another branch of the stream. Now on more gently graded tread, indistinct at times, pass over boulders, stroll through lush vegetation, and hop over another tiny watercourse before following an angling traverse across the slope. The trail becomes more distinct again on the way to the north shore of dramatic Grizzly Lake, where the full breadth of deep, blue Grizzly Lake and the magnificent basin finally lies before you.

Nearly level slabs of granite ease into the water just west of the outlet, offering splendid opportunities for sunbathing, quick dips into the chilly water, or simply admiring the stunning scenery. Mountain hemlocks, red firs, and whitebark pines eke out an existence in cracks and on ledges around the nearly solid granite basin. Lush gardens of wildflowers bloom in tiny meadows long after the blooms of their counterparts have

Grizzly Meadow

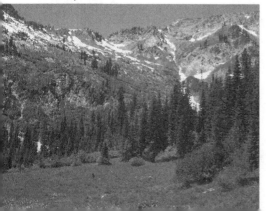

faded in Grizzly Meadow below. Above the first set of cliffs to the southeast, a large, higher cirque and shelf on the north face of jagged, 9002-foot Thompson Peak hold perpetual snowfields and patches of ice that resemble glaciers.

There are a handful of useable campsites sprinkled on the rock slabs along the north shore, and among small groves of conifers on a ridge and peninsula above the northwest shore. If you decide to camp near the lake, don't burn firewood if you even find any. Old-timers in the Trinity Alps may tell tales of taking limits of rainbow trout, all exceeding 12 inches, but heavier visitation has taken a harsh toll on the fish population in Grizzly Lake. Today you'll be fortunate to catch enough pan-sized trout for breakfast.

Rock climbers and scramblers will find an abundance of good vertical and overhanging granite both above and below the lake. For the more prosaic who desire to stand atop the summit of the highest peak in the Trinity Alps, the route up the arcing northwest ridge is a straightforward ascent—you may want an ice ax in early season. From the north shore of the lake, work above the granite cliffs to the southwest. You angle across granite slabs above, which may be covered with snow in early season, to the low point on the ridge leading up to the summit. From there, follow the backside of the ridge to the top, where the far-ranging views are utterly superb.

Cross-Country Route to Lois Lake

For cross-country enthusiasts, the route to diminutive Lois Lake, directly west of the much larger Grizzly Lake, is a short and straightforward endeavor. To reach Lois Lake, climb clefts in the ridge southwest of the north shore of Grizzly Lake until gaining the top of the ridge. Turn left (west) along the ridge and climb to a saddle at the intersection of another ridge from the northwest. Carefully drop down southwest from the ridge to where you can see Lois Lake below, sitting serenely in a rock basin, and then descend about 350 feet to the shore. The ridge above Lois Lake includes a panorama across a 2700-foot-deep cleft of Mt. Shasta in the distant east and excellent views of Thompson Peak.

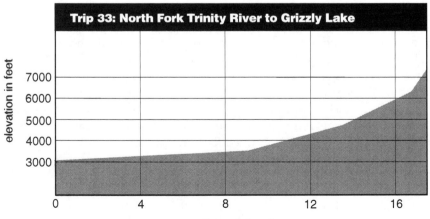

TRIP 34

North Fork Trinity River to Papoose Lake

Papoose Lake is a beautiful gem tucked into a deep cirque rimmed with serrated cliffs.

Trip Type:	Backpack, 3–6 days
Distance:	25 miles round-trip, out-and-back
Elevation Change:	3695 feet, average 296 per mile
Difficulty:	Moderate
Season:	Mid-July to early October
Maps:	USGS *Thurston Peaks, Cecil Lake, Thompson Peak,* and *Mount Hilton*; USFS *A Guide to the Trinity Alps Wilderness*
Nearest Campground:	Hobo Gulch

see map on p. 248

The Rattlesnake Creek Trail to Papoose Lake traverses one of the most intensely mined areas in the entire Trinity Alps. Enormous rock piles, pits, ditches, and mining relics, dating from the early '49er days to the present, litter the first 4 miles of steep-walled Rattlesnake Canyon from the confluence with the North Fork Trinity River all the way to Mill Creek. Somewhere between 50 and 100 Americans and an unrecorded number of Chinese immigrants lived and grubbed here in the mid- to late 19th century. Most of the gold the miners extracted from Mother Nature now lies hidden in vaults, but the evidence of their labor will remain for centuries to come. The scars left behind by the miners should not deter you from taking this trip. Fortunately, present-day mining activity is fairly minimal, although claims are still posted throughout the canyon.

While the mining history of the area will fascinate some, the main feature of this trip is lovely Papoose Lake. Unlike increasingly popular Grizzly Lake, roughly 3 air miles north, Papoose Lake offers a reasonable expectation of solitude, even during peak backpacking season. Opportunities abound for rock climbing and off-trail exploration of the peaks and ridges above the lake. Also, the fishing can be quite good.

Two small notes of caution: Although chances are good that you won't see either, use a bear canister or hang your food properly, as bears are active in this area; watch carefully for snakes, particularly in the lower parts of the canyon—Rattlesnake Canyon is so named for a reason.

Starting Point

The Hobo Gulch trailhead is 17 miles north of the turnoff to the ghost town of Old Helena from Highway 299. Driving west from Weaverville on Highway 299, you top Oregon Mountain Summit at 4 miles and, 0.4 mile farther, pass a historical monument on the left featuring a hydraulic miners "Long Tom." Although nature has done a great deal of healing over the last century, keen eyes can still see where the entire side of the mountain south of the highway was washed down Oregon Gulch by hydraulic mining activity. At 8 miles from Weaverville, you pass through tiny Junction City, dating from the early mining days, beside the Trinity River at the bottom of the Oregon Mountain hill. In 7 more miles you reach a bridge over North Fork Trinity River and, immediately beyond, your turnoff, which is signed OLD HELENA.

Leaving Highway 299, head north of the town site, following a narrow, paved road, which crosses the North Fork and then continues along the East Fork of the North Fork for 2.7 miles to a junction with the Hobo Gulch Road. Turn left at the junction and follow a narrow, very crooked, and sometimes steep gravel road that climbs more than 8 miles to the top of a ridge between the North Fork and East Fork of the North Fork. A steeper downgrade of 5 more miles leads to the trailhead, 0.3 mile above Hobo Gulch Campground.

Large ponderosa pines and Douglas firs shade the primitive Hobo Gulch Campground, placed on a quarter-mile-long flat beside the river, which is the only water source. The free year-round campground has vault toilets but no trash pickup and is often crowded during the height of the season.

Description

The trail starts out almost level through dense mixed forest on the way to a junction with a spur trail from the campground. Beyond the junction, you climb moderately steeply for a short stretch before descending the east slope to cross Backbone Creek, 0.6 mile from the trailhead, where you reach a somewhat confusing three-way junction on the north bank.

Farthest to the right, Backbone Creek Trail 11W07, signed RUSSELL CABIN, heads northeast up Backbone Creek. The trail to the left, leading almost straight beside the river and signed PAPOOSE LAKE—LOW WATER TRAIL, BEAR WALLOW MEADOWS, is the North Fork Low Water Trail, which travels upstream a short distance, fords the North Fork, and then comes to a trail junction, 0.5 mile from this junction. From there, the Whites Creek Trail heads northwest toward Bear Wallow Meadows, and the North Fork Low Water Trail continues north another 0.3 mile, fording the North Fork again and reconnecting with the main trail. The middle trail, your route, signed PAPOOSE LAKE, is the main North Fork Trail, veering slightly to the right and climbing steeply uphill.

The steep climb along the main trail moderates eventually, as you head along a spur ridge between Backbone Creek and the North Fork, and then travel north along the east side of the canyon. Climbing above the canyon, you encounter a very pleasant open forest, which includes madrones, canyon oaks, and an occasional sugar pine, as well as the more common Douglas firs and ponderosa pines. A descent leads to a beautiful flat shaded by incense cedars and Douglas firs. Beyond the flat, you soon drop down to meet the trace of the Low Water Trail, 0.6 mile from Backbone Creek. Seemingly, an entire army could set up camp between here and China Creek and still have an adequate supply of firewood. Another flat with excellent campsites is higher above the river just north of China Creek, 2.3 miles from the trailhead.

At the upper end of the flat, the northern section of the North Fork Low Water Trail veers left down toward the river and more campsites. The main trail on the right climbs up and down several times, passing the remnants of Strunce Cabin on the way. Approximately 0.25 mile past the cabin remnants, you reach the junction of the Rattlesnake Creek Trail to Papoose Lake in a broad flat with plenty of campsites nearby, 4.5 miles from the trailhead.

Leaving the North Fork Trail, you turn northeast and follow the course of an old wagon road across the wide floor of Rattlesnake Creek's lower canyon through a maze of pits, rock piles, and mementos of bygone mining days. Thick growths of alders, willows, and bigleaf maples have gone a long way toward obscuring these old mining scars, as well as blocking views of the tumbling creek.

As the canyon narrows, single-track trail climbs moderately up the southeast slope away from the old road. After a slight detour into Martin's Gulch, the trail rejoins the old road and proceeds to where some large log rounds block further progress along the roadbed. A sign simply marked TRAIL redirects your travel to the left, down through rock debris toward the ford of Rattlesnake Creek, 1.7 miles from the North Fork Trail junction. Immediately past the ford there's a lone campsite along the creek.

Away from the ford, you soon climb up to meet the old road again on the northwest side of the canyon, and then ascend moderately with a few steeper pitches through mixed forest above Rattlesnake Creek, which falls in and out of deep pools through a steep-walled gorge. If you have the extra energy and time to do so, climb down into the gorge past an abandoned 1940s vintage winch and dump truck with some dry flies to try for some surprisingly large rainbow trout from these pools. A long terrace on the opposite side of the canyon is covered with hand-piled boulders for more than a half mile. A short, steep climb leads to a junction with the brutally steep trail up to a ridge above Bobs Farm and back down to Grizzly Creek. Bobs Farm Trail is a rough path and one of the steepest trails in the entire wilderness. Just about anyone who's attempted this route will tell you that traveling the full distance back down the North Fork and then up Rattlesnake Creek is a much better alternative to this "shortcut."

Brown's Mine

It should be easy to recognize Brown's Mine, 1.8 miles from the ford of Rattlesnake Creek. Piles of mining junk are scattered around in all directions near a sign nailed to a Douglas fir. In addition to the usual items—riveted pipe, gears, valves, boiler grates, corrugated iron, bedsprings, and wire rope—a strange welded steel object that resembles a 6-foot guitar case puzzles everyone who passes by.

Past the junction with the Bobs Farm Trail, the Rattlesnake Creek Trail continues east above the creek to a clearing in a grove of manzanita. Here the canyon bends southeast, as you climb steeply, then descend just as steeply to dip down to a crossing of Mill Creek at the lower end of a long cascade from Lois Lake, perched in a high basin to the northeast. There's a single campsite next to the creek.

Above Mill Creek, you climb moderately on good tread through groves of Douglas firs and black oaks and patches of brushy hillside for a half mile to a crossing of Middle Fork Rattlesnake Creek, which combines a boulder hop and a logjam. Another 2 miles of slightly steeper climbing brings you to Enni Camp in a glacial moraine area, 6.3 miles from the North Fork Trail junction. Giant red firs shade campsites, with room for a dozen or more campers. An extremely little-used path leads northeast from the camp up the side of the canyon to Bear Valley Meadows.

The trail to the lake continues on well-defined tread, climbing steeply east of the creek. About 0.75 mile from Enni Camp, you meet some large granite boulders and cross to the south bank of the creek. Ducks show the way east across a sloping bench through ceanothus and manzanita brush and over more boulders. Just to the left of a red fir at the upper end of this bench, you begin a steep climb along the top of a cliff above the creek. At the bottom of a vertical face of metamorphic rock, follow the trail south, and then double back to zigzag up through a crack to a ledge above. Cross this ledge eastward, climbing over granite boulders, and look for ducks leading south to two less vertical faces with a ledge between them. Above the third rock face, continue south along the west edge of a deep gorge, through which the outlet of Papoose Lake falls. Beyond a hump of solid granite, showing some glacial striation and polish, you overlook gorgeous, teardrop-shaped Papoose Lake.

Keen eyes will notice the sharp dividing line running diagonally across the lake's cirque; the southeast

Papoose Lake

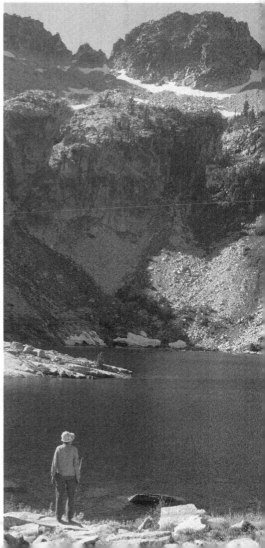

side is composed of granite, while the northeast side is gray metamorphic rock. Seeps and pockets of soil among the rocks around the lake support a marvelous profusion of wildflowers—pink spiraea, Indian paintbrush, wild onion, bistort, multicolored monkeyflowers, leopard lily, mountain aster, and Queen Anne's lace are but a few of the numerous species represented. The sparse conifers around the lake include mountain hemlocks, whitebark pines, and red firs.

A large granite slab slopes gently into the water east of the outlet of Papoose Lake, offering an excellent viewpoint and fishing perch, as well as a great spot to sunbathe and consider inching into the icy waters for a dip. From ledges a little farther along the east shore, you can gaze straight down into the deep water at 12- to 15-inch rainbow trout cruising just out of reach beside the vertical drop-offs. A few of these fish will rise to flies around sundown, if you can find the room necessary to cast. If you catch one, your problem then becomes how to extract them from the water. Catching smaller trout near the outlet should be much easier.

A number of campsites near the outlet may seem overused, but there are better spots with fine views of the lake farther up in the rocks above the northwest shore. Your tent better be freestanding, however, as most of these spots possess only an inch or two of decomposed rock over solid bedrock. Firewood is exceedingly more scarce than soil.

Scramblers will find plenty of opportunities to explore the divide above Canyon Creek, and experienced mountaineers can test their skill on nearby Mt. Hilton, which lies just out of sight from the shoreline to the southeast of Papoose Lake. For the more sedate, Papoose Lake and environs offer marvelous photographic opportunities and a pleasant atmosphere for contemplating life's wonders. The fact that there are no shortcuts to get here, combined with the mass pilgrimage of backpackers to the shores of Grizzly Lake, makes Papoose Lake a relative haven for solitude seekers.

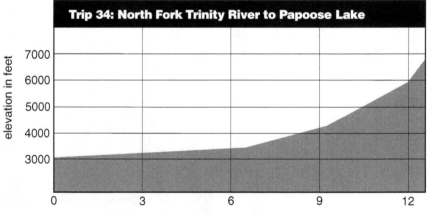

TRIP 35

New River Divide Loop

Views from New River Divide are truly awe-inspiring.

Trip Type:	Backpack, 3–4 days
Distance:	20.5 miles, loop, including side trip to Whites Creek Lake
Elevation Change:	9880 feet, average 481 per mile
Difficulty:	Moderate
Season:	Early July to mid-October (depending on ford of North Fork Trinity River)
Maps:	USGS *Thurston Peaks* and *Cecil Lake*; USFS *A Guide to the Trinity Alps Wilderness*
Nearest Campground:	Hobo Gulch

Nearly guaranteed solitude and incredible scenery are this loop's main attractions. The only time the southern part of the New River Divide Trail sees much traffic is during deer hunting season in late September into early October, with the area virtually deserted during the rest of the year. The same is true of the trail up Whites Creek to Bear Wallow Meadows and Hunters Camp. The section from Rattlesnake Camp down to Morrison Cabin is traveled more often since this is the main route between New River and North Fork Trinity River, but you still won't have to share the trail with many others. However, the 6 miles along the North Fork Trail is a different story—that trail is sometimes referred to as a freeway by people who like to be left alone.

Stunning views include overlooking the entire New River drainage back-dropped by a series of ridges farther west (although this view will more than likely be affected by recent fires). On the east side, the deep chasm of North Fork Trinity River yawns deeply in front of Backbone Ridge, and beyond the ridge are the high Alps near Grizzly and Papoose lakes. Sawtooth Mountain and the high ridge above Canyon Creek make up the skyline farther east.

Evidence of deer and black bears seems to be everywhere along the divide, but the animals in this area are still wild and quite wary, so you probably won't see as many of them as you might in other spots within the Trinity Alps Wilderness. Magnificent forests, ranging in composition from bigleaf maples, alders, and madrones in the bottoms of the canyons to stunted Jeffrey pines and western white pines on the crest, shelter a significant number and variety of songbirds and raptors.

Trails on this loop are well maintained and in surprisingly good condition despite the lack of use. Only one short stretch near Bear Wallow Meadows was hard to follow when I was last there prior to a massive wildfire that swept

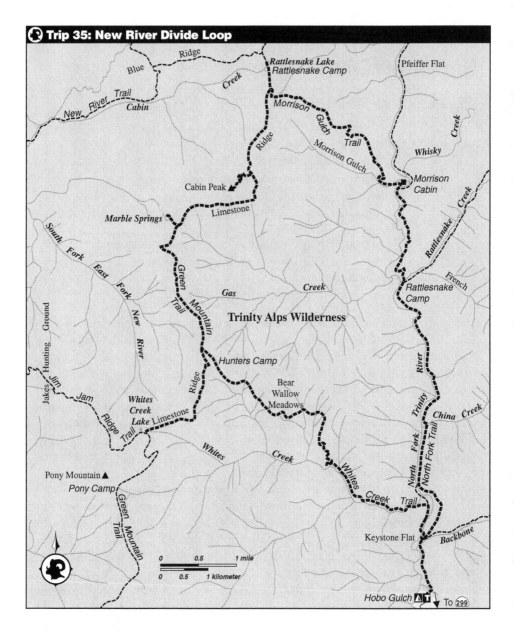

Trip 35: New River Divide Loop

through the area in 2006. You would be wise to check with the U.S. Forest Service on current conditions prior to your trip.

Starting Point

The Hobo Gulch trailhead is 17 miles north of the turnoff to the ghost town of Old Helena from Highway 299. Driving west from Weaverville on Highway 299, you top Oregon Mountain Summit at 4 miles and, 0.4 mile farther, pass a historical monument on the left featuring a hydraulic miners "Long Tom."

Although nature has done a great deal of healing over the last century, keen eyes can still see where the entire side of the mountain south of the highway was washed down Oregon Gulch by hydraulic mining activity. At 8 miles from Weaverville, you pass through tiny Junction City, dating from the early mining days, beside the Trinity River at the bottom of the Oregon Mountain hill. In 7 more miles you reach a bridge over North Fork Trinity River and, immediately beyond, your turnoff, which is signed OLD HELENA.

Leaving Highway 299, head north of the town site, following a narrow, paved road, which crosses the North Fork and then continues along the East Fork of the North Fork for 2.7 miles to a junction with the Hobo Gulch Road. Turn left at the junction and follow a narrow, very crooked, and sometimes steep gravel road that climbs more than 8 miles to the top of a ridge between the North Fork and East Fork of the North Fork. A steeper downgrade of 5 more miles leads to the trailhead, 0.3 mile above Hobo Gulch Campground.

Large ponderosa pines and Douglas firs shade the primitive Hobo Gulch Campground, placed on a quarter-mile-long flat beside the river, which is the only water source. The free year-round campground has vault toilets but no trash pickup and is often crowded during the height of the season.

Description

The trail starts out almost level through dense mixed forest on the way to a junction with a spur trail from the campground. Beyond the junction, you climb moderately steeply for a short stretch before descending the east slope to cross Backbone Creek, 0.6 mile from the trailhead, where a somewhat confusing three-way junction confronts you on the north bank.

Farthest to the right, Backbone Creek Trail 11W07, signed RUSSELL CABIN, heads northeast up Backbone Creek. The middle trail, signed PAPOOSE LAKE, is the main North Fork Trail, veering slightly to the right and climbing steeply uphill. Your trail to the left, leading almost straight beside the river, signed PAPOOSE LAKE—LOW WATER TRAIL, BEAR WALLOW MEADOWS, is the North Fork Low Water Trail, which travels upstream a short distance to a ford of North Fork Trinity River at Keystone Flat.

The crossing of North Fork Trinity River can be very dangerous during high water. If there is any question about the safety of this ford, turn back or perform a rope-belayed crossing. A 150-foot length of climbing rope is generally not something backpackers enjoy carrying for 20-plus miles, but if you need a rope at Keystone Flat you will more than likely also need one for the crossing near Morrison Cabin on the way back.

A beautiful mixed forest of huge Douglas firs, ponderosa pines, incense cedars, black oaks, bigleaf maples, and a few white firs shades Keystone Flat, as you follow nearly level tread north along an old road trace. Camping at this point may seem too early in the trip, but the almost perfect sites along this section are quite tempting. If you decide to take a dip in one of the deep and inviting pools in the river, be advised that the heavily traveled North Fork Trail overlooks the river from high up on the steep east bank, and plenty of anglers

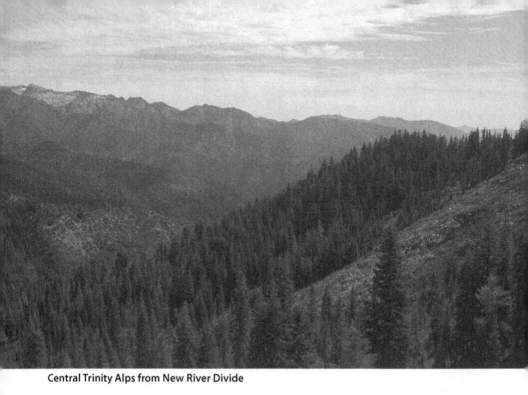

Central Trinity Alps from New River Divide

make their way up here from Hobo Gulch Campground, so skinny-dipping here may be equivalent to a form of exhibitionism. Reach the Whites Creek Trail junction 0.4 mile from the ford of North Fork Trinity River.

From the junction, head northwest across Keystone Flat on the Whites Creek Trail toward Bear Wallow Meadows until the trail turns west up Whites Creek canyon on a shelf above the creek. Narrowing canyon walls push the trail closer to the creek, and you boulder hop to the north bank, 0.5 mile from the Keystone Flat junction. Pools in the small creek above this crossing provide surprisingly good fishing for small, native rainbow trout and an occasional 9- to 10-incher. Just beyond the crossing there's a good campsite.

Extremely lush forest fills the bottom of the canyon—alders and maples along the creek and large Douglas firs farther up the slope. Some poison oak grows beside the trail in dry, open places. Good tread rises gradually except where the narrowing canyon walls force the trail to make short, steep climbs. Beyond one of the narrows, 1.8 miles from Keystone Flat, you climb out into a flinty hillside overlooking a fork in the creek. Both forks fall from pool to foaming pool in deep channels cut into exposed metamorphic rock to meet in a large pool overhung by lush ferns. Unfortunately, a Venturi mining dredge sometimes operates here.

East of the north fork of the creek, you climb steeply north up a rocky hillside over a knob of black rock and across a flat to reenter forest cover. A fine little tributary flows across the trail about 2 miles from Keystone Flat—a good place to acquire water for the steep ascent ahead. Steep switchbacks rise to a rocky point covered with serpentine shards. The trail zigzags to another outcrop, up the nose of a ridge, and around to longer-legged switchbacks up the side of the canyon through open forest and brush. At the top of the switchbacks, you contour west around a shoulder, and then turn back north again far up the east wall of a side canyon. Canyon oaks, black oaks, scrub oaks, and manzanita give way to large Douglas firs and sugar pines after you dip down to cross a seasonal stream that is usually dry by midsummer. However, ice cold, running water resurfaces about 100 feet below the trail.

Bear Wallow Camp appears on the Thurston Peaks quadrangle in the vicinity of two sloping benches a quarter mile from the crossing of the seasonal creek. Apparently, this is a historic site; there are no artificial structures or mining remnants here now, and the two gullies you cross are usually devoid of water. Around the next point, you turn north into another side canyon with the sound of running water ahead. Cross the stream, 3.5 miles from Keystone Flat, and then climb steeply west across a brushy hillside to a wide gully choked with alders and willows. This spot, believe it or not, is Bear Wallow Meadows, not exactly the lush, grassy scene normally associated with the term. The trail turns north beside the "meadow" and then suddenly disappears before reaching treeline above. Don't be too concerned, as you should find defined tread again where the trail crosses a patch of grass at the end of a gully and passes a tree bearing a sign affirming that you're in Bear Wallow Meadows. Two small, fair campsites are near the edge of the trees, west of a spring flowing out of a grass-rimmed pond. Although this is one of the few places within the Trinity Alps Wilderness with plenty of firewood, please use the wood sparingly. Be sure to hang your food well, or use a bear canister—Bear Wallow Meadows does have bears, even if there's not much in the way of meadows.

Above the meadows the trail turns and switchbacks up the hill north of the meadows before turning west over a spur ridge. Next, a long traverse, generally bearing northwest on good tread, travels through some minor ups and downs into side canyons and gullies and around shoulders covered with huckleberry oak and manzanita. Wide views open up behind you down to North Fork Trinity River. You climb steeply north beside a small stream in a gully, 1.8 miles from Bear Wallow Meadows, cross the channel higher up the slope where the streambed is usually dry, and then top out on a flat on a ridge between Whites and Gas creeks. North of the ridgecrest an old sign on a tree beside the trail denotes Hunters Camp, set in a pleasant glade at the head of Gas Creek. The glade offers several excellent campsites and a spring down the hill in a patch of willows is a fine water source.

Beyond Hunters Camp, you rise moderately and turn northwest through open, mature white-fir forest to a junction with the Green Mountain Trail on the crest of Limestone Ridge, 6.1 miles from the trailhead. The parklike forest covering the divide here is as pretty as you will see anywhere, composed almost entirely of white firs, widely spaced on an open floor with patches of pinemat manzanita and ceanothus. However, you're likely to see some evidence of the massive forest fires of 2006 and 2008 from this lofty perch.

Side Trip to Whites Creek Lake

Tiny Whites Creek Lake hangs in a basin at the head of Whites Creek northeast of Pony Mountain. However, without any fishing or swimming, the lake itself is not the main reason to take this side trip. The lake surroundings and the views from the nearly level 1.7 miles of trail along the way are truly outstanding. You can see Hunters Camp below as the trail contours through a magnificent forest away from the Whites Creek Trail junction and around the east side of a hump. Beyond the trees, you traverse south across a steep, brushy hillside, rising gradually to the crest of a spur ridge, 1.2 miles from the junction, and then turn almost directly west toward a ragged peak on the divide north of Pony Mountain. Another half mile, almost level through manzanita and huckleberry oak, brings you around to a shelf below the two peaks. The trail turns south over more open ledges and comes to a junction beyond a small stream, where the Jim Jam Ridge Trail forks west over the crest and eventually goes down to Jakes Hunting Ground and New River.

A nearly solid mass of alders and willows fills a 10- to 15-acre flat west of the trail, and Whites Creek Lake is a half-acre pond buried in the brush at the northeast corner of the flat. The lake's placid surface is a good mirror for the rugged face of Pony Mountain to the south. Other than that, the kindest thing one can say about Whites Creek Lake is that frogs seem to find it a good home. There's a campsite out of the brush beside a small grove of western white pines, an excellent site if not for a pile of rubbish beside an all-too-large fire ring—hopefully it has been cleaned up since I was last there.

The ledge at the east edge of the shelf is a marvelous place to watch the sunrise from behind the vast panorama to the east. The rosy light first touches the tops of the central Alps, from Thompson Peak in the north to Monument Peak and Weaver Bally Mountain in the south. Intervening ridgetops along both sides of Canyon Creek and North Fork Trinity River light up in turn, as the burning orb of the sun clears the ridge on the east horizon. Details soon appear in the gloom of the forested canyons below, and songbirds welcome the new day—all making for an unforgettable experience that's well worth the side trip.

As you head north from the Whites Creek Trail junction on the Green Mountain Trail, the large firs give way to ceanothus, manzanita, and huckleberry oak brush that crowds the path. You have glimpses down into East Fork New River as the trail crosses to the west side of Limestone Ridge. A stately row of Jeffrey pines crowns a knife-edged crest about 0.75 mile from the junction. From a bald summit 0.6 mile farther north, you have your first good view west across the New River drainage, where a series of blue ridges step up to the west horizon beyond the river.

You skirt the east side of a bald knob to the north, and then climb moderately northeast before turning west up the side of a ridge below a chocolate-hued outcrop. The trail ascends to the top of a meadow above this outcrop before turning north again to the brink of a steep drop-off near the top of a low mountain straddling the divide. From this spot, the massive bulk of Cabin Peak rises beyond a deep saddle to the northeast, and you can see the trail contouring around the south side of the peak.

The trail once again dives straight down the north side of the mountain toward a saddle, making one long-legged switchback west and then heading back northeast. A steep and rough section of tread in loose rock and gravel leads to the saddle, where a faint path forks west to run down the side of the ridge a quarter mile to water and campsites at Marble Springs. You may want to make the trip to Marble Springs and fill your water container, as no water will be available along the Green Mountain Trail for the next 4 miles.

Disintegrated rock, almost like volcanic ash, crunches underfoot, as you cross the saddle and start climbing through brush and scattered timber on the slope to the north. The brush soon thins, and you continue climbing north up an open, gravelly slope on the nose of the ridge. The trail turns over to the east side of the ridge, 0.3 mile from the Marble Springs junction, and begins a long traverse east through heavy brush across the south face of Cabin Peak.

At 3.5 miles from the Whites Creek Trail junction is the crest of a spur ridge buttressing the southeast corner of Cabin Peak. The trail turns north from this crest to contour almost level through cool, dense forest, a welcome relief after the mile-long traverse across the hot, brushy south face of the peak. A path to the summit of Cabin Peak branches left a quarter mile into the woods, which once led to a lookout on the peak. The tower is long gone, but the 360-degree view is still there if you don't mind the effort involved. Beyond this junction, you emerge into the open again and turn northwest around a shoulder of the mountain on finely broken, red-rock talus. On the north side of Cabin Peak, the trail turns to descend moderately steeply a little east of north on the crest of the divide.

The ridgetop is generally level beyond the descent from Cabin Peak, but outcrops and knobs along the crest force the trail to climb from one side to the other. A very narrow, brushy section of the crest, 4.4 miles from the Whites Creek Trail junction, offers an unrestricted view southeast down Morrison Gulch all the way to North Fork Trinity River. The trail down to Morrison Cabin marks a trace on the ridge beyond the gulch. A south cutoff to this trail is another 0.4 mile father down the trail. From

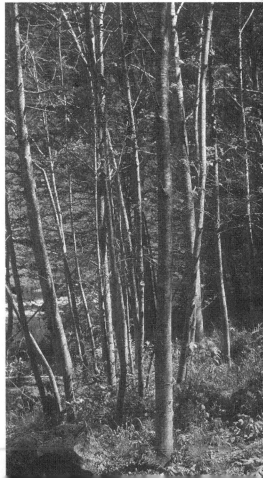

Alders by New River

the junction with the south cutoff below some rock outcrops west of the Green Mountain Trail, you continue north, reaching the north junction of the Morrison Gulch Trail in open forest after 0.3 mile.

Backpackers in need of overnight accommodations will have to proceed north on the Green Mountain Trail, dropping a quarter mile to Rattlesnake Camp on a flat hanging above the canyons of Cabin Creek and East Fork New River. In addition to a sign confirming that this is indeed Rattlesnake Camp, another sign, with an arrow pointing southwest down the hillside, leads to two forks of a spring about 100 yards away. One fork is dry, but a short length of pipe on the other fork runs a pencil-thin stream of clear, cold water into a large enameled basin. Campsites on the flat were littered and overused when I last scouted it, but campers have no other choice for places to camp within 2 or 3 miles—there simply isn't any other source of water along Limestone Ridge. However, the small flat provides an excellent place to watch the sunset behind the ridges beyond New River. Rattlesnake Lake is a murky pond in a brush-filled draw east of the trail 250 yards to the north, whose water is unfit for drinking under any circumstances. A quarter mile beyond the lake, the New River Trail forks west down to East Fork New River. This trail, along with the Morrison Gulch Trail, provides the access for most of the visitors to Rattlesnake Camp.

From the junction of the Morrison Gulch and Green Mountain trails, head south on a moderately steep climb around the west side of a knob on the divide. As the trail turns east around the south side of the knob, you come to a junction with the south cutoff trail, 0.3 mile from the junction. Follow the crest of a razorback ridge farther east, and then circle a knob and zigzag down a wider ridgetop before dropping over the south side of the ridge. On rough, gravelly tread, you descend steeply (very steeply in places) through thick manzanita, scrub oak, and huckleberry oak to turn around the brow of the ridge again and look straight across North Fork Trinity River canyon to the face of the ridge between Grizzly and Rattlesnake creeks.

The next 1.5 miles switchbacks down the ridge, steeply at times, before turning back west through Douglas-fir forest on the side of the canyon above the creek in Morrison Gulch. After a final switchback, follow the creek down to a ford, 3.5 miles from the Green Mountain Trail junction. From the ford, the trail rises to the top of a low ridge between the creek and North Fork Trinity River, then follows the top of the ridge east for 150 yards before turning down toward the river along the edge of a lush, sloping meadow.

Rustic Morrison Cabin

Morrison Cabin is nestled beneath tall Douglas firs and ponderosa pines at the top of the meadow. A family who mined a claim on the river and creek until 1990 occupied the cabin during the summer months. The U.S. Forest Service negotiated abandonment of the claim, and the cabin is now U.S. property. Please treat this historic treasure with the utmost respect.

At a sign below the cabin, you ford the river and then climb up the east bank to a junction with the North Fork Trail, 100 yards up the side of the canyon. From the junction, you are 6 miles north of the Hobo Gulch trailhead. Head downstream along North Fork Trinity River for nearly 2 miles to a ford of Rattlesnake Creek, with good campsites on either side. Just across the creek, you reach a junction with the Rattlesnake Creek Trail heading northeast and then continue downstream along North Fork Trinity River. At Strunce Cabin on the way to China Creek a side trail branches toward campsites along the river.

Beyond China Creek, the main trail proceeds down the river past the north junction of the low water trail. Continue another 0.6 mile to the north bank of Backbone Creek and the south junction of the low water trail on the right and the Backbone Creek Trail heading northeast on the left. Follow the middle trail from the junction across Backbone Creek and then on a short climb above the river before you drop down to the Hobo Gulch trailhead. If you had difficulty at the initial ford of North Fork Trinity River at Keystone Flat, you may find the ford at Rattlesnake Creek challenging as well. Several campsites near the ford and south along the North Fork offer one last night of sleeping out under the stars.

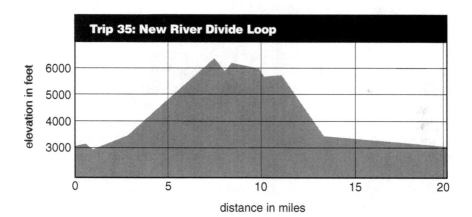

TRIP 36

Green Mountain Trail
to North Fork Trinity River

Solitude, high ridges with expansive views, and deep-green forests thrill on this circuit over Limestone Ridge.

Trip Type:	Backpack, 3–5 days
Distance:	17.6 miles, point-to-point (plus 0.5-mile round-trip to Brushy Mountain and 1.7-mile round-trip to Green Mountain)
Elevation Change:	10,875 feet, average 550 per mile
Difficulty:	Moderate
Season:	Mid-July to mid-October
Maps:	USGS *Jim Jam Ridge* and *Thurston Peaks*; USFS *A Guide to the Trinity Alps Wilderness*
Nearest Campground:	Hayden Flat

The U.S. Forest Service is so firmly convinced about the Green Mountain Trail's lack of use that there isn't enough space to park more than a couple of vehicles anywhere near the trailhead. This lack of attention is certainly not deserved from a scenery standpoint, as the views down into the lush green canyons, and up to Limestone Ridge, Thurston Peaks, and the central Trinity Alps are superb.

This route leads you to only one lake, Whites Creek Lake, which is no more than a murky pond. Even so, plenty of water should be available in creeks and streams along the way. Camping is somewhat limited to specific locations as well, but the camps that do exist are more than adequate for the number of backpackers who use this trail. One, Pony Camp, is set in one of the most scenic basins you could hope to find.

Wildflowers abound in many of the areas during peak season, including some more infrequently seen varieties. A side benefit of the 2008 Buckhorn Fire in this area will likely be an immediate increase in the numbers of flowers growing in the recovering areas. Wildlife should be plentiful as well, but since human contact is relatively light, you're more apt to see their droppings than the animals themselves.

Make sure you bring plenty of water to start the trip, as there isn't an easily accessible source until after 3.5 miles of mostly uphill hiking. If a lack of water at the beginning is a problem, too much water near the end could pose an even more formidable obstacle: The ford of North Fork Trinity River near Keystone Flat can be dangerous during high water—check with the Forest Service about current conditions before embarking on this trip.

Trip 36: Green Mountain Trail to North Fork Trinity River

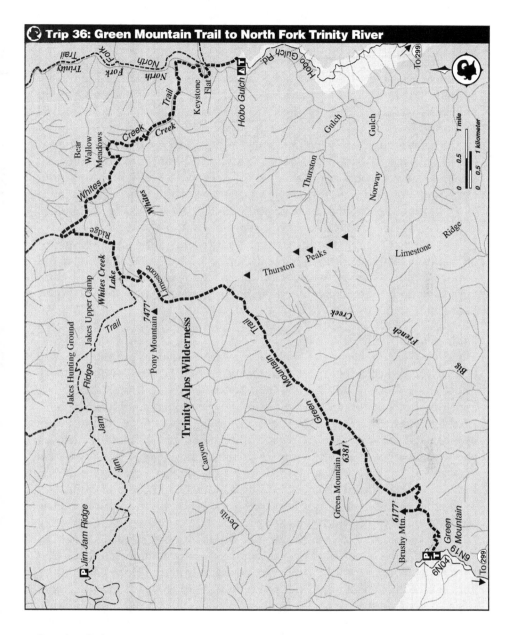

Starting Point

Approximately 29 miles west of Weaverville (6 miles west of Big Bar Ranger Station), Forest Service Road 5N13 turns north from Highway 299, just past a sign marked BIG FRENCH BAR. Traveling from the east, the turnoff is past the end of a guardrail, not at the wide shoulder just after the sign. Shortly after the turnoff, another sign reads FRENCH CREEK TRAILHEAD 3, GREEN MOUNTAIN TRAILHEAD 13. Off to the right, keen eyes may notice the old abandoned highway bridge that used to span French Creek. At 0.5 mile, Road 5N20 veers right and heads down to the water, but you remain on 5N13 straight ahead, slowly climbing above the west bank of Big French Creek. Pass the French Creek trailhead at 2.7 miles from Highway 299, beyond which the road switchbacks and continues climbing past some well-marked side roads and a few clear-cuts on the way up Barnum Ridge. At about 6.5 miles, you reach a clearing and the first glimpse of Limestone Ridge to the west. Reach a major intersection at 9.2 miles, past an old corral.

Continue straight ahead from the intersection, now on Road 6N04, following a sign marked GREEN MOUNTAIN TRAILHEAD 4. At 12.4 miles you reach another signed intersection and turn right onto the narrow track of Road 6N19 (prior to the fires, this road was crowded by vegetation and little used). After 0.5 mile you pass the signed trailhead and continue another 0.1 mile to a wide shoulder, where parking should be available for about a half dozen vehicles.

Hayden Flat Campground is along the north bank of the Trinity River just off Highway 299, 0.3 mile west of the turnoff onto Road 5N13. The year-round campground has running water, vault toilets, and a beach area. Reservations are accepted for 14 campsites by calling Big Bar Ranger Station (530-623-6106). Per night cost in 2009 was $20.

Ending Point

The Hobo Gulch trailhead is 17 miles north of the turnoff to the ghost town of Old Helena from Highway 299. Driving west from Weaverville on Highway 299, you top Oregon Mountain Summit at 4 miles and, 0.4 mile farther, pass a historical monument on the left featuring a hydraulic miners "Long Tom." Although nature has done a great deal of healing over the last century, keen eyes can still see where the entire side of the mountain south of the highway was washed down Oregon Gulch by hydraulic mining activity. At 8 miles from Weaverville, you pass through tiny Junction City, dating from the early mining days, beside the Trinity River at the bottom of the Oregon Mountain hill. In 7 more miles you reach a bridge over North Fork Trinity River and, immediately beyond, your turnoff, which is signed OLD HELENA.

Leaving Highway 299, head north of the town site, following a narrow, paved road, which crosses the North Fork and then continues along the East Fork of the North Fork for 2.7 miles to a junction with the Hobo Gulch Road. Turn left at the junction and follow a narrow, very crooked, and sometimes steep gravel road that climbs more than 8 miles to the top of a ridge between the North Fork and East Fork of the North Fork. A steeper downgrade of 5 more miles leads to the trailhead, 0.3 mile above Hobo Gulch Campground.

Large ponderosa pines and Douglas firs shade the primitive Hobo Gulch Campground, placed on a quarter-mile-long flat beside the river, which is the only water source. The free year-round campground has vault toilets but no trash pickup and is often crowded during the height of the season.

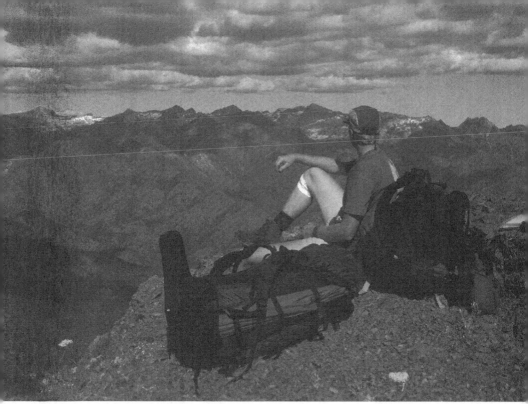
View from Green Mountain Trail near Limestone Ridge

Description

Start up the road from the parking area to the trailhead and begin hiking on the course of an old road heading steeply uphill. The first 100 yards are out in the open alongside canyon oaks before you come under the cover of partially burned fir forest. After climbing steeply for a mile, you reach the top of a ridge, make a brief descent, and come to a junction with an old road leading to the top of Brushy Mountain, 1.25 miles from the trailhead.

Side Trip to Brushy Mountain

You'll quickly notice that Brushy Mountain is very well named. The trail up to the summit is short, not at all steep, but crowded by a preponderance of thick brush. If few souls hike the Green Mountain Trail, even fewer seem inclined to make the quarter-mile ascent to the top of Brushy Mountain. You may have to beat back some of the brushy vegetation, but the superb view from the summit more than compensates for the minor inconvenience. A nearly uninterrupted 360-degree panorama awaits you at the top: east to the spine of Limestone Ridge and the peaks of the central Trinity Alps, north to the Salmon Mountains, and west and south to an endless sea of ridges and canyons of the western Alps. You may even catch a glimpse of one of the many species of raptors that frequent this area.

Back on the main trail, you make a short climb and then begin a long, moderate descent. An abundance of wildflowers appear alongside this part of the old roadbed through midsummer, despite an apparent lack of surface water. As the trail bends north, you have periodic views toward Green Mountain and the steep climb along the exposed southern flank. At 2.5 miles from the trailhead, you reach the saddle between Brushy and Green mountains, as predominantly fir forest gives way to oak and manzanita.

The ascent up the side of Green Mountain is both steep and rocky and, if the sun is out and the day is warm, hot as well. Once this obstacle has been surmounted, the trail heads back into the trees, crosses a pair of rivulets, and then crosses the main channel of the creek flowing down into Willow Gulch, the first reliable source of water in the first 3.5 miles. The trail ascends moderately along the east bank of the creek, crosses to the west bank 0.5 mile farther up amid an array of wildflowers, and then shortly passes Stove Camp on the opposite bank.

Fighting the 2008 Buckhorn Fire

Tragically, the Green Mountain Trail saw a great deal of use in 2008, as a helicopter crash just below Limestone Ridge on August 6 took the lives of a pilot, a U.S. Forest Service employee, and seven firefighters who were battling the Buckhorn Fire. Four others fortunately survived the crash. The Buckhorn Fire was one of several fires started by lightning strikes on June 21 that made up the Iron/Alps Complex. Total costs for fighting these fires exceeded $81 million over several weeks and ultimately burned more than 105,000 acres.

Emergency personnel and recovery crews regularly used the section of the Green Mountain Trail from the trailhead to the crash site between Green and Pony mountains. Since this segment of the trail had to be brushed wide enough for pack stock to haul out debris from the wreckage, trail users will reap the somber benefit of a well-maintained trail for the immediate future. The extensive fire damaged a huge swath of forest from the crest of Limestone Ridge west to the Green Mountain crest, a grim site that will surely be noticeable on the drive to the trailhead and for much of the initial route of the trail.

Stove Camp is the first flat spot large enough for a decent size campsite within the first 4 miles of the Green Mountain Trail. Only one established site occupies a broad, slightly sloping area surrounded by towering firs. If you should happen to encounter the rare possibility of a party already camped here, there are other potential places to camp at Stove Camp, but please restore them to their natural condition upon your departure. An abundance of bear scat makes hanging your food securely a reasonable precaution—better yet, carry a bear canister. Fortunately, bears in this part of the wilderness still remain quite skittish around humans.

About 0.25 mile above Stove Camp, after crossing the diminishing creek a third time, you crest the ridge and reach a junction with an old road heading west toward the summit of Green Mountain.

Side Trip to Green Mountain

The trail to the top begins climbing moderately through a continuation of fir forest until about halfway up the mountain, where the grade levels out and the vegetation becomes predominantly manzanita. Unlike the trail to Brushy Mountain, this trail requires no bushwhacking and is quite easy to follow. Continue up the road along the top of a ridge to reach the summit. The view from Green Mountain is partially occluded by trees to the north and south, but offers magnificent vistas of Limestone Ridge, Thurston Peaks, and Jim Jam Ridge, plus a fairly comprehensive look at the route ahead, which undulates over peaks and through saddles to surmount the crest of Limestone Ridge.

From the Green Mountain junction, the trail follows a series of roller-coaster romps northeast up minor peaks and into the saddles in between. In one of these minor saddles, 1.25 miles from the Green Mountain junction, you come upon an interesting geologic formation in a large outcrop of dark, green rock. This particular rock is serpentine, igneous in origin, but subducted, exposed to cool temperatures and metamorphosed into its current state. Views are often quite impressive along this stretch of old road, as you stroll along the crest of the ridge connecting Green Mountain to Limestone Ridge.

In the next to the last of the saddles, 5.9 miles from the trailhead, you see the first sign of civilization since the beginning of the trip, a wood sign attached to a ponderosa pine that reads PONY CAMP with an arrow pointing straight ahead and LADDER CAMP pointing downhill to the left. The faint path down to Ladder Camp soon disappears, and the only more difficult task than locating the trail becomes finding Ladder Camp. If you want to camp there, I can only wish you good luck, as I never found it in my scouting efforts.

Proceed ahead on the old road for another 0.3 mile from the junction to where the route becomes a bona fide single-track trail for the first time in 6.2 miles. The trail ascends the side of the last bump on the ridge and drops you at a saddle separating Green Mountain ridge from Limestone Ridge. At this point the views are stunningly impressive, including the route of the trail north up to the crest of Limestone Ridge just below Pony Mountain. Follow a level traverse around the head of a basin for 0.7 mile to the crossing of a delightful creek that drops through Devils Canyon, cascading down narrow rock clefts and bordered by moss-covered rocks and lush foliage.

From the creek, the trail continues traversing until you ascend the side of Limestone Ridge. Well-graded tread crosses a barren slope and, just before you encounter some rocks, climbs a series of switchbacks to a notch in a satellite ridge. From there, the trail descends briefly, and then makes an ascending traverse to the crest of Limestone Ridge. One odd geologic note is that the green rock found along this section of Limestone Ridge is not limestone at all, but a type of metamorphosed plutonic rock. The 7000-foot-plus apex of the ridge is the high point of your journey, with correspondingly spectacular views east to the highest of the Trinity Alps peaks. Below you, a quarter mile away, is Pony Camp cradled in a cirque basin.

One switchback and a steady descent of 250 vertical feet brings you to Pony Camp, tucked into a sloping meadow blanketed with colorful wildflowers below 7477-foot Pony Mountain. A spring meandering through the meadowland assures the availability of water. The main campsite in the area nestles beneath some old Douglas firs, with other sites scattered around the basin. The view from the main camp plunges down the hillside to the lush green canyon below and then rises up to the snow-clad granite spires of the central Alps above. For an even grander view, you can easily ascend the southeast slope of Pony Mountain. Considering all the marvelous attributes of Pony Camp, including an almost ironclad guarantee of solitude, the one drawback the site is cursed with is hard to fathom—an inordinate amount of debris left behind by horse packers. Hopefully, a trail crew has cleaned up this mess since I was last there, but there is no report of any recent maintenance this far up the Green Mountain Trail. If the trash remains, please consider hauling out at least a portion of the debris, thereby helping to restore the camp to a pristine state.

Leaving the pleasant environs of Pony Camp, you begin the long descent toward North Fork Trinity River. Away from the camp, the trail drops around a hillside into the cover of fir forest, switchbacks twice, and continues descending along the spine of a ridge. At the end of the ridge, the trail switchbacks sharply and descends moderately around the head of a minor basin and out to a crossing of flower-lined Whites Creek, 1.3 miles from Pony Camp. Thirty yards prior to the creek is an unsigned junction with the Jim Jam Ridge Trail heading west toward Jakes Upper Camp.

Side Trip to Whites Creek Lake

Tiny Whites Creek Lake hangs in a basin at the head of Whites Creek northeast of Pony Mountain. However, without any fishing or swimming the lake won't make anyone's list of top 10 lakes in the Trinity Alps. A nearly solid mass of alders and willows fills a 10- to 15-acre flat west of the trail, and Whites Creek Lake is a half-acre pond buried in the brush at the northeast corner of the flat. The lake's placid surface is a good mirror for the rugged face of Pony Mountain to the south. Other than that, the kindest thing one can say about Whites Creek Lake is that frogs find it a good home. There's a campsite out of the brush beside a small grove of western white pines, an excellent site if not for a pile of rubbish beside an all-too-large fire ring—hopefully this mess has been cleaned up since I was last there.

The ledge at the east edge of the shelf is a marvelous place to watch the sunrise from behind the vast panorama to the east. The rosy light first touches the tops of the central Alps, from Thompson Peak in the north to Monument Peak and Weaver Bally Mountain in the south. Intervening ridgetops along both sides of Canyon Creek and North Fork Trinity River light up in turn, as the burning orb of the sun clears the ridge on the east horizon. Details soon appear in the gloom of the forested canyons below, and songbirds welcome the new day—all making for an unforgettable experience that's well worth the side trip.

From the crossing of Whites Creek, the trail ahead is visible, cutting north-northeast across a manzanita-covered hillside. You follow this traverse around the nose of a ridge and then drop more steeply to the north through shady fir forest with an occasional incense cedar. Continue the steady ascent to a junction with the Whites Creek Trail, 1.8 miles from the crossing of Whites Creek. A lone campsite is near the junction, but there's no water anywhere close by.

Leaving the Green Mountain Trail behind, turn right (southeast) at the junction and follow Whites Creek Trail on a wandering descent, still through predominantly fir forest. Cross three tributaries to a clearing, where you can gaze west toward Limestone Ridge and Pony Mountain. From there, a very short climb leads to the top of a ridge overlooking Bear Wallow Meadows, with a fine view of the central Alps and Limestone Ridge as well. A steep and winding descent leads down to the meadows. There are two small, fair campsites near the edge of the trees, west of a spring flowing out of a grass-rimmed pond. This is one of the few places within the Trinity Alps Wilderness with plenty of firewood, but please use it sparingly. Be sure to hang your food well, or use a bear canister. Bear Wallow Meadows does have bears, even if there's not much in the way of actual meadows.

After a short climb that crosses a trio of tributary streams, you descend, steeply at times, toward the main stem of Whites Creek, where a more moderate descent follows the narrow canyon generally east downstream toward North Fork Trinity River. Reach a junction with the North Fork Low Water Trail in Keystone Flat, with excellent campsites nearby. Turn right to follow the Low Water Trail downstream to the ford of the river, and then climb up the far bank to meet the main North Fork Trail at a three-way junction with the Backbone Creek Trail heading northeast. From there, continue downstream on the North Fork Trail 0.6 mile to the Hobo Gulch trailhead.

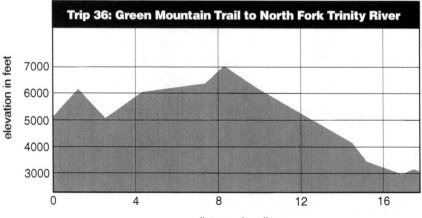

TRIP 37

New River and Slide Creek to Historic Mining District and Eagle Creek

Solitude combined with a taste of Trinity Alps mining history make for a rich experience indeed.

Trip Type:	Backpack, 3–6 days
Distance:	24 miles, loop
Elevation Change:	7740 feet, average 323 per mile
Difficulty:	Difficult
Season:	Mid-May to early November
Maps:	USGS *Jim Jam Ridge* and *Dees Peak*; USFS *A Guide to the Trinity Alps Wilderness*
Nearest Campground:	Denny

Seeing another soul on the greater New River and Slide Creek route, one of the more remote trails in the western Trinity Alps, is highly unlikely. Old mining towns and related sites abound in the Historic Mining District, including Old Denny, where, around the turn of the 20th century, 500 residents once lived and worked. Nowadays, the old town site may not see that many visitors in a hundred-year span. Rich with history, other town sites, such as Marysville and White Rock City, invite explorers to discover the treasures of the past. While most of the Alps mining was hydraulic or placer, this route passes near the Sherwood and Hunter mines, two of the area's very few examples of hard-rock mining. The more modern-day "agricultural miners" who grew illegal crops of marijuana in this area in the 1970s and '80s have been rooted out. During the pot-growing heyday, recreational enthusiasts entering this part of the wilderness were placing their safety and even their lives in jeopardy. If you happen to see any suspicious activity in this area, please report it to the Big Bar Ranger Station.

You'll travel alongside the cascading streams and deep green pools of Slide and Eagle creeks. Most of the trail is below 4000 feet, a prime environment for mixed forests of deciduous trees, such as live oaks, canyon oaks, madrones, and bigleaf maples, and the primary conifers in the area, Douglas firs. Higher up pines and firs become the dominant species in pockets of dense coniferous forest. Occasional wildflower displays add color in early summer.

Summer temperatures can be quite hot at these elevations, which makes late spring and early fall the best times to enjoy this part of the Trinity Alps. However, an excellent network of connecting trails allows you to alter your route into the cooler temperatures of the higher elevations near the crest of the

Trip 37: New River and Slide Creek to Historic Mining District and Eagle Creek

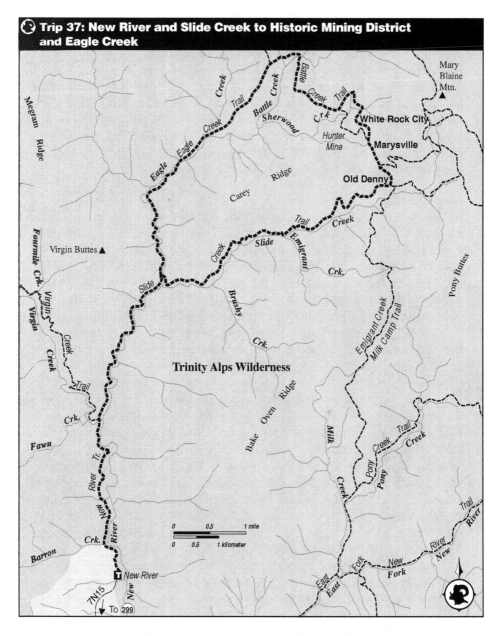

Salmon Mountains. Even though the upper reaches of the trail may be free of snow by the first part of May, the amount of runoff rushing down Virgin Creek at a ford, 3 miles from the trailhead, may keep you from progressing. Check with the U.S. Forest Service about the condition of this crossing before your trip. The lower elevations pose some additional potentially adverse possibilities: Poison oak is prevalent but easily avoided alongside much of the trail, rattlesnakes are common, and all food should be hung well away from any uninvited dinner guests. Fishing is quite good in Slide and Eagle creeks, but anglers should check with the Department of Fish and Game for the current fishing regulations, as the Trinity River and its tributaries are closely monitored.

Due to the area's remote nature, a lack of funding resulting in little or no trail maintenance, and a 2006 wildfire that burned a significant portion of the New River drainage, this trip is for seasoned hikers only. Beyond the first 3 miles of trail, maintenance has been nonexistent for several years, so be prepared to do some route-finding and possibly some bushwhacking. Topographic maps, a compass, a GPS receiver, and the knowledge to use them are absolute essentials for this circuit through these isolated and rugged lands.

Starting Point

The first step is reaching the settlement of Denny, which is a long way up the canyon of New River. County Road 402 branches away from Highway 299 at Hawkins Bar, 46 miles west of Weaverville and 10 miles east of Willow Creek. Beyond a high bridge over the Trinity River, you travel 0.25 mile to an intersection, where you turn back west and then north beside Hawkins Creek, passing several houses and a subdivision to the next intersection. Turn right and begin a long, twisting climb generally east up the side of Trinity River canyon.

At 6.3 miles from Hawkins Bar, beyond some unbelievably tight hairpin turns, a dirt road forks left to Happy Camp and points farther north. Another 1.2 miles leads to the end of the climb at a point on a spur ridge dividing the drainages of Trinity River and New River. Narrow pavement snakes down the east side of the ridge, and then turns northeast through a gap in a spur ridge to a cluster of homes among neat orchards on a flat far above New River. Eventually the road draws near to the river at Panther Creek, 14.5 miles from Hawkins Bar.

Denny Campground straddles the road 0.3 mile farther up the canyon, with Denny Forest Service Guard Station out of sight above the upper part of the campground. A Forest Service employee is usually available to provide a wilderness permit or information on the current state of the trails. At 1400 feet, the free year-round campground is fairly large and quite pleasant, with vault toilets but no potable water or trash pickup.

The community of Denny begins about 0.7 mile above the campground, and is strung out along the road for the next half mile or so. Continue on paved road past Denny and Quinby Creek to a signed junction with Road 7N15 on the left.

Turn onto the gravel surface of Road 7N15, which doubles back from the paved Denny Road and climbs away from the river. The road turns north, then east around the shoulder of a ridge, and then north again on the west side of New River canyon across from the East Fork. At 4.7 miles from County Road 402, having passed forks with three or four lesser roads, veer right at a signed intersection, remaining on Road 7N15, and proceed to another junction at 5.4 miles. Turn left here, as the surface turns from gravel to dirt, which may be impassable during wet weather. Continue to the trailhead at the end of the road, with plenty of parking space and a stock tie area.

Description

Single-track trail descends 0.4 mile to the wilderness boundary, merges with the trace of an old road, and then returns to single track on the way down a short, steep pitch to Barron Creek in an alder thicket. A footlog below the ford is available during periods of high water, but the crossing is usually problem-free. As you climb moderately out of the creek bed, tall Douglas firs, madrones, and a few tanoaks grow above an understory of vine maples, ceanothus, redbuds, and dogwoods on the hillside. A few blackberry vines in slide areas provide a welcome treat in season. You can hear New River in the bottom of the canyon to the east.

A short distance away from Barron Creek you reach and then follow the west bank of New River for 250 yards. After a moderate climb up the canyon wall, the trail stays away from the river across steep hillsides, flats, and ledges. Good tread follows the contour of an old mining ditch in places. A spring flows across the trail at 0.7 mile from Barron Creek.

Beyond the spring, the trail rises more steeply to a rocky point, around which the river roars in a horseshoe-shaped curve at the base of a steep-sided gulch cut into dark metasedimentary rock. You descend north of this point through rock piles left over from an old mining site, and pass a large campsite on a flat between the trail and the river. A well-used trail turning left alongside an old ditch leads to a mining claim on the south bank of Virgin Creek. The trail north crosses the ditch and drops to a flat, 2.8 miles from the trailhead, where Virgin Creek Guard Station once stood before burning to the ground. Beyond a wide bed of boulders north of the flat, you reach Virgin Creek, 200 yards east of the confluence of Slide Creek, where the two creeks merge to form New River.

Just past the ford of Virgin Creek is a trail junction, signed SOLDIER CREEK to the left (west) and OLD DENNY to the right (east). Your trail toward Old Denny climbs east above the roar of the creek through mixed forest of bigleaf maples, Douglas firs, tanoaks, and canyon oaks, which thickens as the trail rounds a curve to the northeast. Ascend to the top of a shoulder of a ridge dividing the drainages of Slide and Virgin creeks and then drop into the canyon of Slide Creek, catching glimpses along the way of the channel the rushing waters of the creek has cut over time through the metasedimentary rock. The descent continues until the trail is only a few feet away from and directly above the creek.

Beyond a clearing, a switchback leads away from the banks of the creek up to a bench with a campsite. Apparently this site was home to a structure from a bygone era, as the presence of a 20-foot rock wall clearly indicates. A hundred feet up the trail is a rivulet drifting across the path. About 2 miles from Virgin Creek, the trail becomes steep, switchbacks a couple of times, and climbs over a hill to a gully with a seasonal stream. Another 0.75 mile leads to the junction of Slide and Eagle creeks, 0.15 mile upstream on Eagle Creek from the confluence of the two creeks. This junction is the beginning of the 12.25-mile loop that continues up Slide Creek, crosses Carey Ridge through the Historic Mining District, and then returns down Eagle Creek.

Following signed directions to Old Denny and Mary Blaine Meadows to the right (east), you follow a short-legged switchback down to a boulder hop across Eagle Creek. In high water, look for a footlog 150 feet upstream. The creek is a good place to replenish your water supply, as the next 3 miles of trail are dry. Little-used campsites are on the east side of the ford.

The trail climbs steeply away from the Eagle Creek ford, switchbacks, and comes around a ridge dividing the two drainages to Slide Creek again. Under cool and shady mixed forest, the trail traverses the slope high above the level of the creek, at times nearly out of earshot, until an ascent leads up to a flat, the site of an old cabin and quite a bit of debris.

From the cabin site, the well-graded trail gently rolls up and down without gaining or losing much elevation and remains high above the creek. Approximately 2.4 miles from the ford of Eagle Creek and 8.2 miles from the trailhead, you drop down to a large flat next to the creek with several good campsites. Plenty of old mining paraphernalia is scattered about the flat, including an intact wood and metal hand truck. With an abundance of firewood, the camp is a fine destination for backpackers who desire a moderate first-day's hike.

Following a moderate ascent away from the camp, the trail climbs past a seasonal stream, up a steep hillside to an open area, and then winds down to a flowing stream bordered by lush vegetation. Step over the stream and follow the trail into a grassy meadow to a somewhat confusing junction, 0.2 mile from

New River and Slide Creek mining artifacts

the camp. The temporary confusion is quickly alleviated once you proceed on the left-hand trail trending northeast, where, 40 feet from the junction, a sign posted on a pine informs you that the other path, the combination Emigrant Creek and Milk Camp Trail, leads to Milk Camp and Pony Creek.

From the sign, the trail heads up and away from the meadow, as the vegetation transitions to predominantly evergreen forest. The trail soon becomes steep and dry, remaining so for much of the distance to Old Denny. A clearing on the way allows for views up to the crest of the Salmon Mountains. Trailside mining debris becomes more prevalent well before you reach Old Denny. Heading through a dry ravine, you reach the town site and a junction in a grove of second-growth forest, 10.3 miles from the trailhead. A crude, hand-lettered sign marked simply WATER points the way to the right (east) to a spring near a meadow.

Since Old Denny once supported such a large number of people, you should be able to find any number of places to pitch your tent, spread out over the width and breadth of the old town. Please give the area your utmost respect and leave it in good condition. Oddly enough, there are a few private inholdings upstream from Denny, where modern-day residents attempt to maintain cabins on a seasonal basis. Please respect those sites as well, if you happen to come upon any.

Old Denny

Many artifacts remain in Old Denny, despite the number of years that have passed since the former town's heyday (although the extent of damage from recent fires is unknown). The ground is littered with all manner of debris, including cast-iron skillets, metal pots, mining equipment, rubber shoe parts, tin cans, bottles, and pottery shards. Once upon a time, 500 people lived and worked here as permanent residents. Looking around the old town site, it's hard to believe that this area could have supported so many people. A bustling mining town did, in fact, exist here during a period that spanned nearly 40 years, but time has erased much of the evidence. The miners left long ago and their buildings, some as high as three stories, have been replaced by a mature, second-growth forest.

Tattered old signs pass on tidbits of information about the town: Old Denny was founded by Clive Clements in 1883, and was originally named New River City. New River was named when discovered after all of the surrounding country had been explored except for the rugged terrain around the river. The quest for gold eventually lured humans to search for every possible location of the precious ore, which led to the discovery of the last river in the area, hence the appellation "New River." The last permanent residents left Old Denny in 1920, and decades later only a small number of temporary visitors pass through where once so many lived and worked. Modern-day explorers can while away many hours, if not days, poking around the old town site and uncovering the rich history.

Turn north from the junction to the spring in Old Denny in the direction of a sign attached to a fir that reads MARY BLAINE MEADOW, CINNABAR MINE. The trail climbs steeply away from Old Denny on little-used tread covered with leaves. Two long-legged switchbacks lead to the top of a divide separating the waters of Slide and Eagle creeks and a junction, 0.35 mile from Old Denny.

From the junction, a fine trip extension continues up the Slide Creek Trail to Cinnabar Mine, Mary Blaine Meadows, and connects with the Summit Trail, with a return to the loop via the north section of the Battle Creek Trail. However, the route described here descends northwest on the Battle Creek Trail, as the vegetation changes to predominantly fir forest. After 0.3 mile, you reach the old town site of Marysville but, unlike Old Denny, there's little left to show the modern-day traveler that this was once a bustling community.

A short distance from the site of Marysville, you pass an even more infrequently traveled trail on your left to the ruins of the old Hunter Mine. The main trail heads uphill, steeply at times, through mixed forest and eventually breaks out of the trees just before gaining the top of a ridge. The site of White Rock City is a short distance farther, 0.3 mile from the junction of the trail to Hunter Mine, 1.1 miles from Old Denny, and 11.4 miles from the trailhead. The level ground around the old town site offers lots of opportunities for setting up camp, with plenty of firewood, and water available from Sherwood Creek, 0.2 mile away.

White Rock City

White Rock City is more aesthetically pleasing for backpackers than the environs around Old Denny. Set on the side of a ridge, the old town site has views out to the west and north to the crest of the Salmon Mountains. The wide, level town site is set pleasantly beneath cedars and pines, and is graced by cool mountain breezes. Even fewer humans get to White Rock City than Old Denny, which may account for artifacts of greater number and superior quality. Some of the debris from the buildings that once stood here is scattered about as well. The function of an unusual looking, 75-foot-diameter circular pit near the trail is a mystery.

Leaving White Rock City, you head down to a crossing of Sherwood Creek, climb away from the far bank, and follow a 0.3-mile traverse through firs and cedars to a spring. Above the spring on the far side next to a seep sits a lone campsite with a fire pit and a few old relics. From the spring, the trail starts a descent into more of a mixed forest. Poison oak, which has been absent since the slope above Old Denny, reappears in sporadic clumps. As the descent becomes steeper, you start to hear the roar from Sherwood Creek in the canyon below. Alert eyes may spy a large, unnatural hump on the steep slope below signifying the closed entrance to the Sherwood Mine. Down the slope about 50 to 75 yards is the buried opening to the mine, along with an old ore cart, rails, and ties. Soon after the mine, you come upon a sign attached to a tanoak identifying the northwest junction of the trail to Hunter Mine, 2 miles from Old Denny.

Leaving the Historic Mining District behind, the trail makes a gentle ascent beneath ponderosa pines and incense cedars that becomes steeper just before rising to the top of a ridge. A descent from the ridge leads through cool and shady fir and pine forest before eventually returning to a predominantly oak forest. Rounding a bend, the track narrows and makes a somewhat tedious descending traverse of a rocky hillside. Returning to mixed forest, the path widens again, which makes for easier travel. On the approach to Battle Creek, you enter a zone of much denser vegetation that threatens to overgrow the trail in places. Up to this point, the trail was easy to follow, but this particular section runs the risk of becoming lost to the forest understory, especially without any recent trail maintenance.

About 13.4 miles from the trailhead and 3.1 miles from Old Denny, you hop across the main branch of Battle Creek, a cool and refreshing stream beneath dense Douglas-fir forest cover. Climbing away from the creek, you soon reach a tributary amid dense vegetation, which quickly opens up again where you reach a dry, rocky slope dotted with ponderosa pines and incense cedars. The tread narrows across this slope and becomes a bit unstable, but soon widens again under mixed forest. Ascending to the top of a ridge, you reach a junction with the Eagle Creek Trail, 3.9 miles from Old Denny. A sign attached to a cedar points north toward Rock Lake.

Leaving the Battle Creek Trail, you turn left and head southwest past a sign on a ponderosa pine marked SLIDE CREEK. Immediately past this sign, the trail turns sharply left (south) and heads down away from the ridge across a dry and rocky slope. Through forest of Douglas firs, incense cedars, ponderosa pines, and digger pines, you head down and then up again to the top of another ridge, which divides the drainages of Eagle and Battle creeks. Cross the ridge and descend southwest into Eagle Creek canyon under a canopy of primarily Douglas firs and incense cedars.

Descending steeply at times, you reach a clearing where the trail angles toward the right, following a sweeping horseshoe bend, switchbacking twice, and then heading west into the trees at the bottom of the slope. Watch for cairns through this clearing. Continuing ahead, the trail proceeds toward Eagle Creek and shortly becomes almost impossible to follow. However, once you reach a dry open hillside, you can easily descend to the east bank and pick up the trail again paralleling the creek. Alongside the stream the tread becomes distinct and the grade eases, as you travel under tanoaks, canyon oaks, and Douglas firs. Soon after passing an old campsite, you come to a boulder hop of Eagle Creek, 15.4 miles from the trailhead.

This stretch of Eagle Creek is delightful, with deep green pools suitable for swimming and fishing. The creek rushes down the canyon along a much steeper route than does the trail, which is a dirt path covered with pine needles, gently graded and quite pleasant to walk upon, passing beneath a primarily Douglas-fir forest next to lush trailside vegetation. Eventually the trail becomes a rolling, up-and-down affair, coming near the creek and climbing away several times. Good campsites are few and far between along Eagle Creek, which is too bad because the environment around the creek is quite pleasant. However, if your desire to camp becomes too great to ignore, you could find passable sites with a little effort. After the rolling descent down Eagle Creek, a short climb leads to the junction of Slide and Eagle creeks and the close of the loop section. From there, retrace your steps 5.75 miles to the New River trailhead.

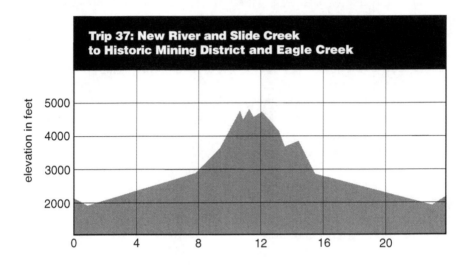

TRIP 38

New River and Virgin Creek to Salmon Summit and Devils Backbone

Solitude, magnificent forests, and incomparable views are this trip's primary rewards.

Trip Type:	Backpack, 5–9 days
Distance:	40 miles, loop
Elevation Change:	22,120 feet, average 553 per mile
Difficulty:	Difficult
Season:	Mid-July to early October
Maps:	USGS *Jim Jam Ridge*, *Dees Peak*, *Trinity Mountain*, *Salmon Mountain*, and *Youngs Peak*; USFS *A Guide to the Trinity Alps Wilderness*
Nearest Campground:	Hobo Gulch

This trip provides a good conversation piece: How many people do you know who have hiked up Virgin Creek to Salmon Summit, or the trail along Devils Backbone—or who have driven the road to Denny, for that matter? Although some gold miners may be working legitimate claims on Virgin Creek, meeting anyone at all along the trail once you start up Virgin Creek beyond the New River junction is highly unlikely. Virgin Creek lives up to its name beyond the confluence of Soldier Creek, as virtually no one travels the rest of the way up the steep, wooded canyon to Salmon Summit or out to Devils Backbone.

Except for stretches along Devils Backbone and a few open, dry hillsides where canyon and Oregon oaks flourish, most of the trip travels through dense forest. Live oaks, tanoaks, madrones, bigleaf maples, and Douglas firs line the canyon bottoms. Magnificent, dense forests of ponderosa pines, sugar pines, Jeffrey pines, black oaks, and white firs carpet the upper basin of Virgin Creek and the slopes of Salmon Summit. This is one of the few places in the Trinity Alps with plenty of firewood. Also, an amazing variety of wildflowers bloom in the many different habitats found along the way. Anglers should stay abreast of the fishing regulations for New River and its tributaries, which occasionally result in closures. Fishing should be fair in both Rock and Red Cap lakes for eastern brook trout.

Due to the low elevation, early-season hikers can travel a long way up Virgin Creek before encountering any of the lingering snow patches that keep the upper mountains inaccessible until summer. However, during spring, the condition of the access road to the trailhead and the ability to successfully make the ford of Virgin Creek may be more limiting factors than the snow higher up

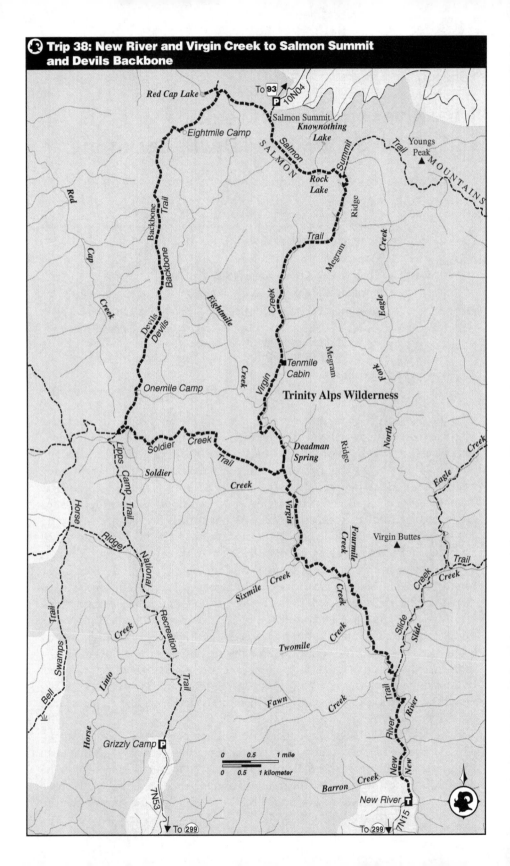

in the mountains. As with much of the backcountry in the western Trinity Alps, some of this route passes through areas burned in a wildfire in the 1990s.

Starting Point

The first step is reaching the settlement of Denny, which is a long way up the canyon of New River. County Road 402 branches away from Highway 299 at Hawkins Bar, 46 miles west of Weaverville and 10 miles east of Willow Creek. Beyond a high bridge over the Trinity River, you travel 0.25 mile to an intersection, where you turn back west and then north beside Hawkins Creek, passing several houses and a subdivision to the next intersection. Turn right and begin a long, twisting climb generally east up the side of Trinity River canyon.

At 6.3 miles from Hawkins Bar, beyond some unbelievably tight hairpin turns, a dirt road forks left to Happy Camp and points farther north. Another 1.2 miles leads to the end of the climb at a point on a spur ridge dividing the drainages of Trinity River and New River. Narrow pavement snakes down the east side of the ridge, and then turns northeast through a gap in a spur ridge to a cluster of homes among neat orchards on a flat far above New River. Eventually the road draws near to the river at Panther Creek, 14.5 miles from Hawkins Bar.

Denny Campground straddles the road 0.3 mile farther up the canyon, with Denny Forest Service Guard Station out of sight above the upper part of the campground. A Forest Service employee is usually available to provide a wilderness permit or information on the current state of the trails. At 1400 feet, the free year-round campground is fairly large and quite pleasant, with vault toilets but no potable water or trash pickup.

The community of Denny begins about 0.7 mile above the campground, and is strung out along the road for the next half mile or so. Continue on paved road past Denny and Quinby Creek to a signed junction with Road 7N15 on the left.

Turn onto the gravel surface of Road 7N15, which doubles back from the paved Denny Road and climbs away from the river. The road turns north, then east around the shoulder of a ridge, and then north again on the west side of New River canyon across from the East Fork. At 4.7 miles from County Road 402, having passed forks with three or four lesser roads, veer right at a signed intersection, remaining on Road 7N15, and proceed to another junction at 5.4 miles. Turn left here, as the surface turns from gravel to dirt, which may be impassable during wet weather. Continue to the trailhead at the end of the road, with plenty of parking space and a stock tie area.

Description

Single-track trail descends 0.4 mile to the wilderness boundary, merges with the trace of an old road, and then returns to single track on the way down a short, steep pitch to Barron Creek in an alder thicket. A footlog below the ford is available during periods of high water, but the crossing is usually problem-free. As you climb moderately out of the creek bed, tall Douglas firs, madrones, and a few tanoaks grow above an understory of vine maples, ceanothus, redbuds, and dogwoods on the hillside. A few blackberry vines in slide areas provide a welcome treat in season. You can hear New River in the bottom of the canyon to the east.

A short distance away from Barron Creek you reach and then follow the west bank of New River for 250 yards. After a moderate climb up the canyon wall, the trail stays away from the river across steep hillsides, flats, and ledges. Good tread follows the contour of an old mining ditch in places. A spring flows across the trail at 0.7 mile from Barron Creek.

Beyond the spring, the trail rises more steeply to a rocky point, around which the river roars in a horseshoe-shaped curve at the base of a steep-sided gulch cut into dark metasedimentary rock. You descend north of this point through rock piles left over from an old mining site, and pass a large campsite on a flat between the trail and the river. A well-used trail turning left alongside an old ditch leads to a mining claim on the south bank of Virgin Creek. The trail north crosses the ditch and drops to a flat, 2.8 miles from the trailhead, where Virgin Creek Guard Station once stood before burning to the ground. Beyond a wide bed of boulders north of the flat, you reach Virgin Creek, 200 yards east of the confluence with Slide Creek, where the two creeks merge to form New River.

The ford of Virgin Creek shouldn't be a problem by early to midsummer, but may be dangerous during periods of high water earlier in the year. Forest Service personnel at Big Bar may be able to update you on the current condition of the crossing. Just past the ford of Virgin Creek, 3 miles from the trailhead, is a trail junction signed SOLDIER CREEK to the left (west) and OLD DENNY to the right (east). Several excellent campsites on a flat north of Virgin Creek will tempt overnighters.

Veer to the left and follow the Virgin Creek Trail west from the junction, across the hillside above the large flat. You won't be close to Virgin Creek again for the next 4 miles, with the first easily accessible water in Fourmile Creek, 2.8 miles away. After 300 yards of steep climbing, you round a shoulder, turn north to follow the canyon on a moderate ascent, and then contour across steep, bare slopes and open forest. Beside a mining claim sign posted to a tree, 1 mile from the junction, a side trail forks left down the side of the canyon. As you climb over a steep point, 0.25 mile farther, you may spy a two-story house built of lumber, not logs, which is the first destination along the side trail. The house seems quite out of place, perched on a shelf on the far side of Virgin Creek. The side trail also leads up to the site of the old Barritt Cabin beyond Twomile Creek. You can see the log cabin from Virgin Creek, which seems quite at home amid the surroundings.

Continuing up the Virgin Creek Trail, you round a shoulder and descend into the side canyon of Fourmile Creek, 2.8 miles from the New River junction. The tread is generally good across the steep, open slope, except where some small slides have run across the trail in a few places. The cool shade and cold, clear water are especially welcome on the typically hot summer day. Before you drop down to cross the creek, there's a good small campsite on a bench.

A little more than a mile farther up the canyon, Virgin Creek makes an oxbow bend around a narrow, rocky point, where Sixmile Creek flows into Virgin Creek directly across the canyon. A moderate climb west leads to the top of this point, from where the trail turns back northeast to traverse an almost sheer rock wall before descending to a small flat beside Virgin Creek, 4.2 miles from the New River junction.

The trail follows the east side of the canyon to a crossing at the confluence of Soldier Creek. At the lower end of a large flat just prior to the crossing, you come to the end of the Soldier Creek four-wheel-drive road, which has a locked gate at the wilderness boundary that supposedly blocks entry to all but legitimate claim holders. The immediate area was heavily mined in the past, but only a few miners still hold claims, and more stringent mining regulations have considerably limited activity. You shouldn't see any miners and hopefully not too much evidence of their previous work. If you're in need of overnight accommodations, the flat has some excellent campsites.

The road turns to cross both Virgin and Soldier creeks almost at their confluence, 5.4 miles from the New River junction. The Virgin Creek Trail follows the track of an old road, branching right between the two creeks. Keep left at a fork, 100 yards farther on, just past a miner's camp, and look for a trail turning uphill just beyond a blazed tree on the right. A sign 20 feet up the trail confirms that this is the Virgin Creek Trail.

Back on single-track trail, you ascend steeply northwest for 0.4 mile, with the aid of a couple of zigzags, and then turn back east around the shoulder of a ridge between Soldier and Virgin creeks. A few more zigzags north bring you to the top of a hump on the side of the ridge and a junction with your return trail from Devils Backbone and Trinity Summit. The Soldier Creek Trail will return you to this spot after nearly 22 miles. At the junction a sign points north to Salmon Summit and south back toward New River.

Remaining on the Virgin Creek Trail, you trace a contour for the next 1.7 miles along the side of the canyon, descending to Eightmile Creek through a uniquely beautiful forest. Douglas firs are the predominant tree, but the forest includes very large sugar pines, Jeffrey pines, incense cedars, madrones, bigleaf maples, tanoaks, and canyon oaks. In open spaces, Washington lilies nod their pale lavender, speckled heads. The trail ducks in and out of lush little gullies that harbor fugitive flowers from the Cascade Range—pipsissewas, mahonias, twinflowers, and saxifrages. At their confluence, Eagle Creek is larger than Virgin Creek. Both are stunningly scenic streams, with umbrellalike leaves of Indian rhubarb vibrating above the currents. Large boulders beside the streams are decorated with intricate patterns of mosses and ferns, and delicate fronds of goat's beard wave in the breeze in more open spots. You'll find a good campsite with an elaborate rock fireplace on a little flat between the two creeks; a fine spot if the trash left behind by previous parties has been removed. Eager little steelhead fry pop up in every pool in Virgin Creek—just the right size for breakfast.

From Eightmile Creek, you climb the west side of the canyon and continue north, with some ups and downs well away from the creek. After a mile, you descend to a series of ledges beside the creek again. At one point, the trail runs down to the creek and threatens to cross to the far bank, but instead continues up the west side. A large bench, 2 miles north of Eightmile Creek, offers excellent campsites, although there is little evidence that many have camped here previously. The canyon narrows above the bench, forcing the trail up the hillside once more.

Another half mile up the trail, the two-room Tenmile Cabin, framed with poles and walled and roofed with hand-split shakes, perches on a narrow shelf below the trail and overlooks a 10- to 15-foot waterfall. The roof is mostly intact, although you probably won't want to sleep here unless you're hit with a cloudburst—the interior is quite messy. A better place to pitch your tent is beside the remnants of another cabin on a site dug out of the hill above the trail. Jumbo Mine, a large hard-rock gold-mining operation, was in the canyon above the cabins, but little trace of it remains today. Only one prospect hole across the creek is visible from the trail. Rumor suggests that the remnants of a 40-foot waterwheel and extensive diggings are in a side canyon, but we were unable to locate them.

Three short, steep switchbacks beyond Tenmile Cabin lead to the brink of some cliffs overlooking the creek. After skirting the tops of these cliffs, the trail climbs again, and then levels off through dense forest to a brushy slope, where a small stream tumbles down the hillside. Head back into lush forest again and pass two falls in the creek, 0.8 mile from the cabin. In a grove of beautiful, tall alders, you cross Virgin Creek and then turn up the creekbed 150 yards to cross back to the west bank. From there, you begin a steep climb as the creek bends east.

The trail crosses back to the south side of the creek, 1.6 miles from Tenmile Cabin, and makes a very steep ascent with a few switchbacks through heavy brush. As you climb higher, the brush is replaced with dense forest, which now includes red firs. The trail turns north, then west to another crossing of Virgin Creek. One final crossing of the diminishing creek below a mass of willows and alders brings you to the base of the final climb to Salmon Summit through magnificent red-fir forest, with queen-cup lilies and bunchberries blooming on the open forest floor. After two switchbacks, you round a shoulder and suddenly stand on top of a view-packed ridge, 16.25 miles from the trailhead.

From this aerie, the Marble Mountains appear on the horizon north of the deep trench of the Salmon River. Off to the southeast, the central Trinity Alps around Thompson Peak raise snowcapped peaks against the backdrop of a cobalt sky. Much more distant, Mt. Shasta floats above a series of forested ridges. Closer up, the red-dirt trace of a trail across the brush-covered face of Youngs Peak is directly east across the upper canyon of North Fork Eagle Creek.

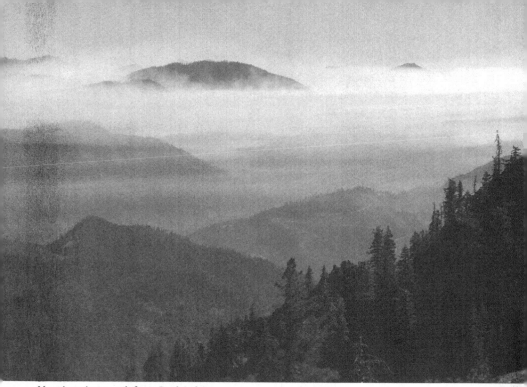

Morning view north from Rock Lake

As you follow the trail north around the east side of a mountain, forest gives way to tall ceanothus brush. Push on through tough going for about 300 yards to a junction with the Salmon Summit Trail on a knob in open forest, where the only sign points to Virgin Creek, back the way you came.

The trail on the right heads downhill 0.3 mile to Salmon Summit Mine and then over to Slate Gap, eventually connecting with the Eagle Creek Trail. Your route turns left from the junction, climbs up a mountain, descends along the north side of the summit, and arrives at lovely, little Rock Lake, 0.6 mile from the junction.

Rock Lake is almost perfectly round, sitting right under the precipitous north face of a granite mountain. Granite talus falls into the water on the south side, but metamorphic rock slopes rise up from the rest of the shoreline. The formation of this cup is hard to fathom, appearing as a glacial cirque, but there exists no evidence of glaciation along this stretch of the Salmon River Divide. One good campsite and a few fair ones under scattered red firs and western white pines occupy spots above the east shore. Late in the season, the water drops below the level of the outlet and the lake loses some of its aesthetic appeal. Fishing is good for eastern brook trout up to 10 inches. Red newts may surprise you by rising to the surface to breathe, but they won't take flies. The top of a spur ridge east of the lake offers breathtaking views of sunrises and sunsets over the Salmon River canyon. Coastal fog often creeps up the canyon at sunrise to set a series of ridges adrift in a pink sea.

From the lake, the Salmon Summit Trail crosses the willow-lined outlet stream and follows a descending traverse around the head of a valley to a gorgeous little meadow in a saddle just over the ridgecrest, where a profusion of sulfur flowers and naked eriogonums bloom in midsummer. You continue the descent for a quarter mile, first through brush and groves of incense cedars, and then through more meadows, before the trail climbs steeply back to the top of the ridge. After climbing along the ridge, steeply at first, you eventually begin a gently descending traverse across the east side of Peak 6305, amid open fir forest floored with grass and low brush. After the traverse, drop down more abruptly to a junction with the High Point Trail in the open grassy saddle of Salmon Summit, 1.5 miles from Rock Lake. The High Point trailhead is 0.7 mile to the northeast.

A point-to-point trip between the New River and High Point trailheads is certainly possible, however, the transportation logistics are horrendous. Driving just one-way between the two trailheads would require more than half a day. If arrangements could be made, a better plan would be for a group to start from each trailhead and exchange car keys in the middle of the trip. Another alternative might be to start at the High Point trailhead and then turn around at any point along Virgin Creek—a better plan early in the season when the ford of Virgin Creek might be hazardous.

Heading northwest away from Salmon Summit, the track of the Salmon Summit Trail may not be clearly evident in the tall grass, but an obvious old roadbed almost immediately heads down from the saddle around the upper edge of the Eightmile Creek basin through wide meadows dotted with clumps of ceanothus and willows and carpeted with wildflowers. The road is washed out in a gully farther down the slope, and then becomes discernible again where the grade levels out. There's a good campsite beside a little stream that has cut through the road, 0.5 mile from Salmon Summit.

Raw red dirt, which appeared as a mine dump from farther up the hill, turns out to be a massive slide at the head of Eightmile Creek, as you rise slightly and reach the edge. You have to climb up the east side of the slide to get across and then drop back down to the road again on the west side. Continue a moderate rise northwest across the head of the basin above a mass of willows, and then climb more steeply through red-fir forest to the ridgecrest and a junction with the Devils Backbone Trail, 1.2 miles from Salmon Summit. From the junction, the old road along the top of the ridge runs north toward Salmon Mountain, reaching a junction with the trail down to Red Cap Lake after 200 yards.

Side Trip to Red Cap Lake

Head north on the road along the ridge to a junction with the seldom-used and rarely maintained trail heading west, and plunge steeply down the hillside 0.3 mile to the east shore of Red Cap Lake. Meadows, carpeted with colorful wildflowers, caress a fair part of the shoreline, the lush grasses occasionally attracting wary wildlife out of the neighboring forest. Along the south shore, rugged slopes and cliffs rise up to the ridgeline above, with light forest around the rest of the shoreline shading several good campsites. Perhaps the best site is in a grove of trees at the southeast edge of the lake, just beyond the meadows. Thanks to the area's remoteness, you should have your pick

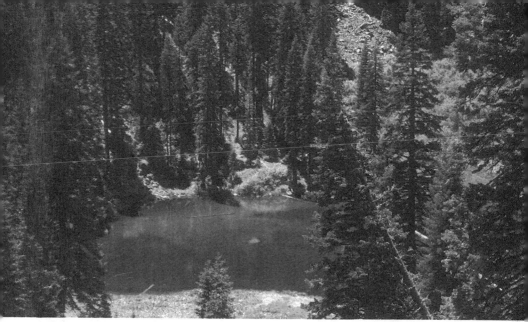

Red Cap Lake

of campsites almost any time you visit Red Cap Lake. A spring on the southwest side of the lake provides a fine source of running water. The shallow lake has a mud bottom and is crisscrossed with numerous dead snags, making it unsuitable for swimming, but large eastern brook trout reportedly inhabit the shallow waters.

From the junction of Devils Backbone and Salmon Summit, you turn left and head south along the ridge, ascending through fir forest to the top of a knoll, marked 6555 on the USGS 7.5-minute *Salmon Mountain*, where the path breaks out into the open in a large, grassy meadow.

Just as you drop away from the top of the knoll, the tread becomes indistinct and difficult to follow in the tall grass. Where three white firs grow close together on a small hummock, the route veers left (southwest)—watch for cairns leading through the meadow and into the trees, where the trail becomes distinct again. The descent becomes steeper under white and red firs until you wind your way out to the ridgecrest once more, next to a metasedimentary rock knob with a sheer north face overlooking the steep hillside below. A short downhill jaunt from the knob leads to Eightmile Camp, adjacent to another flower-covered meadow, 1.2 miles from the Salmon Summit Trail junction and 20.5 miles from the New River trailhead.

Eightmile Camp is a remote site nestled beneath tall firs and overlooking a grassy meadow filled with colorful wildflowers. Partial views of the distant terrain, including Devils Backbone, can be had through gaps in the trees. Many of the previous visitors, although few and far between, must have been hunters, as there are cables to hang meat, places to tie stock, and lots of log rounds upon which to sit. A short, boot-beaten path leads away from the camp about 25 yards to a spring surrounded by lush vegetation, where there's a small pool just the right size for easily acquiring water. Firewood is plentiful, but you may have to scout around a bit.

The correct route away from Eightmile Camp can be confusing. Just below the camp, the trail makes a hairpin turn and then follows a faint track east across an overgrown meadow to the east side, immediately above a thicket of alders. A blaze on a fir tree at the far end of the meadow marks the resumption of distinct tread. The trail heads steadily downhill through lush vegetation of ferns and wildflowers beneath a dense canopy of firs. Approximately 0.5 mile from Eightmile Camp, you first hear and then cross a gurgling tributary of Eightmile Creek. After following the west bank for a short distance, you climb up to a little-used campsite next to scattered deadfalls. Although the trail appears to stop right in the middle of the campsite, the route proceeds straight ahead for 50 to 75 feet over the deadfalls to where distinct tread can be picked up again. Continue downhill through a predominantly white-fir forest until a bend in the trail leads to an open traverse across a hillside covered with ponderosa pines, incense cedars, white firs, and manzanita brush. At the conclusion of the traverse, you reach the spine of Devils Backbone, 0.75 mile from Eightmile Camp.

Devils Backbone was so named for a pronounced lack of shade and water, and nothing has changed. The trail along the crest can be described as an undulating, rollercoaster trek headed due south, with unobstructed, incomparable views west to the coast range and east to the central Trinity Alps. Devils Backbone is definitely not the place to be during the middle of a very hot summer day! Along the way, you'll probably see more bear scat than boot prints.

Ascending south, the trail skirts just below the ridge's high point (5725 feet) and then makes a steep descent, briefly interrupted by a level stretch, to a saddle. Views east to the snowcapped peaks of the central Alps and west to the wild, wooded ridges of the coast mountains are nearly constant companions.

From the saddle, a steep climb leads to the summit of a knob, followed by a short descent to a very small, but welcome, grove of Douglas firs and knobcone pines. A slight descent from this grove and some level walking through a broad saddle bring you to the base of a rounded peak, 2 miles from the start of the route along Devils Backbone. Instead of climbing up the rounded peak, the trail traverses the west side in open forest.

A gently undulating traverse, in and out of light forest shade, leads to a long stretch of forest shade and thick vegetation below the crest. A 25-foot section is even overgrown with vine maple—a stark contrast to the sparse, dry vegetation seen previously along the crest. The pleasant stroll through cooler forest is abruptly interrupted by an extremely steep turn upward that soon returns you to the ridgetop. The first half of this ascent is mercifully shaded, but the second half is fully exposed.

Another traverse along the ridge leads to some shrub-covered metasedimentary rock cliffs with a spectacular view of the central Alps. A steep descent to the next low spot along the ridge leads to a short, shaded section of Douglas firs before a climb on rocky trail through manzanita and ceanothus brings you to the crest once more. A long, brushy descent is briefly suspended by a short climb up a little knob, and then resumes, eventually coming under cool,

Douglas-fir forest. Proceeding through the forest, the trail switchbacks twice, and then heads down a hillside to Onemile Camp on a large, wooded flat, 5.2 miles from Eightmile Camp.

Onemile Camp is a relatively large camping area, with plenty of firewood, fire pits, and artifacts scattered around. Water is available quite a way down the hillside from a spring: Faint tread leads downhill from the south end of the camp next to two large firs, where you'll notice a large downed timber with a section cut out for the trail to pass through. A long, fairly steep descent along this trail eventually leads you to Onemile Spring, the first water close to the trail for the last 5 miles since crossing the upper tributary of Eightmile Creek.

Away from Onemile Camp, the trail climbs steeply through mixed forest, then levels off, traversing the hillside south before another steep, short climb leads back to the ridgecrest. A general descent brings you to a junction in a broad, densely forested saddle, from where the Soldier Creek Trail down to Virgin Creek heads northeast, 0.75 mile from Onemile Camp. Nailed to a western yew, an old metal sign covered with pitch drippings points the way down very faint tread. Although a pair of cairns marks the junction, this intersection could be easily missed, so pay very close attention on the approach. Otherwise you could conceivably end up at the Grizzly Camp trailhead, a good distance away from your intended destination.

The Soldier Creek Trail between the junction and Virgin Creek is probably the least-traveled section of one of the least-traveled trails in the entire Trinity Alps. Fortunately, the trail was reconstructed in 2000 (although the trail has not been maintained since 2005). The first 3 miles generally traverses the ridge east above Soldier Creek, followed by 1.5 miles of a steep, winding descent that drops 1500 feet down to Virgin Creek. You arrive at the junction with the Virgin Creek Trail, 4.4 miles from the Devils Backbone Trail junction.

Taking a cool dip in the pools of Virgin Creek might be a good idea before retracing your steps 9.1 miles down the canyon to the New River trailhead.

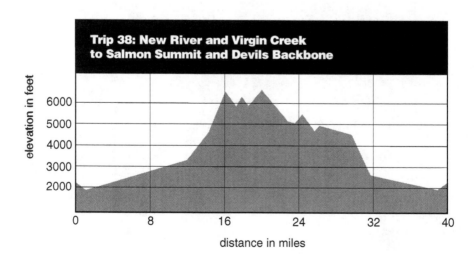

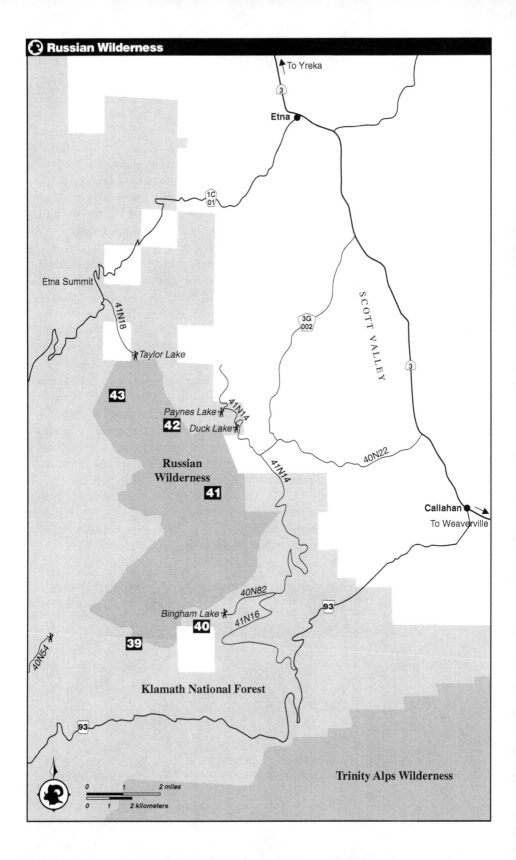

To Yreka

3

Etna

1C
01

Etna Summit

41N18

Taylor Lake

43

SCOTT VALLEY

3G
002

Paynes Lake

42

41N14

Duck Lake

Russian
Wilderness

41

41N14

40N22

3

Callahan
To Weaverville

40N82

Bingham Lake

40

41N16

93

39

40N54

Klamath National Forest

93

Trinity Alps Wilderness

0   1   2 miles

0   1   2 kilometers

CHAPTER 6

Trips in Russian Wilderness

The 12,000-acre Russian Wilderness may be small compared to the much larger Trinity Alps Wilderness to the south, but its amazing biological diversity makes up for its smaller size. The range is comprised of north-south trending granitic ridge incised by glacier-carved valleys, with elevations ranging from around 5000 feet to 8196 feet at the summit of Russian Peak. Most recreational enthusiasts visit the Russian Wilderness during the summer months. Occupying a small chunk of a remote section of Northern California, the Russian Wilderness is a lightly used area.

This chapter includes five trips that are equally well suited to dayhikes or backpacks, leading to 9 of the 19 named lakes within the wilderness. Because of the relatively low elevation, hikers and backpackers can enjoy snow-free trails in the Russian Wilderness by late spring or early summer, although most visits occur during the main part of summer. Wilderness permits are not required for overnight stays in the Russian Wilderness.

Similar to the Trinity Alps to the south, this area offers additional recreational opportunities to hiking and backpacking the outstanding trails. The Scott and Salmon rivers, both tributaries of the Klamath River, provide excellent white-water rafting, with stretches of Class IV and V rapids. One of the few free-flowing rivers left in California, the Salmon River is an important fishery for salmon, steelhead, and trout. Although there are no campgrounds in the immediate vicinity of the Russians, several Forest Service campgrounds are strung out along both the Scott and Salmon rivers.

TRIP 39

Waterdog and Russian Lakes

A short hike to two pretty lakes

Trip Type:	Dayhike or 2-day backpack
Distance:	9 miles, out-and-back
Elevation Change:	1600 feet, average 355 per mile
Difficulty:	Moderate
Season:	Mid-June through October
Maps:	USGS *Tanners Peak* and *Eaton Peak*; USFS *A Guide to the Marble Mountain Wilderness & Russian Wilderness*
Nearest Campground:	Trail Creek

Although popular by Russian Wilderness standards, scenic Waterdog and Russian lakes should provide the wilderness traveler with plenty of picturesque scenery without having to rub elbows with a high number of fellow recreational enthusiasts. While the relatively short distance of 4.5 miles and the general lack of excellent campsites make this trip better suited for dayhikers, weekend backpackers who aren't too particular will find the area quite appealing as well.

Starting Point

Drive on Highway 3 to the small community of Callahan and immediately north of town, turn left at the junction of Forest Road 93, heading toward Cecilville, Forks of Salmon, and Somes Bar. Climb 11.7 miles on Road 93 to Carter Meadow Summit and the signed Pacific Crest Trail parking area on the left, and then continue westbound down the canyon of East Fork of South Fork Salmon River for about 8 miles to a right-hand turn onto Forest Road 93. A steady, winding 8-mile climb on Road 93 leads to a junction with Forest Road 39N58. Turn right at the junction and continue another 2 miles to the Deacon Lee trailhead on a large, open, flat knoll that provides primitive, waterless camping.

Description

From the parking area, follow the continuation of the old road along a view-packed ridge, where the snowcapped peaks of the central Trinity Alps can be seen to the south, with the more remote Marble Mountains visible to the north. Eventually the road is left behind as single-track trail leads farther along the ridge. Where the trail leaves the ridge and starts to arc across the head of the Sixmile Creek drainage, a forest of red firs and western white pines shelters the

Trip 39: Waterdog and Russian Lakes

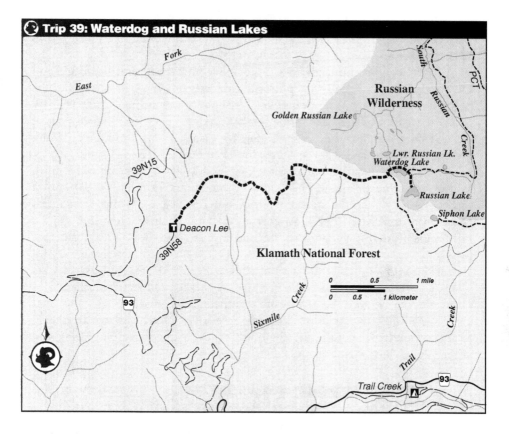

East Fork

Russian Wilderness

Golden Russian Lake

39N15

Lwr. Russian Lk.
Waterdog Lake

Russian Lake

Siphon Lake

Deacon Lee

39N58

Klamath National Forest

93

Sixmile Creek

| 0 | 0.5 | 1 mile |
| 0 | 0.5 | 1 kilometer |

Trail Creek

93

South Russian Creek

PCT

trail and limits the views. Around 1.8 miles, the trail crosses the south ridge of Peak 7667 and enters the main canyon of Sixmile Creek. According to maps of the area, in a dry gulch, 2.4 miles from the trailhead, is a junction with a secondary trail that climbs over a saddle and drops into East Fork White Gulch, but I found no evidence of a trail there when I scouted the area.

Beyond the gulch, the trail soon crosses a number of nascent Sixmile Creek's trickling rivulets, along with some pretty pocket meadows. Around the 3.5-mile mark the trail climbs more steeply into an open area covered with scattered granite boulders. In this open area you reach

Russian Lake

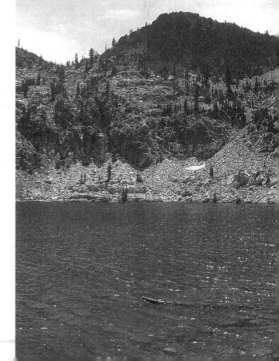

a signed junction with the continuation of the trail on the right to Siphon Lake and a connection to the Pacific Crest Trail, and your route to the left to Waterdog Lake.

A short, steep climb leads to a ridge above and a partial, filtered view of the lake below. An equally steep drop soon leads down to the outlet and the north shore of lovely Waterdog Lake. A couple of fair to poor campsites are tucked beneath the trees above the north shore and up the hill farther above the east shore. Anglers can ply the waters for eastern brook and rainbow trout. Swimming will be chilly in the nearly 7000-foot lake until mid-August.

To reach the much larger Russian Lake, follow the trail around the north side of Waterdog Lake and bear right on the use trail around the far end of the lake. A very short distance down this shoreline use trail, watch for a much fainter path that heads uphill away from the lake. A steep climb through the trees leads around the edge of a lush meadow and over to the north shore of Russian Lake.

Tucked into a basin at the base of rugged Peak 7731, 5-acre Russian Lake offers a more mountainous ambiance than its smaller and shallower neighbor. Campsites on the northwest shore are cramped and exposed to the winds that characteristically swoop down from the peak. Fair-sized rainbow trout will tempt any anglers in your group. Swimming is even more refreshing than usual at this higher, larger, and deeper lake.

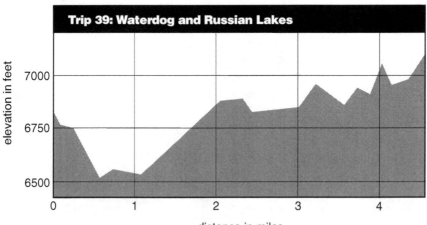

TRIP 40

Bingham Lake

A short hike with an incredibly steep section leads to a beautiful lake at the base of Russian Peak.

Trip Type:	Dayhike
Distance:	2.5 miles, out-and-back
Elevation Change:	780 feet, average 624 per mile
Difficulty:	Moderate
Season:	Mid-June through October
Maps:	USGS *Eaton Peak* and USFS *A Guide to the Marble Mountain Wilderness & Russian Wilderness*
Nearest Campground:	Trail Creek

Reaching Bingham Lake requires only an hour of your time but a gallon of your sweat. Most of the route is along the mild to moderate grade of an old road with excellent views much of the way. Although short, the last section to the lake is one of the steepest climbs and even steeper descents on a maintained trail you'll ever hope to see. Plus, you'll have to reverse the whole process in order to get back to your vehicle. Despite this inconvenience, the lake receives a fair share of visitors, so don't expect to be alone.

The lake itself is quite scenic, occupying a steep-sided bowl beneath the 8196-foot hulk of Russian Peak, the highest summit in the Russians and a straightforward, off-trail climb from the lakeshore.

Bingham Lake

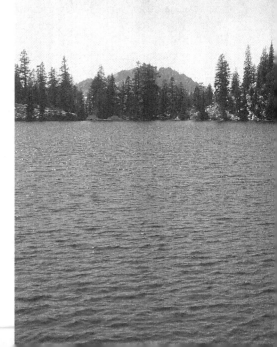

Starting Point
Follow Highway 3 to the small community of Callahan, and immediately north of town, turn left at the junction of Forest Road 93, heading toward Cecilville, Forks of Salmon, and Somes Bar. Climb 5.7 miles on Road 93 and turn right onto Forest Road 41N14. Reach a Y-junction after 1 mile and veer right, remaining on Road 41N14. At 5 miles from Road 93 is another Y-junction, where you follow Road 40N82 climbing uphill on

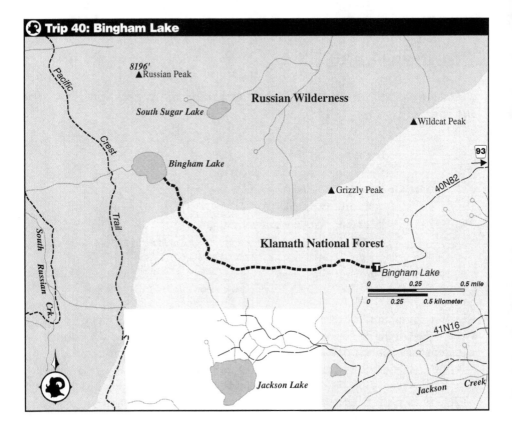

Trip 40: Bingham Lake

the right. Continue on Road 40N82 at an intersection with gated Road 40N83 on the left, after rounding a corner at 6.5 miles. After another 0.3 mile of climbing you reach a large, open parking area near the Bingham Lake trailhead.

Description

From the parking area, you climb steeply up the continuation of the road, which is blocked by boulders after a short distance. The open topography allows good views of the surrounding terrain, including Jackson Lake down the steep hillside 800 feet below. Light forest eventually limits the views, as the grade has eased to more of a mild to moderate climb along the old roadbed. Farther on, you break out of the trees again to expanding views to the north of 8196-foot Russian Peak. Soon back in previously logged forest, you reach the end of the road 1 mile from the trailhead.

From the end of the road, veer right onto single-track trail and climb very steeply up the hillside toward a saddle in the ridge above. After a brutal 0.4-mile climb, catch your breath at the saddle, which sits on the Russian Wilderness boundary, and gaze straight down the hillside about 350 vertical feet to the shimmering surface of your destination, Bingham Lake. The trail plunges even more steeply, if possible, from the saddle down to the lakeshore in 0.2 mile, an almost unbelievably steep descent.

Bingham Lake is perched in a steep-walled cirque, broken only by the narrow cleft of the outlet pouring out of the lake on the west side, headed toward the South Russian River 1200 feet below. The topography is too steep for decent camping—not that anyone in their right mind would want to haul a backpack up to the saddle above the lake and back down again. Anglers, carrying a pole and some tackle, can fish for small- to medium-sized rainbow trout. After the steep climb, swimmers will find the chilly waters of the lake quite tempting.

Those with unlimited energy may opt to climb nearby Russian Peak by heading around the east shore to the north side of the lake. From there, ascend directly north 1000 feet to the boulder-covered summit and an incredible view, including Mt. Shasta, the Trinity Alps, and the Russian Wilderness.

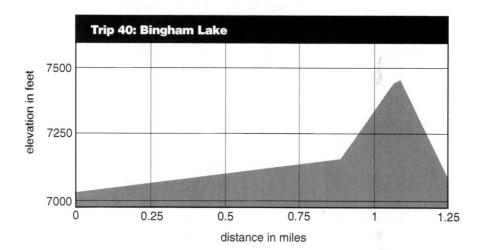

TRIP 41

Big Duck, Little Duck, and Horseshoe Lakes

These three lakes beautifully represent the best of the Russian Wilderness.

Trip Type:	Dayhike or 2- to 3-day backpack
Distance:	10 miles, out-and-back (plus 3 miles round-trip to Horseshoe Lake)
Elevation Change:	2660 feet, average 532 per mile (plus 805 feet to Horseshoe Lake, average 537 feet per mile)
Difficulty:	Moderate
Season:	Late June through October
Maps:	USGS *Eaton Peak* and USFS *A Guide to the Marble Mountain Wilderness & Russian Wilderness*
Nearest Campground:	Hidden Horse

Big Duck and Little Duck lakes, along with nearby Horseshoe Lake, are some of the prettiest lakes in the Russian Wilderness. Although the distance from the trailhead to the lakes is minimal, much of the grade is stiff and hikers should be well conditioned to fully enjoy this trip. Trail use is generally light in the wilderness, but you're likely to see at least one other party on this trip if you're here on a weekend. The lakes themselves are quite scenic, lined with forest and backdropped by granite cliffs, offering campers, anglers, and swimmers some fine opportunities.

Starting Point
Turn west from Highway 3, 8.2 miles north of Callahan and 4.1 miles south of Etna, onto French Creek Road. Follow paved road past ranchland into forest on the east side of the Russian Mountains for 5.4 miles, where the surface changes to gravel and then dirt. Just past an unsightly clear-cut and a sign marked END OF COUNTY MAINTAINED ROAD, you enter national forest land and reach an intersection with Forest Road 41N22. Turn right, following signed directions for the Duck Lakes and Eaton Lake trailhead, and proceed another 1.6 miles to a T-junction. Turn right onto Forest Road 41N14 and continue another 1.3 miles to a left-hand turn into the signed parking area for the trailhead.

Description
Through a mixed forest of incense cedars, Jeffrey pines, Douglas firs, and a few sugar pines, you head away from the trailhead along the course of an old road on a moderate climb. Soon you follow a series of long-legged switchbacks

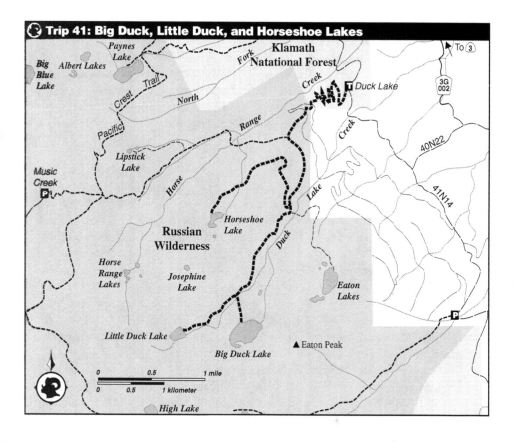

Trip 41: Big Duck, Little Duck, and Horseshoe Lakes

Paynes Lake

Big Blue Lake

Albert Lakes

Klamath Natational Forest

Fork

Klamath

Creek

Duck Lake

To ③

3G 002

Pacific Crest Trail

North

Range

Creek

40N22

41N14

Lipstick Lake

Music Creek

Horse

Russian Wilderness

Horseshoe Lake

Lake

Duck

Horse Range Lakes

Josephine Lake

Eaton Lakes

Little Duck Lake

Big Duck Lake

▲ Eaton Peak

0   0.5   1 mile
0   0.5   1 kilometer

High Lake

that zigzag back and forth toward the southeast lip of the canyon carrying the waters of Horse Range Creek. Farther up the slope, the forest lightens, which allows filtered views to the east of Scott Valley. In the midst of the switchbacking ascent, you cross the signed Russian Wilderness boundary and continue climbing moderately to moderately steeply. Eventually the trail ascends straight up the crest of a ridge to a junction with the trail to Lipstick Lake on the right, 1.7 miles from the trailhead.

From the junction, proceed ahead toward Duck Lake, as the grade mercifully eases and the shade of the forest returns—both welcome after the previously steep and exposed climb.

Duck Lake

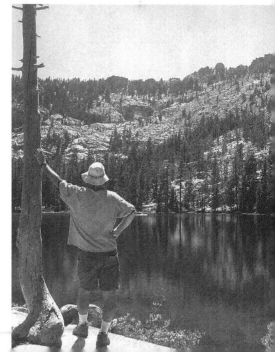

After a brief respite, the grade increases to moderate again and then to steep where the route leaves the old roadbed and, after a short stretch of single-track, merges with the course of another old road. Fortunately, gentler tread leads generally south and then southwest on a rising traverse across the hillside on the way toward the canyon of Duck Lake Creek. Along this traverse, the forest occasionally parts just enough to allow good views of distant Mt. Shasta and Scott Valley below. At 2.4 miles you reach a junction with the trail to Horseshoe Lake.

Side Trip to Horseshoe Lake

Whether you choose to do so on your way toward or on the return trip from the Duck Lakes, a visit to Horseshoe Lake is a worthy endeavor. From the junction with the trail to Duck Lake, turn right and begin a moderate climb along an old road bed through Douglas-fir forest with a trailside understory of manzanita and tobacco brush. The trees thin a tad as you round the nose of the ridge dividing the Duck Lake Creek and Horse Range Creek drainages. As you bend around into Horse Range Creek canyon, the forest transitions to primarily white firs and western white pines. With the roar of the tributary from Horseshoe Lake in your ears, the road becomes quite steep and rocky on the way to a crossing of the alder-lined stream. The stiff climb continues beyond the crossing, finally easing where you crest the lip of Horseshoe Lake's basin and make a short stroll to the northwest shore.

The 6.1-acre lake has a solemn ambiance, encircled by the brooding boughs of white firs, mountain hemlocks, and western white pines that fill the lake's basin. A couple of fair to good campsites near the outlet seem sufficient to handle the few who haul their backpacks up this trail. With a depth of 21 feet, the lake harbors a good population of eastern brook and rainbow trout. Swimmers will find the waters enticing enough for a swim by late July.

Horseshoe Lake

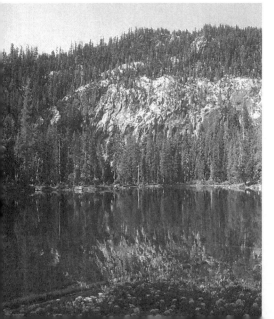

From the Horseshoe Lake junction, you leave the roadbed behind and follow single-track trail on a moderate climb through scattered to light forest. In midsummer, more open areas on the forest floor are sprinkled with the blossoms of paintbrush, lupine, wild rose, and thimbleberry. The grade increases and the tread becomes rockier for a stretch as you switchback through shady forest with a lush understory of ferns and alders. Shortly after stepping over a trickling side stream, you reach a junction with the lateral to Big Duck Lake, 3.7 miles from the trailhead.

Turning left (southeast), you boulder hop Duck Lake Creek and then make a short, winding climb up a boulder-studded slope to the crest of the lip of Big Duck Lake's basin and a view through the trees of the 26-acre lake. From there, a very short descent leads to the north shore.

Picturesque Big Duck Lake has a shoreline rimmed by light forest and towered over by rugged granite cliffs forming the Russian Wilderness crest. The northwest shore has several spacious campsites, as the lake seems to be the preferred destination of most backpackers setting off from the Duck Lake trailhead. Anglers can test their skill, or luck, on the eastern brook and rainbow trout that inhabit the 27-foot-deep lake. After the stiff climb, swimmers will find the temperature of the lake quite refreshing.

To reach Little Duck Lake, return to the junction and head upstream on a mild to moderate climb. Pass a small, murky pond on the left and then break out of the forest to views of the granite cliffs at the head of the upper lake's cirque.

You soon reach Little Duck Lake, where granite slabs run down to the shore and lodgepole pines find footholds in cracks between the slabs. At 5.2 acres and a depth of 18 feet, Little Duck is much smaller than its neighbor and attracts fewer visitors. Consequently, campsites are not as abundant or as developed, but the prospect of more solitude may influence your choice to camp here. At 6700 feet, Little Duck should be warm enough for decent swimming by late July. Fair-sized eastern brook trout will entice any anglers in your party.

The decent network of connecting trails on the east side of the Russian Wilderness allows you to make forays to other lakes in the area. However, be forewarned that trails to Eaton and Lipstick lakes are in very poor condition and difficult to follow. The route to Paynes Lake is much more defined, especially once you reach the Pacific Crest Trail.

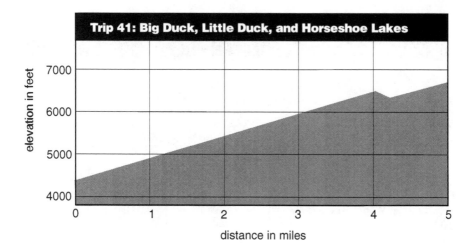

TRIP 42

Paynes Lake

A short but grueling climb leads to a picturesque lake below the crest of the range.

Trip Type:	Dayhike or 2-day backpack
Distance:	4.2 miles, out-and-back
Elevation Change:	2100 feet, average 1000 feet per mile
Difficulty:	Difficult
Season:	July through October
Maps:	USGS *Eaton Peak* and USFS *A Guide to the Marble Mountain Wilderness & Russian Wilderness*
Nearest Campground:	Hidden Horse

Paynes Lake is a beautiful body of water backdropped by rugged cliffs of the Salmon Mountain divide, a worthy destination for backpackers and hikers alike. While the majority of visitors reach the lake along the longer but mellower Pacific Crest Trail from Etna Summit, this description takes the direct approach up the steeper Paynes Lake Creek Trail. The 2.1-mile trail leads up the creek's canyon through mostly thick forest all the way to the lake, where fantastic scenery awaits, along with good camping, fishing, and swimming opportunities. Competent off-trail hikers can find plenty of diversions as well, including the Albert Lakes and nearby Big Blue Lake.

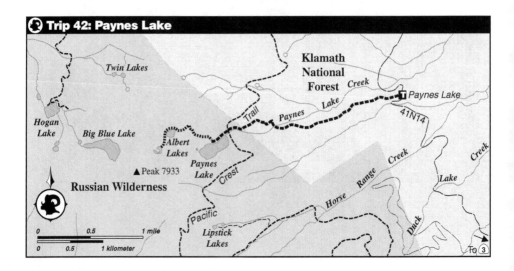

Starting Point

Turn west from Highway 3, 8.2 miles north of Callahan and 4.1 miles south of Etna, onto French Creek Road. Follow paved road past ranchland into forest on the east side of the Russian Mountains for 5.4 miles, where the surface changes to gravel and then dirt. Just past an unsightly clear-cut and a sign marked END OF COUNTY MAINTAINED ROAD, you enter National Forest land and reach an intersection with Forest Road 41N22. Turn right, following signed directions for the Duck Lakes and Eaton Lake trailhead, and proceed for 1.6 miles to a T-junction. Turn right onto Forest Road 41N14 and continue another 2.6 miles, passing by the Duck Lake trailhead on the way, to a large parking area at the signed trailhead.

Description

Through predominantly Douglas-fir forest, you start out climbing stiffly from the trailhead, reaching a set of switchbacks after a quarter mile along the south lip of Paynes Lake Creek canyon. The creek remains out of sight at the bottom of the steep canyon for the first mile or so, before the trail suddenly stops climbing to descend past the signed wilderness boundary to a crossing of Paynes Lake Creek at 1.4 miles.

Beyond the crossing of the creek, the stiff climb resumes, switchbacking away from the creek through the dense cover of a mixed forest of white firs, western white pines, and mountain hemlocks. After 0.4 mile the trail heads back to the creek and follows the tumbling stream more closely on a winding climb up the hillside. A rocky section of tread across an open hillside provides your only views along this trail of Scott Valley below and Mt. Shasta on the east horizon. Back under forest, you proceed up the slope to a junction with the wide and well-traveled track of the Pacific Crest Trail.

A short walk from the PCT junction leads upstream to 17-acre Paynes Lake, reposing majestically in a glaciated cirque below the Salmon Mountain crest.

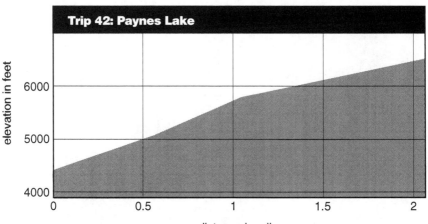

Scattered conifers grace most of the shoreline, with talus slides and granite cliffs rising up to craggy Peak 7933 above the far end of the lake. A short but steep essentially cross-country route runs up to diminutive Albert and Upper Albert lakes near the crest of the divide. There are a number of fair campsites spread around the lake, a favorite stopping place for backpackers on the PCT. Anglers can ply their craft on both eastern brook and rainbow trout that seem to flourish in the 50-foot-plus deep waters. At 6450 feet, the water temperature will be chilly until the first part of August.

Experienced cross-country enthusiasts can climb over the ridge from the Albert Lakes to visit Big Blue Lake. By hiking north on the PCT, Taylor Lake would be an easier off-trail scramble over the crest, but the easy, half-mile hike from the Taylor Lake trailhead ensures that the lake receives a high number of visitors.

TRIP 43

Taylor, Hogan, and Big Blue Lakes

Choose from an easy stroll to Taylor Lake, a moderate hike to Hogan Lake, and a rugged off-trail route to Big Blue Lake.

Trip Type:	Dayhike or 2-day backpack
Distance:	8.6 miles, out-and-back to Big Blue Lake
Elevation Change:	3000 feet, average 698 feet per mile
Difficulty:	Moderate
Season:	July through October
Maps:	USGS *Eaton Peak* and USFS *A Guide to the Marble Mountain Wilderness & Russian Wilderness*
Nearest Campground:	Idlewild

Just about every recreational enthusiast will find something to enjoy on this excursion into the northern Russian Wilderness. The trip to Taylor Lake is wheelchair accessible, and short and easy enough for families with small children to handle with little complaint. The lake offers a chance to fish for eastern brook trout, swim in the refreshing waters, or set up an easy overnight camp. The short and easy trail even allows boaters to haul in a canoe, kayak, or rubber raft with a little effort. A straightforward cross-country route east of the lake offers the more adventurous access to the Pacific Crest Trail along the crest of the range.

Ratcheting up a notch, the moderate, 3.75-mile hike to Hogan Lake leads to a scenic body of water beneath sparkling granite cliffs highlighted by a beautiful cascade spilling down the face. The hike back to the trailhead is the most strenuous part of the trip, as you must gain back more than 1000 feet of lost elevation from the lake to the top of a divide. Hogan Lake is a fine spot for a base camp, with ample opportunities to fish and swim in the lake, or scramble up the nearby cliffs.

For the super-adventurous, off-trail routes beyond Hogan Lake to Neil and Big Blue lakes, and over the ridge to Albert and Paynes lakes are attractively challenging. By following the Pacific Crest Trail north from Paynes Lake, a loop trip is possible by dropping off the crest back to Taylor Lake.

Starting Point

First, you must get to Etna just west of Highway 3, about 26 miles south of Yreka and 12 miles north of Callahan. From Highway 3 head toward the center of town on Main Street/Sawyers Bar Road to a stop sign and turn right. Remaining on Sawyers Bar Road, you drive out of town and follow the road on a winding climb 10.3 miles to Etna Summit, on the Scott River/North Fork

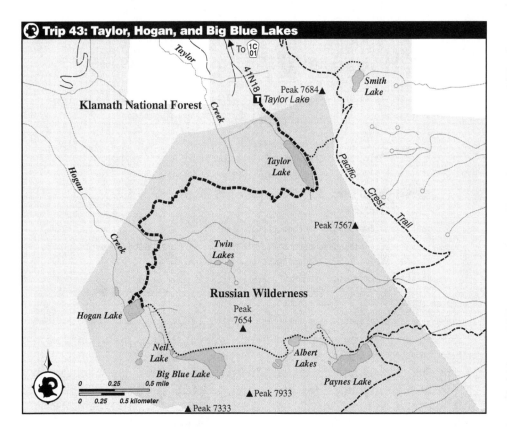

Trip 43: Taylor, Hogan, and Big Blue Lakes

Salmon River divide. At Etna Summit there is a large gravel parking area for the Pacific Crest Trail trailhead, on the left-hand side of the road near the base of a communication tower.

Continue down Sawyers Bar Road from the summit for another 0.3 mile to a left-hand turn onto Forest Road 41N18, signed TAYLOR LAKE TRAILHEAD. Follow the gravel and dirt road, with sections of pavement on the steeper parts, for 2.3 miles to the paved parking lot at the trailhead. The trailhead area, by far the most developed trailhead for the Russian Wilderness, is equipped with a modern vault toilet, striped parking, and handicapped access.

Description

The wide, well-graded, handicapped accessible tread of the old road leading to Taylor Lake is so easy to walk that you'll likely cover the half-mile distance before you break a sweat. Strolling through a mixed forest of white and red firs, western white pines, incense cedars, and lodgepole pines, you reach the long, narrow lake in short order. At the lower end of the lake, a path on the right crosses the outlet and heads around the north shore and partway along the west shore before dead-ending in a tangle of brush.

There are no campsites on this side of the lake, but the path provides access to the lakeshore for anglers. Backpackers will find passable campsites above the northeast side of the lake, although the easy access may deter those looking for anything close to solitude from camping here. Meadows and patches of shrubs border the far end of the lake, which is otherwise encircled by conifers.

Side Trip to Smith Lake

Competent off-trail hikers can follow the course of an abandoned trail from the halfway point along the lake steeply up the slope to meet the Pacific Crest Trail in a saddle on the crest. Smith Lake is accessible from there by heading northbound on the PCT and dropping down cross-country along a descending ridge to the north shore. The 6-acre, 56-foot-deep lake, just outside the wilderness boundary, is cradled in a compact, deep cirque beneath Peak 7684. Although campsites are severely limited, the lake will tempt anglers to fish for eastern brook, rainbow, and brown trout.

The main trail continues ahead above the east shore of Taylor Lake below a rugged granite ridge forming the crest of the Russian Wilderness. Climbing west away from Taylor Lake, you follow switchbacks through mostly fir forest and open areas, the trees thinning the higher up the slope you travel, allowing for fine views of the surrounding terrain and the lake below. Thicker forest returns as you gain the crest of a ridge, 1.8 miles from the trailhead.

After 0.2 mile of gently graded trail along the north flank of Peak 7077, you begin a moderate, protracted descent into the canyon of Hogan Creek, with filtered views into the deep gorge below. Breaks in the forest allow the views to improve on occasion, as the steady descent continues, aided by a number of switchbacks. Just beyond a pretty little meadow filled with grasses and corn lilies, you make a short climb up to the crossing of a small stream and then soon

Taylor Lake

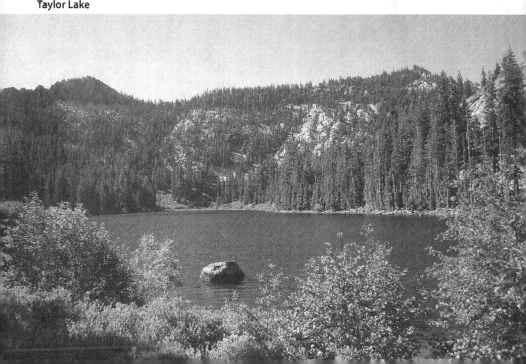

come to a second meadow, where the tread momentarily disappears in the lush vegetation. Defined track reappears at the far end of the meadow and continues down the hillside. After a while the trail skirts an even larger meadow carpeted with small plants and corn lilies, where the track disappears once again. By heading straight across the meadow you find defined tread again at the edge of the trees. Beyond the meadow the trail drops down and bends over to the north shore of Hogan Lake, 3.75 miles from the trailhead.

A dense forest of firs, western white pines, mountain hemlocks, and a few incense cedars borders the near side of the 7.4-acre lake. The far side of the lake is backdropped by rugged granite cliffs rising steeply up from the south side above scattered trees and patches of shrubs. A beautiful cascade threading its way down through the rock from the lakes adds a very picturesque touch to the subalpine scene. A few fair to good campsites nestle beneath the trees near where the trail meets the lake. Anglers can fish for eastern brook and rainbow trout inhabiting the 26-foot-deep lake. At an elevation of 5950 feet, the water temperature is usually warm enough for comfortable swimming by mid- to late July.

Tarn above Hogan Lake

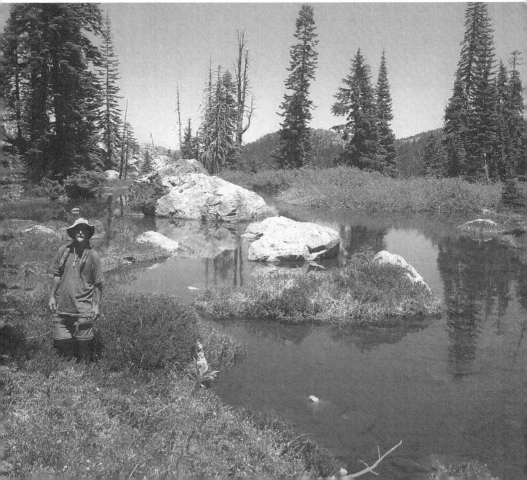

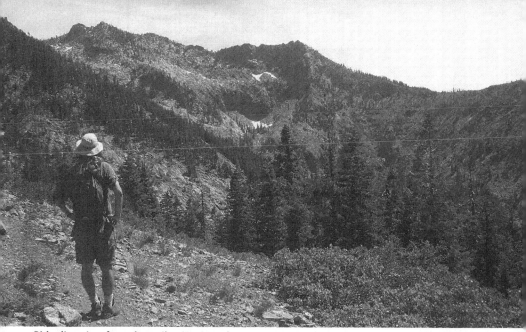

Ridgeline view from the trail to Hogan Lake

Rugged cross-country routes avail themselves to the adventurous from Hogan Lake up the rocky, brush-filled slopes to the southwest. First you have to negotiate your way through the thick forest and dense shrubs bordering the lakeshore. From there, you can head straight up the slope to two small tarns, or slightly more southeast to tiny Neil Lake and much larger Big Blue Lake, 4.3 miles from the trailhead. A saddle in the crest directly northeast of Big Blue Lake provides access to Albert and Paynes lakes on the east side of the crest. From Paynes Lake you could head northbound on the Pacific Crest Trail and drop down from the saddle on the crest above Taylor Lake to create a fine loop trip.

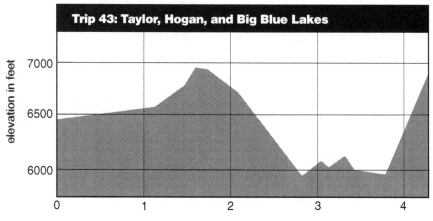

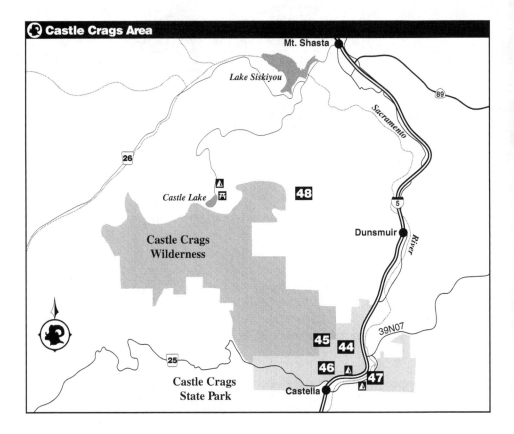

CHAPTER 7

Trips in the Castle Crags Area

The granite spires of Castle Crags provide a recognizable landmark for travelers on nearby Interstate 5, but they also offer some excellent hiking opportunities for people willing to leave the highway. Castle Crags State Park, at 6216 acres, and the adjoining 10,500-acre Castle Crags Wilderness are a hiker's haven. A wide variety of elevations, from around 2000 feet along a stretch of the upper Sacramento River to a high point of 6544 feet at the highest of the crags, provide an environment for a wide variety of plant life as well.

Of the five described trips, the first four originate in Castle Crags State Park, offering a couple of short hikes to Root Creek and the Sacramento River, a stiff climb to the base of the crags, and a loop trip through the lower elevations of the park. The last trip originates on the north side of the wilderness from Castle Lake and travels to the site of an old lookout on top of Mt. Bradley. With the exception of the trip to Mt. Bradley, which should be done in summer, the hikes in the Castle Crags area are best during spring or fall.

Wilderness permits are not currently required for overnight stays in Castle Crags Wilderness, and registration is not required for hiking in Castle Crags State Park as well. Forest Service campgrounds at Castle Lake and Gumboot Lake, on the north and west side of the wilderness, respectively, offer primitive camping. More developed camping is available in Castle Crags State Park, although the 50-plus sites are tucked into a narrow canyon in close proximity to Interstate 5 and a set of frequently used railroad tracks. The park offers more secluded tent camping at a couple of environmental sites along the banks of the river and Castle Creek. Anglers can easily access the Sacramento River from the park. In addition to hiking, camping, and fishing, Castle Crags State Park has a picnic area at Vista Point, from where visitors can enjoy a meal with a fine view of the towering crags.

TRIP 44

Root Creek

Stroll through cool forest to a tumbling stream lined with beautiful foliage.

Trip Type:	Dayhike
Distance:	2.2 miles, out-and-back
Elevation Change:	250 feet, average 227 feet per mile
Difficulty:	Easy
Season:	April through November
Maps:	USGS *Dunsmuir* and *Castle Crags State Park* by California State Parks
Nearest Campground:	Castle Crags State Park

A cool, forested journey on gently graded tread leads to lovely Root Creek just inside the southeast corner of Castle Crags Wilderness. Springtime hikers will delight in the colorful wildflowers, including columbines, lady slippers, tiger lilies, western azaleas, and several varieties of orchids. Flowering dogwoods offer additional color, from changing leaves in autumn to white flowers in spring. Root Creek is a fine spot for a picnic lunch or for simply admiring nature's handiwork.

Starting Point
From Interstate 5 south of the town of Dunsmuir, take the Castella exit (#724) and head west on Castle Creek Road past a conveniently placed general store and snack bar to a right-hand turn into Castle Crags State Park, which charges an entrance fee. Just past the entrance station, turn right again, head past the campground entrance, and then follow narrow, steep, paved road to Vista Point, 1.8 miles from the park entrance. The large parking area is equipped with modern vault toilets and picnic tables.

Description
Follow a path from the parking area down to the beginning of the Crags Trail on the north side of the road, where a trailhead sign reads CRAGS TRAIL, ROOT CREEK 1.0, INDIAN SPRINGS 1.6, CASTLE DOME 2.7. A wide, nearly level track leads away from the road through a second-growth, mixed forest of Douglas firs, incense cedars, white firs, ponderosa pines, bigleaf maples, alders, and black oaks. Although poison oak grows trailside, the extra wide track of the trail should allow you to successfully avoid brushing up against this plant. After a quarter mile of gentle walking, you reach a junction with the Crags Trail toward Castle Dome on the left and your route to Root Creek ahead.

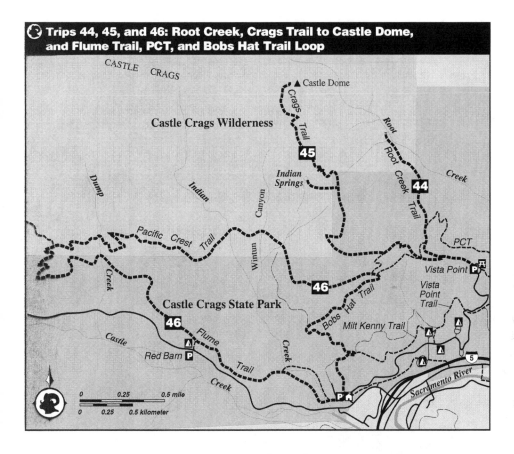

Trips 44, 45, and 46: Root Creek, Crags Trail to Castle Dome, and Flume Trail, PCT, and Bobs Hat Trail Loop

CASTLE   CRAGS

▲ Castle Dome

Castle Crags Wilderness

Crags Trail

45

Indian Springs

Root

Root Creek Trail

Creek

44

Dump

Indian

Canyon

Pacific   Crest   Trail

Wintun

PCT

Creek

Vista Point **P**

Vista Point Trail

46

Castle Crags State Park

Bobs Hat Trail

Milt Kenny Trail

46

Castle

Flume

Red Barn **P**

Creek

Trail

Creek

Sacramento River

5

0   0.25   0.5 mile
0   0.25   0.5 kilometer

Root Creek

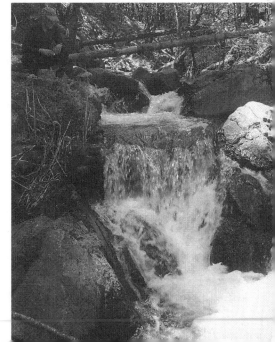

From the Crags Trail junction, your trail continues through mixed forest briefly before passing across the wide cut below a major transmission line. Away from this eyesore, you head back into the trees and proceed a short distance to a junction with the Pacific Crest Trail on the left. From the junction, continue ahead, now technically on the PCT for a brief stretch, on pleasantly graded, slightly rising tread. Just after crossing a bridge over a seasonal tributary, you soon reach yet another junction, where the PCT veers away to the right and the Root Creek Trail resumes its forward journey.

Away from the PCT, a mild climb leads across a forested slope toward the drainage of Root Creek, with dogwoods spicing up the mixed forest with pretty white flowers in spring and colorful leaves in autumn. Hop across a thin rivulet lined with alders and lush foliage and continue toward the increasing roar of the creek ahead. A cool, forested stroll leads alongside tumbling Root Creek, passing an old iron pipe from a bygone era and continuing a short distance to the end of the trail. The shady environs of Root Creek produces a fine display of foliage along the banks.

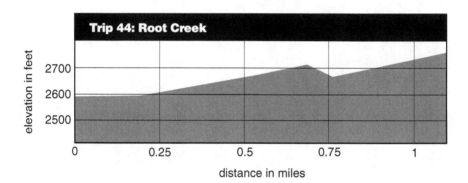

TRIP 45

Crags Trail to Castle Dome

A close-up of the spectacular Castle Crags

Trip Type:	Dayhike
Distance:	6 miles, out-and-back
Elevation Change:	2635 feet, average 941 feet per mile
Difficulty:	Difficult
Season:	Mid-April through mid-November
Maps:	USGS *Dunsmuir*
	and *Castle Crags State Park* by California State Parks
Nearest Campground:	Castle Crags State Park

see map on p. 319

The dramatic, well-named Castle Crags are seen by thousands of disinterested motorists streaming down Interstate 5 every day. Far, far fewer souls turn off the highway to take a closer look, and only a fraction of those spend the time and energy to hike the 3-mile, moderately steep trail for an even better view of this majestic formation of towering spires. Castle Crags is one of northern California's more impressive natural features, and the Crags Trail to the base of Castle Dome is the preeminent trail within the namesake park and adjoining wilderness area.

Beginning at the Vista Point in Castle Crags State Park, the Crags Trail starts out at a gentle grade but after 0.25 mile attacks the steep terrain with a vengeance. The steep section is relatively short at 2.75 miles, but strenuous. Dense forest shades most of the lower half of the trail, while the upper half winds through mostly rocky terrain with incredible views of Castle Crags, Mt. Shasta, and the Sacramento River and Castle Creek canyons along the way. The climax of the trip occurs at the trail's end, where fortunate visitors stare down a steep rock cleft out toward distant Mt. Shasta.

Numerous climbers' trails run toward the base of the pinnacles and domes, offering plenty of diversions for those with the extra time and energy to explore the nooks and crannies of the southeastern Castle Crags. A side trip to Indian Springs is a short and easy quarter-mile traverse from the midpoint of the Crags Trail to a lovely set of springs bubbling out of a granite face bordered by ferns and moss—a refreshing haven well worth the 15-minute out-and-back hike.

Starting Point

From Interstate 5 south of the town of Dunsmuir, take the Castella exit (#724) and head west on Castle Creek Road past a conveniently placed general store and snack bar to a right-hand turn into Castle Crags State Park, which charges an entrance fee. Just past the entrance station, turn right again, head past the campground entrance, and then follow narrow, steep, paved road to Vista Point, 1.8 miles from the park entrance. The large parking area is equipped with modern vault toilets and picnic tables.

Description

Follow a path from the parking area down to the beginning of the Crags Trail on the north side of the road, where a trailhead sign reads CRAGS TRAIL, ROOT CREEK 1.0, INDIAN SPRINGS 1.6, CASTLE DOME 2.7. A wide, nearly level track leads away from the road through a second-growth, mixed forest of Douglas firs, incense cedars, white firs, ponderosa pines, bigleaf maples, alders, and black oaks. Although poison oak grows trailside, the extra wide trail should allow you to successfully avoid brushing up against this plant. After a quarter mile of gentle walking, you reach a junction with the Crags Trail toward Castle Dome on the left and the trail to Root Creek ahead.

Remaining on the Crags Trail, you immediately start gaining the 2000-plus-feet necessary to stand below the spires and domes of Castle Crags. A set of switchbacks leads shortly to the top of a ridge and the obnoxious looking set of transmission lines above a swath of clear-cut forest and a signed junction with the famed Mexico-to-Canada Pacific Crest Trail.

Continue ahead on the unrelenting climb toward the Crags, as another set of switchbacks takes you across a dry drainage swale in an otherwise unremarkable stretch of forest to a three-way junction with the Bobs Hat Trail.

From the Bobs Hat junction, the trail continues the steady ascent, passing briefly into the wilderness where the trail arcs around the nose of a ridge. From there, you quickly exit the wilderness and bend north. Intermittent gaps in the now mostly evergreen forest allow brief tastes of the dramatic scenery that waits farther up the trail. The grade eases a bit across the west slope of a hill on the way to a saddle and a junction with the lateral to Indian Springs, 1.5 miles from the trailhead. There is a crude, dry campground near the junction.

Side Trip to Indian Springs

Don't miss the short excursion to Indian Springs, whether you detour on the way up to or back down from Castle Dome. From the junction at 1.5 miles from the trailhead, head west and traverse across the slope, initially through predominantly oak forest before breaking out onto an open slope with fine views of the surrounding terrain and some of the craggy cliffs above. As you start to hear the sound of running water, you head into mixed forest and soon reach the babbling brook emanating from Indian Springs in a cool, shady nook lined with ferns. A sign near this lovely oasis indicates the springs are the water source for the campground below. This enchanting grotto is hard to leave.

The steep climb resumes beyond the Indian Springs junction, passing through a light, deciduous forest with trailside shrubs. Soon the forest parts along the side of a hill, which allows a fine view northeast to Mt. Shasta and up to Castle Dome, with the fire lookout on top of Mt. Bradley positioned between these two striking features. The trail switchbacks and then swings around to

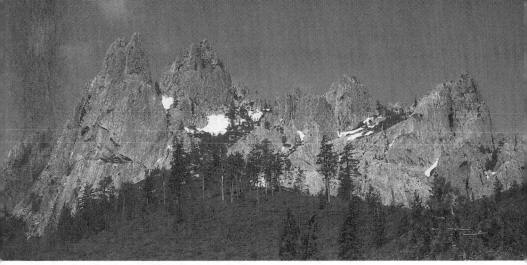

Some of the Castle Crags from the Crags Trail

the west side of a ridge, where a tight set of switchbacks leads up rocky terrain before crossing back to the east side of the ridge and more views of Shasta and Castle Dome above. As you wind up among the rocks, numerous climber trails veer off in a number of directions, but the main route is generally obvious at all junctions. After a winding section of trail weaving among the rocks, the tread returns to dirt for a while under light forest cover.

More switchbacks take you farther up the slope to an open ridgecrest carpeted with manzanita and dotted with an occasional pine, which allows for stunning views of the Castle Crags as you approach them. Maintained trail ends near a wire fence that protects visitors from plunging down into a deep, rocky gorge northwest of Castle Dome. Out this dramatically deep cleft, you have a marvelous view of snowcapped Mt. Shasta. Although the official trail ends at this overlook, numerous use trails allow those with additional time and energy to further explore the strikingly beautiful Castle Crags. There are poor to fair campsites scattered around the area, but prospective campers will have to pack in all of their water.

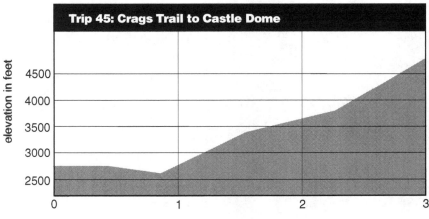

TRIP 46

Flume Trail, PCT, and Bobs Hat Trail Loop

A fine sampler of the Castle Crags area

Trip Type:	Dayhike
Distance:	7 miles, loop
Elevation Change:	2800 feet, average 400 feet per mile
Difficulty:	Moderate
Season:	April through November
Maps:	USGS *Dunsmuir* and *Castle Crags State Park* by California State Parks
Nearest Campground:	Castle Crags State Park

see map on p. 319

The trails highlighted in this trip are most popular with thru-hikers on their way from Mexico to Canada on the Pacific Crest Trail. Otherwise, these trails don't receive much attention, which is unfortunate, as the loop combination of the Indian Creek Nature Trail, Flume Trail, Pacific Crest Trail, and Bobs Hat Trail provides visitors to Castle Crags State Park a representative sample of the area's many treasures.

Springtime hikers will see a surprising array of blooms on azaleas and dogwoods and a wide variety of wildflowers, including several species of wild iris. Various spots along the trail offer fine views of the pinnacled Castle Crags thousands of feet above, as well as views of the Gray Rocks to the northwest, and sweeping vistas down into the Sacramento River and Castle Creek canyons. The loop also travels through several different vegetative zones such as oak woodland, mixed coniferous forest, chaparral, and riparian. There's even some history along the way, where the Flume Trail follows the course of an old flume used to carry water from Indian Creek to the town of Castella, which, interestingly enough, was the center of alcohol production in northern California during Prohibition.

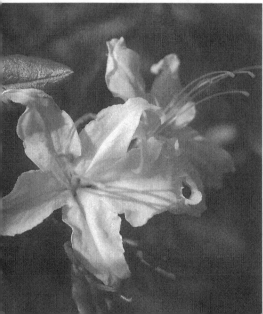

Azalea blossoms on the Flume Trail

Starting Point

From Interstate 5 south of the town of Dunsmuir, take the Castella exit

(#724) and head west on Castle Creek Road past a conveniently placed general store and snack bar to a right-hand turn into Castle Crags State Park, which charges an entrance fee. Find the trailhead at the large parking area west of the entrance station.

Description

You head away from the Visitor Center parking lot on the needle-covered track of Indian Creek Nature Trail, a mile-long interpretive trail with numbered posts corresponding to a park leaflet about the natural history of the Castle Crags area. Soon reach a junction with the nature trail's loop portion and veer left, following signed directions for the Flume Trail. Drop down immediately to a bridged crossing of Indian Creek and head upstream, passing below the transmission lines that slice an unsightly path through the park. Through very brief gaps in the forest you have fleeting views of the granite crags looming thousands of feet above. The trail soon moves away from the creek and the riparian foliage lining the banks into the more drought-tolerant vegetation of manzanita beneath Jeffrey pines, incense cedars, white firs, and oaks. A short, moderate ascent leads to a junction near the half-mile mark, where you forsake the Indian Creek Trail and head west onto the Flume Trail.

After a stretch of minor ups and downs, you cross the bed of the old flume with the roar of the Sacramento River to your left and follow the flume's former course into a forest dense enough to prevent much ground cover from growing. Soon the trail crosses back over the remnants of the flume and passes some discarded machinery. Farther along the trail, a more intact section of the wood flume gives you a glimpse into the past, when it provided the water supply for the town of Castella along the banks of the Sacramento River. Where the hillside becomes steeper, the trail climbs correspondingly for a brief stretch, levels out, and then drops down to cross a seasonal drainage on a wood-plank and rail bridge. Continue along the course of the flume to a junction, 1 mile from the trailhead. Here a very short path leads down to Red Barn Environmental Campsite at the edge of a grassy meadow. The campsite is

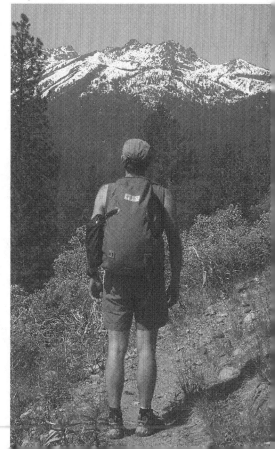

Gray Rocks from the Pacific Crest Trail

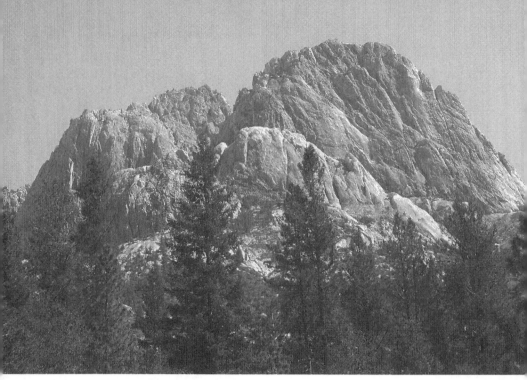

Some of the Castle Crags from the Pacific Crest Trail

equipped with a vault toilet, picnic tables, a bear box, and a fire ring; the fee was $15 in 2009. Across paved Forest Road 25 is the red barn for which the camp is named.

Continuing ahead from the junction, the trail regains the course of the flume for a while and then follows a steady ascent into more open forest, with views of Gray Rocks to the northwest and some of the Castle Crags above. The trail bends into a side canyon, crosses a bridge over a seasonal swale, curves around through oaks, dogwoods, azaleas, and seasonal wildflowers, including irises, tiger lilies, and yellow peas. Wind around to the crossing of a second drainage, where you can usually hear water above but the stream is usually dry below the bridge. After a traverse of a dry hillside, you reach the lower junction of the shortcut between the Flume and Pacific Crest trails near the edge of perennial Dump Creek, 2 miles from the trailhead.

From the junction, proceed ahead on the Flume Trail across a bridge over the flower- and azalea-lined creek and travel a short distance to a bridge over a usually dry side channel. The trail continues through predominantly oak woodland to a series of switchbacks that climb an open hillside to the top of a knoll. Along the way you have fine views of Gray Rocks and Castle Crags, and eventually leave behind the state park lands to enter Castle Crags Wilderness. At 2.8 miles you intersect the Pacific Crest Trail at a signed junction.

Turn right onto the well-trod PCT and make a switchbacking descent east into a canyon and over to Dump Creek, with a deep pool and a picturesque 10-foot cascade plunging into a smaller, upper pool. A short way past the creek a PCT post reading FLUME TRAIL with an arrow pointing downhill marks the otherwise indistinct, upper junction with the shortcut trail down alongside Dump Creek, 3.25 miles from the trailhead.

Away from the junction, the PCT climbs on moderately rising tread almost all the way to the next drainage before switchbacking up the slope. A long traverse follows through mostly open terrain with good views down into the canyons below and up to Gray Rocks and Castle Crags. After a grove of forest, you emerge out onto open, granitic slopes again, cross a seep, and then follow a mildly rising traverse toward Indian Creek. Forest cover returns on the approach to Indian Creek, which picturesquely tumbles down a rock-and boulder-filled canyon. You wrap around the nose of a ridge into Wintun Canyon and cross a bridge over the next tributary of Indian Creek gracefully sliding down steep rock slabs. Around the nose of the next ridge you come to the branch of Indian Creek spilling forth from Indian Springs. After hopping over this maple-lined stream, you soon encounter No Name Creek with a scenic waterfall. Pass a little-used campsite just beyond the last stream crossing and head back into Castle Crags State Park. A traverse across forested slopes leads to a pair of close junctions. Proceed to the farthest junction, about 25 yards from the first and 5.6 miles from the trailhead, where a sign reading in part BOBS HAT TRAIL, STATE PARK HQ 1.5 KM points downhill to the left.

Turn left and head downhill away from the PCT on Bobs Hat Trail via switchbacks to a junction with a fire road. Following a sign for park headquarters, take the wide track of the fire road down the hillside past a road angling in from behind on the right and beneath a set of power transmission lines to a three-way junction. Turn right at the junction and walk a short distance past a post marking the Milt Kenny Trail and continue down the hillside to a post marking a single-track trail toward park headquarters. Finally leaving the road behind for good, the trail winds down steeply and then levels out beneath dense, shady forest on the way to a crosswalk across the campground access road near the Visitor Center and the parking lot beyond.

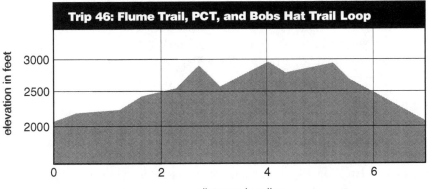

TRIP 47

River Trail

A fine stroll along the Sacramento River in a section of Castle Crags State Park

Trip Type:	Dayhike
Distance:	3.0 miles, out-and-back
Elevation Change:	50 feet, average 33 feet per mile
Difficulty:	Easy
Season:	Late March through November
Maps:	USGS *Dunsmuir* and *Castle Crags State Park* by California State Parks
Nearest Campground:	Castle Crags State Park

This easy stroll along a stretch of the Sacramento River is a pleasant way to spend a couple of hours enjoying the river and the riparian habitat along the south bank. Anglers have plenty of spots along the way to drop a line. During hot summer afternoons the river will entice swimmers, although the water temperature is usually chilly.

Starting Point

You have two options for accessing the River Trail. If you plan to camp in the main campground at Castle Crags State Park, from Interstate 5 south of the town of Dunsmuir, take the Castella exit (#724) and head west on Castle Creek Road past a conveniently placed general store and snack bar to a right-hand turn into Castle Crags State Park, which charges an entrance fee. The trail begins near campsite #13, which is on the first campground loop on the right. Otherwise, you can head in the opposite direction from the Castella exit and turn left onto Frontage Road. After 0.2 mile, turn right across a bridge over the Sacramento River and turn left onto Riverside Road. Proceed 0.3 mile to the entrance into Riverside Campground and Day-Use Picnic Area, where the trail begins on the east side.

Description

From campsite #13, follow closed, paved road below a large grassy clearing, pass through a gate in a cyclone fence, and walk through a pedestrian tunnel beneath Interstate 5. Immediately beyond the far end of the tunnel, you squeeze through a gap in a fence and turn left, following an arrowed sign marked RIVER TRAIL, to walk along the edge of Frontage Road near a wire fence for 0.2 mile. At the second opening in the fence, leave the side of the road and follow another sign down rocky tread to cross underneath the railroad tracks into a cool, mixed

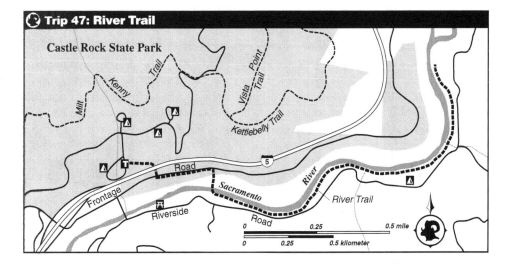

Trip 47: River Trail

Castle Rock State Park

Kenny Trail

Milt

Vista Point Trail

Kettlebelly Trail

5

Road

Frontage

Sacramento River

River Trail

Riverside Road

0   0.25   0.5 mile
0   0.25   0.5 kilometer

forest. Soon cross over the long suspension bridge spanning the Sacramento River and immediately intersect the trail from Riverside Campground at a signed junction (this junction is just a short walk east from the picnic area).

Head upstream following the course of the wide river through predominantly Douglas-fir forest with a smattering of oaks and a lush trailside understory that includes ferns, alders, maples, and a host of wildflowers in early spring. The roar of the river is almost enough to drown out the nearly continuous din

Sacramento River from the River Trail

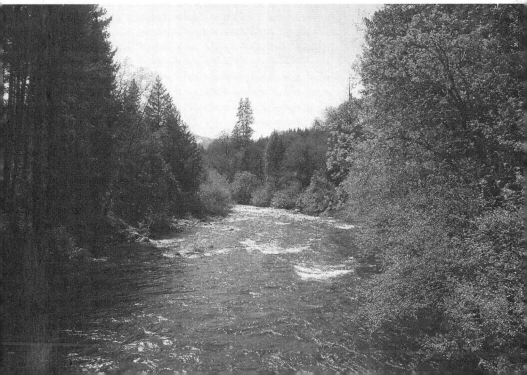

of vehicle noise from Interstate 5 on the opposite side of the river reverberating through the canyon. Continue upstream as a number of wood bridges provide crossings of the trickling side streams flowing into the river. Just before the river makes a bend to the north, you pass below a meadow with an environmental campsite nearby. The trail follows the course of the river through the sweeping bend to where the path suddenly dead-ends at the state park boundary, where a short side trail leads down to the river's edge. Across the river is an impressive rock wall, built for who knows what purpose.

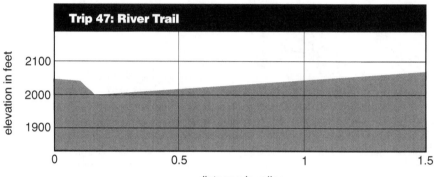

TRIP 48

Castle Lake Trail to Mount Bradley Lookout

A trio of pretty lakes and plenty of dramatic views offer tantalizing rewards.

Trip Type:	Dayhike or 2-day backpack
Distance:	11 miles round-trip, out-and-back
Elevation Change:	2400 feet, average 218 per mile
Difficulty:	Moderate to difficult
Season:	Mid-June to mid-October
Maps:	USGS *Seven Lakes Basin* and *Dunsmuir*; USFS *A Guide to the Mt. Shasta Wilderness & Castle Crags Wilderness*
Nearest Campground:	Castle Lake

This trip is one of extremes. Beautiful Castle Lake, at the beginning of the trip, draws hordes of fervent worshippers who drive the paved road every summer day to boat, fish, or swim in the water, or camp and picnic around the shoreline. Mt. Bradley, at the end of the trip, is a lonesome spot; only a relative few make the journey all the way to the old lookout near the summit. In between are two attractive lakes, scenic Heart Lake perched below Castle Lake's dramatic head-wall, and pastoral Little Castle Lake occupying a meadow-filled flat near the head of Ney Springs Creek. The long ridge route leading to the lookout beyond the lakes is blessed with nearly constant, extremely stunning views that take in a wide portion of northern California, culminating in the jaw-dropping vista from the old lookout.

Although this trip is perhaps best suited for dayhikers, backpackers can squeeze into the small, poor campsites around Little Castle or Heart Lakes. Anglers will find the fishing to be fair at best for small- to medium-sized trout in both of those lakes, with the best camping, fishing, and swimming in the area at road-accessible Castle Lake.

Starting Point

Follow Interstate 5 to the Central Mt. Shasta exit and go west, curving around shortly to a stop sign. Turn left onto South Old Stage Road and drive 0.25 mile to a Y-junction, bearing right onto West Barr Road. After 0.6 mile, continue straight ahead on West Barr Road at a four-way stop with West Ream Avenue. Pass the Mt. Shasta Resort, the east side of Siskiyou Lake, and Box Canyon Dam on the way to a junction with Castle Lake Road, approximately 3 miles from Interstate 5.

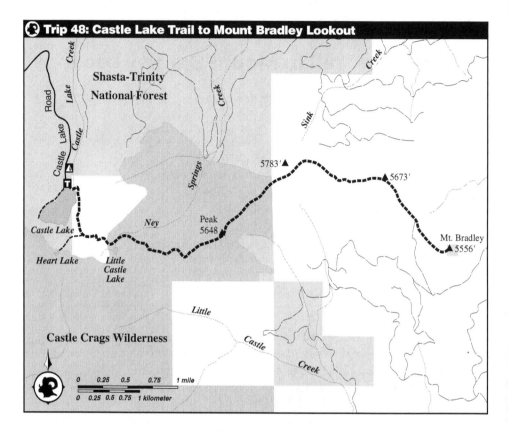

Trip 48: Castle Lake Trail to Mount Bradley Lookout

Turn left and follow Castle Lake Road 7.25 miles to the end and the parking lot near the north shore of Castle Lake. A modern vault toilet is just below the parking area and along the outlet are a number of walk-in campsites that don't have running water, picnic tables, fire pits, or trash pickup. Back down the road a quarter mile, an unsigned dirt road to the east leads shortly to a free campground along Castle Lake Creek with 6 sites that have picnic tables, fire pits, and primitive pit toilets but don't have access to running water or trash pickup.

Description

From the parking area, veer off to the east on single-track trail past a number of walk-in campsites to where you cross the lake's outlet on a combination of boulders, concrete walls, and a wood plank. Beyond the last campsite on the far side of the outlet, an old sign attached to a fir marked CASTLE LAKE TRAIL, LITTLE CASTLE LAKE, MT. BRADLEY LO ("LO" here is short for *lookout*) heralds the beginning of the trail that rises steadily above the east shore of Castle Lake. Passing through a light forest with a shrubby understory and a sprinkling of seasonal wildflowers, follow the trail on a moderate to moderately steep climb up the slope. Farther up the trees are left behind as the climb continues up open, rocky slopes before leveling off in a small basin with a seasonal pond.

Side Trip to Heart Lake

At the near edge of the tiny basin holding a seasonal pond, look for signs of a faint path on the right occasionally marked by ducks, which is the unmaintained trail toward Heart Lake. Scamper over some rocks to a view ahead of the open slope rising up to form the headwall of the Castle Lake cirque. Although a number of faint paths have been formed over the years, the most direct route to the lake proceeds initially southwest and then bends west to the north shore of the 0.75-acre, roughly heart-shaped lake. Anglers can ply the 11-foot-deep waters for small eastern brook trout, but the real gem to be found here is the stunning view of the lake backdropped by the snowy summit of Mt. Shasta. For more wide-ranging views, work your way around the shoreline to the south side and scramble up the north-facing wall of the cirque to the top of the ridge above. Not only will you have an unobstructed view of Shasta, but northeast to Oregon's Mt. McLaughlin as well.

From the vicinity of the seasonal pond, the Castle Lake Trail drops into the drainage of Ney Springs Creek through open terrain covered with shrubs, principally manzanita. Fine views of Mt. Shasta accompany you as the descent becomes steeper on rocky tread leading to a wildflower-sprinkled meadow in a small flat and an unmarked junction, 1 mile from the trailhead. The trail on the right leads a very short distance down to Little Castle Lake, a 2-acre, 9-foot-deep body of water bordered by dense shrubs on the near shore and backdropped

On the way to the Mt. Bradley Lookout

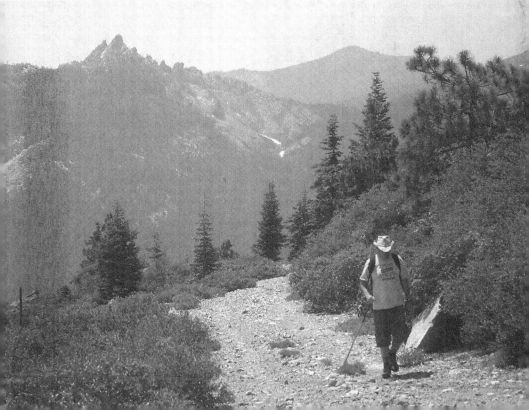

by rocky cliffs on the far shore. Fishing is fair for medium-sized eastern brook trout but the thick brush inhibits access around much of the shoreline. A pretty cascade spilling down the cliffs provides some visual interest.

From the junction, the main trail soon crosses Ney Springs Creek, follows the south bank downstream for a short distance, and then makes a descending traverse across an open slope with fine views of Mt. Shasta and Shastina along the way. Entering forest cover, the tread falters in places but only for short stretches. After a while the trail starts climbing and emerges from the forest onto the open slopes of a ridgecrest, 1.9 miles from the trailhead, with fine views of Castle Crags to the south—the first of many such views to come.

Heading northeast, you follow the open, shrub-covered ridge through a sprinkling of colorful wildflowers in early summer. Thick manzanita threatens to overgrow the trail in places—you may wish you had brought along a pair of hedge clippers. The continuous views of Castle Crags are quite stunning as you make a moderate ascent up the southwest ridge of Peak 5648. At the top of this knob, 14,162-foot Mt. Shasta springs into view along with 6325-foot Black Butte, a cinder cone directly south-southwest of Shasta.

Drop away from Peak 5648 into a saddle, climb over a bump on the ridge, drop into the next saddle, and proceed across the unmarked boundary of Castle Crags Wilderness. Now on private lands, you follow a rising traverse across the southeast slope of Peak 5783 through a light forest that inhibits the grand views and into another saddle. Here the trail turns southeast through diminishing forest to follow the ridge over the next high point, across a broad saddle, and up to the top of Peak 5673. From this aerie you have a supreme view across the deep hole of Strawberry Valley, the City of Mt. Shasta, and Interstate 5's ribbon of pavement to the lofty summit of Mt. Shasta, bordered by the satellite cone of Shastina directly west, and the black volcanic slopes of Black Butte near the base of the massive mountain's west flank.

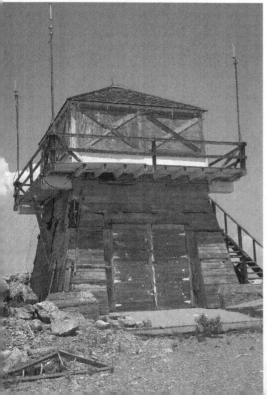
Old lookout on top of Mt. Bradley

Pressing on toward the lookout atop Mt. Bradley, the trail now veers southeast to descend a steep, rocky slope through open, shrub-covered terrain on the way to the next saddle. Unlike the hill you're descending, the slope of Mt. Bradley ahead is cloaked with a mantle of dense forest. After a significant loss of elevation, you stand in the saddle, 5 miles from the trailhead, where a well-traveled road bends around toward the lookout and the top of Mt. Bradley, 300 feet above.

After the seemingly wild and remote nature of the journey to this point, the well-graded road ahead is an affront to the sensibilities of the typical wilderness wanderer. Nevertheless, you press on, passing around a closed steel gate to climb steeply up the road through mixed forest. The trees progressively diminish farther up the hillside on the way to a split in the road. The left-hand road provides access to the communication equipment on top of the peak, while the right-hand road wraps around to the lookout.

As with the vast majority of old fire lookouts, the one on top of Mt. Bradley hasn't been used for some time. Fortunately, the view is still intact, with much of northern California visible from the decks of the old lookout. Dunsmuir, 3000 feet below along the banks of the upper Sacramento River, appears to be close enough to hit with a rock. Regal Mt. Shasta, completely dominating the landscape to the northeast, doesn't feel much farther away. The slopes of more distant Lassen Peak glimmer to the southeast, while the Sacramento Valley spills away in the southern distance. Immediately south, the nearby Castle Crags sparkle in the customary sunshine, and the peaks known as The Eddys appear directly west. What a rewarding daily view for the rangers who once staffed the lookout.

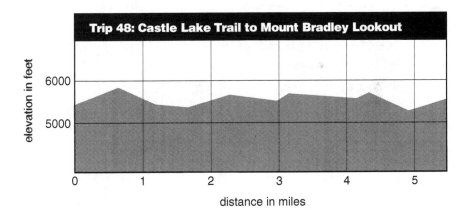

Recommended Reading

Agee, James K. *Steard's Fork: A Sustainable Future for the Klamath Mountains*. Berkeley: University of California Press, 2007.

Arnold, Mary Ellicott, and Mabel Reed. *In the Land of the Grasshopper Song*. Lincoln: University of Nebraska Press, 1957.

Beffort, Brian. *Joy of Backpacking*. Berkeley: Wilderness Press, 2007.

Heid, Matt. *101 Hikes in Northern California*. 2nd edition. Berkeley: Wilderness Press, 2008.

Johnston, Verna R. *California Forests and Woodlands*. Berkeley: University of California Press, 1994.

Most, Stephen. *River of Renewal, Myth, and History in the Klamath Basin*. Portland: Oregon Historical Society Press, 2006.

Schaeffer, Jeffrey P. *Pacific Crest Trail: Northern California*. 6th edition. Berkeley: Wilderness Press, 2003.

Selters, Andy, and Michael Zanger. *The Mt. Shasta Book*. 3rd edition. Berkeley: Wilderness Press, 2006.

Stienstra, Tom. *California Camping*. 15th edition. Emeryville, CA: Avalon Travel Publishing, 2007.

———. *Northern California Camping*. 1st edition. Emeryville, CA: Avalon Travel Publishing, 2007.

——— and Stephani Stienstra. *Northern California Cabins and Cottages*. 1st edition. Emeryville, CA: Avalon Travel Publishing, 2002.

Wallace, David Rains. *The Klamath Knot*. 20th anniversary edition. Berkeley: University of California Press, 2003.

Index

About the Author

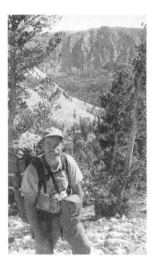

Mike White was born and raised in Portland, Oregon. He learned to hike, backpack, and climb in the Cascade Mountains and further honed his outdoor skills while obtaining a B.A. from Seattle Pacific University. After college, Mike and his wife, Robin, relocated to the high desert of Reno, Nevada, where he was drawn to the majesty of the Sierra Nevada.

In the early 1990s, Mike began writing about the outdoors, expanding the third edition of *The Trinity Alps*. His first solo publication for Wilderness Press was *Nevada Wilderness Areas and Great Basin National Park*. Fifteen more titles followed, including the *Snowshoe Trails* series, books about Sequoia, Kings Canyon, and Lassen Volcanic national parks, *Backpacking Nevada* and *Afoot & Afield Reno-Tahoe*. Two of his books have won national awards, *Top Trails Lake Tahoe* and *50 Classic Hikes in Nevada*. Mike has also contributed to *Sierra South, Sierra North,* and *Backpacking California*. In addition to his book projects, Mike has written articles for *Sunset, Backpacker,* and the *Reno Gazette Journal.* A former community college instructor, Mike is a featured speaker for outdoor groups.

Mike lives in Reno with his wife. His two sons, David and Stephen, and his daughter-in-law, Candace, live in the area as well.